Herbs for Health and Healing

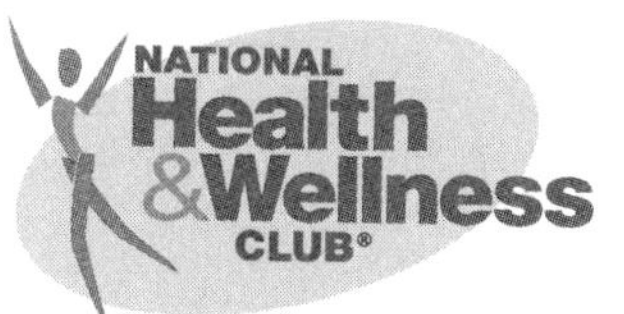

About the Author

Sarah Harding Laidlaw, M.S., R.D., M.P.A., is a Registered Dietitian with a nutrition consultation practice in Western Colorado. She has worked in the field of nutrition for 25 years. Her interest in herbal medicine and dietary supplements began as an undergraduate student, and both topics have been focal points of her career since then. She is editor of Nutrition In Complementary Care, the newsletter for the Dietetic Practice Group (DPG) within the American Dietetic Association. Gardening has been a passion of Sarah's for many years and as a result, she has an herb garden that contains many of the supplements she describes in this book. She balances her family's food choices with well-researched supplements, choosing wisely for wellness and specific conditions as appropriate.

Herbs for Health and Healing

The nutritional and health information presented in this book is based on an in-depth review of the current scientific literature. It is intended only as an informative resource guide to help you make informed decisions; it is not meant to replace the advice of a physician or to serve as a guide to self-treatment. Always seek competent medical help for any health condition or if there is any question about the appropriateness of a procedure or health recommendation.

1 2 3 4 5 6 7 8 9 10 / 07 06 05 04 03 02

ISBN: 1-58159-191-8

National Health & Wellness Club
12301 Whitewater Drive
Minnetonka, MN 55343
www.healthandwellnessclub.com

Tom Carpenter
Creative Director

Heather Koshiol
Managing Editor

Laura Holle
Book Development Assistant

Bill Nelson Creative, Inc.
Illustration, Book Design & Production

Photo Credits
Front Cover: NHWC Photo Archives; ©Index Stock Photography/Frank Siteman; Rim Light/Photolink/Getty Images; Ryan McVay/Getty Images; ©Index Stock Photography/Peter Scholey; Jim Franco/Getty Images.

Back Cover: NHWC Photo Archives; Ryan McVay/Getty Images; Quill/Getty Images; NHGC Photo Archive.

Special thanks to: Terry Casey, Janice Cauley, Nadine Trimble, Veronica Young and Sandy Zilka.

CONTENTS

Introduction

In recent years, herbs have enjoyed a renaissance as interest in taking responsibility for one's own health and self-care has taken hold. Instead of buying medicines and foods, growing and preparing them at home is gaining popularity. People wishing to return to a more natural time are finding a fascination with herbs as varied as their scents, colors and flowers.

The purpose of this book is to neither promote nor discourage self-medication with herbs and botanicals. The information herein is presented for educational purposes represented by the author's diligence in providing the most current information on the safe and appropriate use of herbal products. Although herbs and botanicals have been part of traditional medicine through time and between cultures, some information has not been verified by adequate research. The dietary supplement industry is making strides toward ensuring a product's quality, safety and effectiveness, but the industry remains, for the most part, self-regulated. Many current-day prescription and over-the-counter drugs have a botanical history. These, because they are proprietary medicines, have undergone safety and effectiveness testing prior to their marketing.

Botanicals grown in your garden or purchased in bulk from herbalists may suffer some of the same

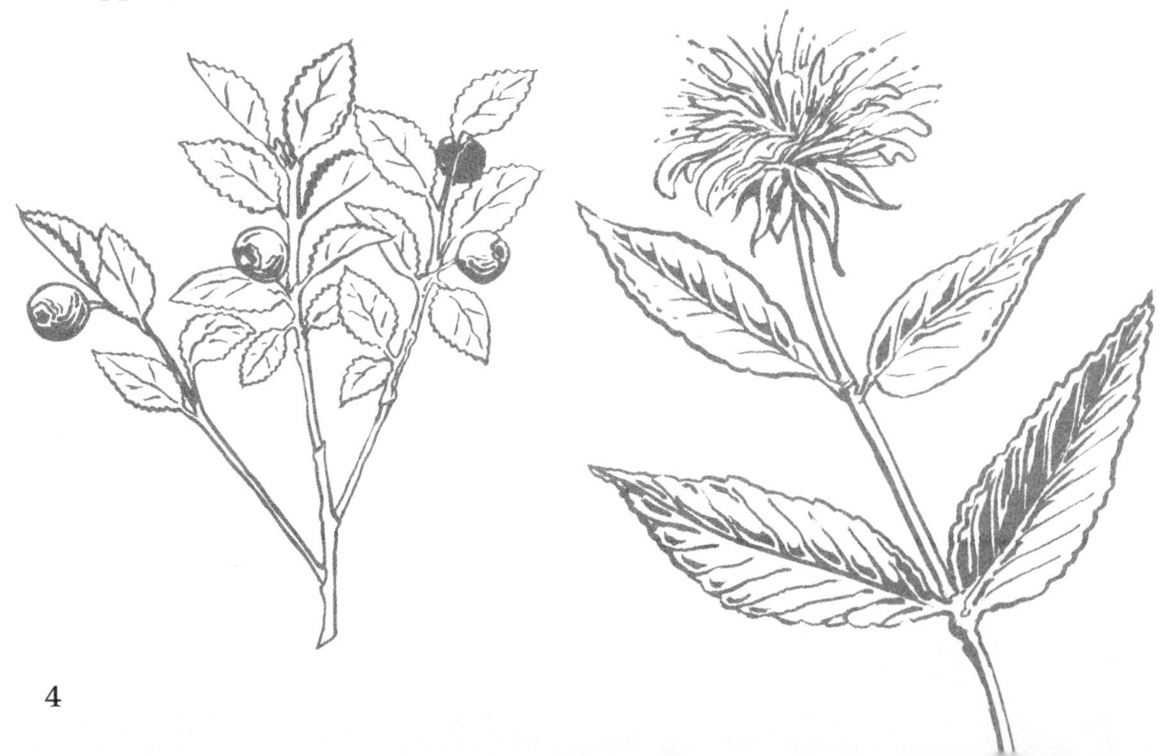

problems as prepared ready-to-take supplements—lack of known purity and effectiveness. In this book you will find information to help assure you of quality, purity and effectiveness in those botanicals you choose to grow or purchase. The book will also aid you in knowing which preparations are considered most effective for particular conditions and how to prepare and use them safely.

Numerous herbs have medicinal and culinary uses. Whether you want fresh herbs for cooking, self-care, or just want more information about them, you will find the basic information you need to get you started on the road to using herbs for health and healing.

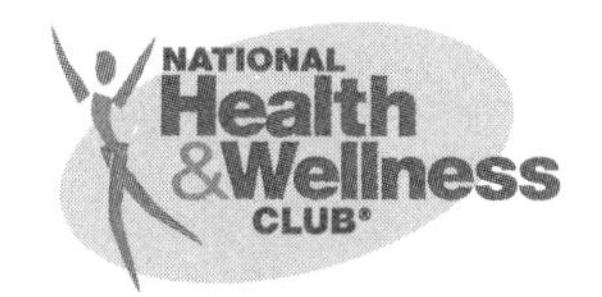

Why Aren't Herbs Tested Like Drugs?

- Herbs can't be patented like drugs—herbs can't be made chemically unique, which allows them to be sold as brand name or generic drugs for specific uses, and for more money.
- They are available in nature, and thus available to everyone regardless of their health condition.
- They are considered dietary supplements rather than drugs, so they fall under a different set of regulations.

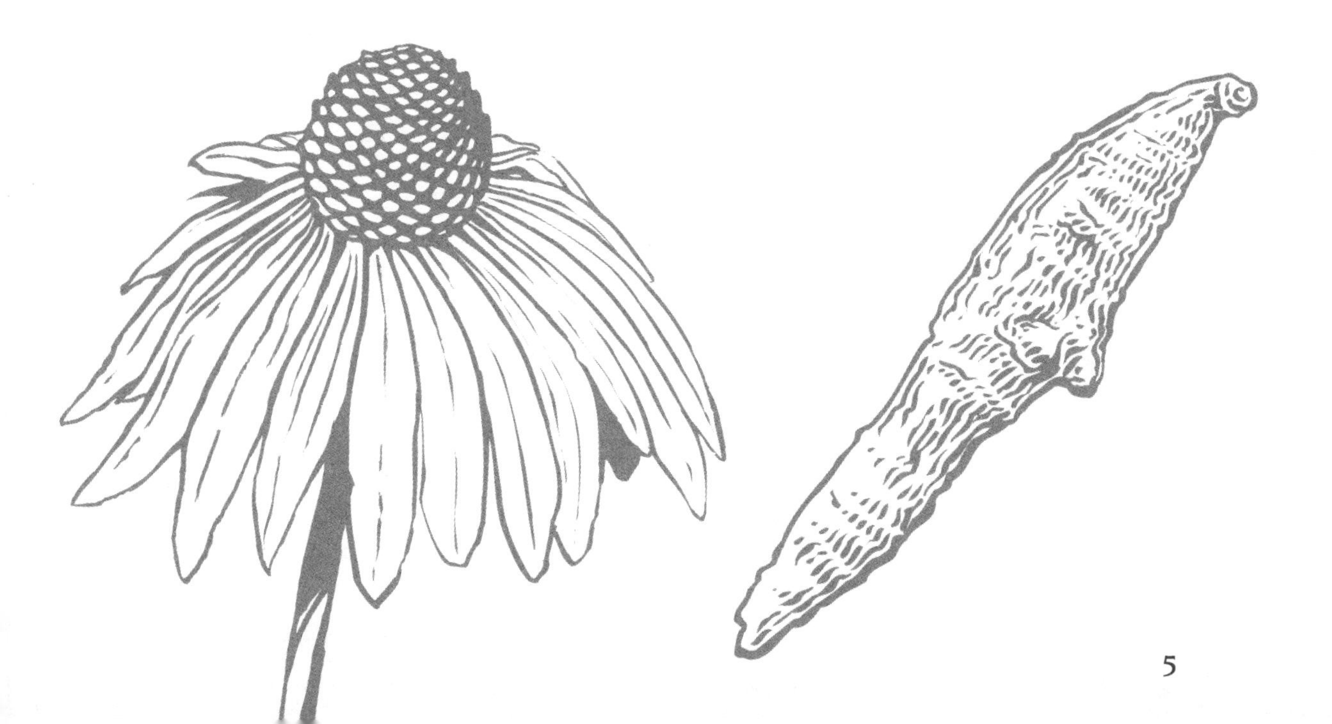

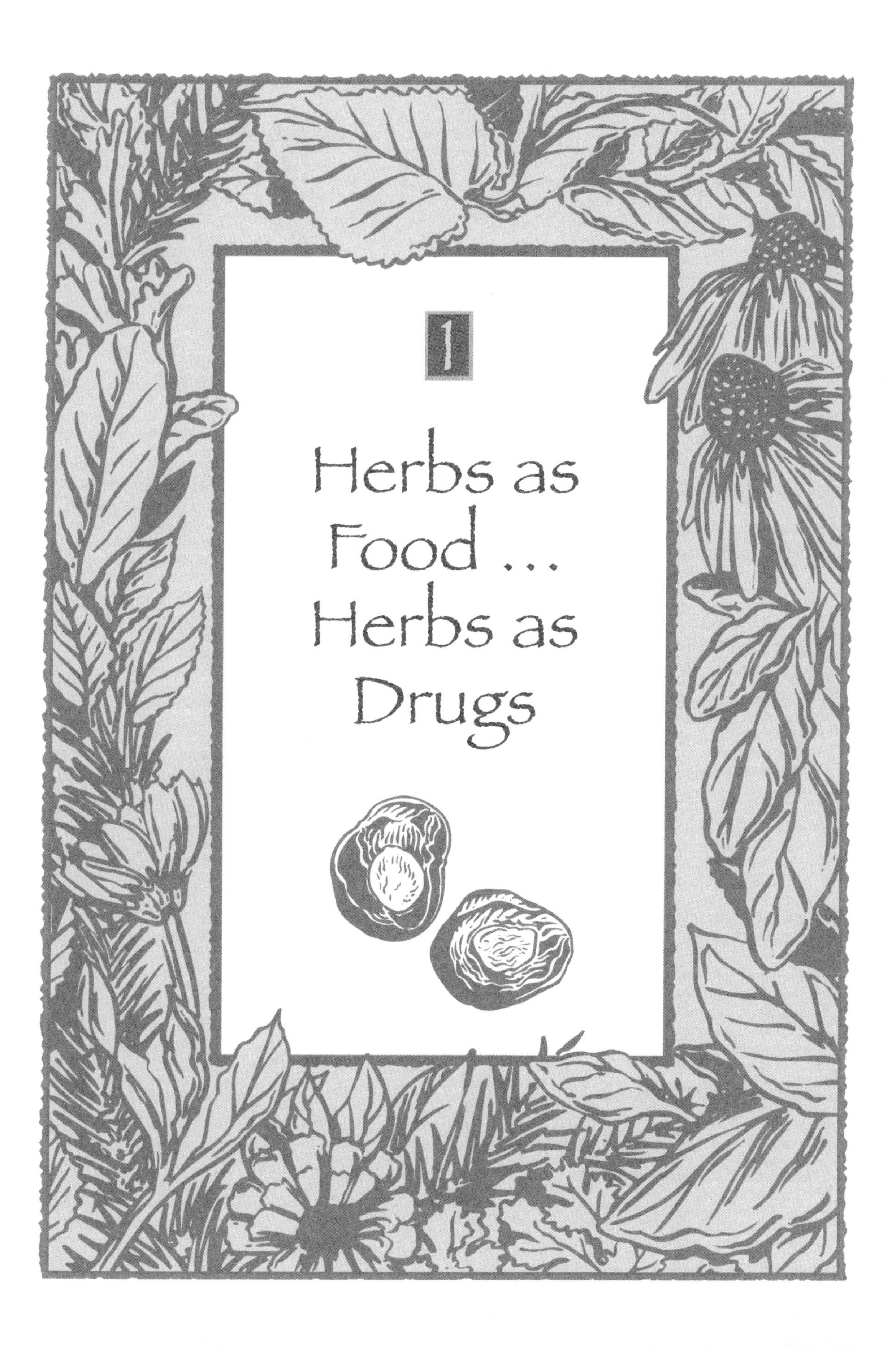

1

Herbs as Food ... Herbs as Drugs

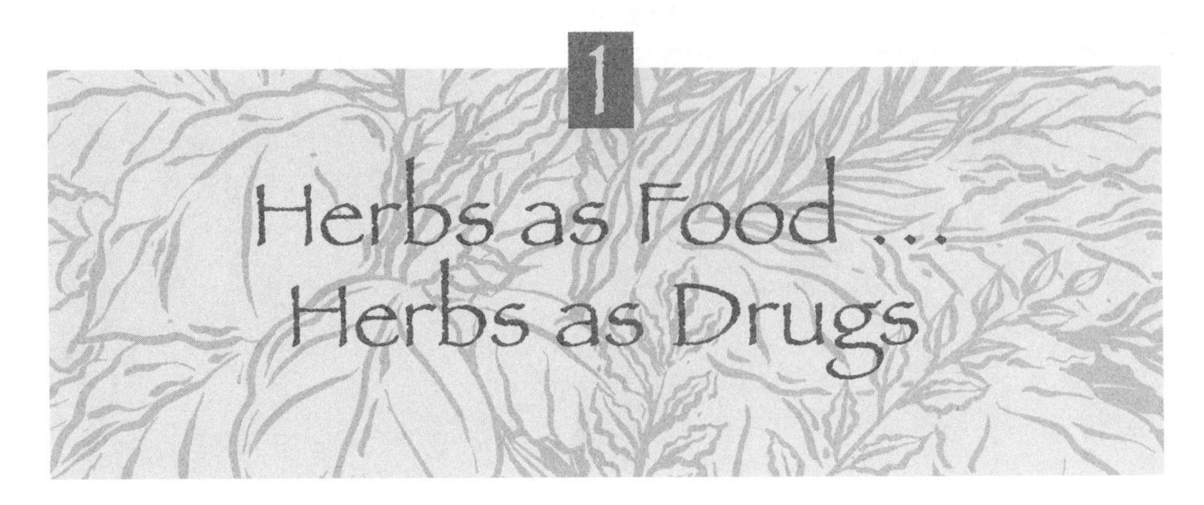

Herbs as Food ... Herbs as Drugs

What Are Herbs?

There are many ways to define herbs, depending on their intended use and whom you ask. Some herbs are roadside and lawnscape menaces—dandelions, chicory, chickweed and stinging nettle. Others are prized for their scent or colorful foliage and flowers—lavender, roses, flax and echinacea. Still more are valued for their culinary properties—basil, thyme, parsley and rosemary. When you know that thousands of plants are included in the definition, it is easy to understand that many herbs can have multiple uses.

An herb may be defined as a seed-producing, non-woody plant that dies in winter, such as parsley or angelica. They also include, however, woody plants like Siberian ginseng and *ginkgo biloba*. Herbs are plants that have medicinal and/or culinary uses. Herbs come from cold or tropical environments and they are not necessarily green. Barks, roots, mushrooms, shrubs, vines, flowers, roses and trees can offer some medicinal value in their most colorful or colorless parts.

Names & Definitions

Herbs have many definitions and many names.

Botanicals is the term the Food and Drug Administration prefers for herbs. It allows for the broader definition consisting of plant-based products including trees, shrubs and herbs.

Herbal Medicinals are products derived from plant parts that have a pharmacologic effect. (This term is sometimes incorrectly used interchangeably with phytopharmaceuticals.)

Phytopharmaceuticals are plant-based medicines that have been standardized for key compounds, or active constituents, and adjusted to ensure that the level of these compounds is consistent.

Herbs in Action

Some herbalists believe that herbs have specific actions. They are considered to be Specifics or Tonics depending on the symptoms the herbs treat or the health enhancement properties they hold. Herbs with the prefix "anti" fight against particular conditions or symptoms, while there are a whole host of other action-type herbs that are believed to have particular benefits. Although not all herbs will be labeled with their specific actions, these are worth mentioning as they are commonly seen in advertising, health publications and literature from manufacturers. Some herbs may have several uses, depending on the desired outcome.

Specifics are for a particular condition and should be taken only for a short time, just as a prescription medicine might be used.

Tonics are for general health enhancement and are taken for longer periods of time, sometimes with a break.

Antispasmodics help relieve spasms and are often used for respiratory and intestinal problems.

Antioxidants will be discussed in more detail in the next column on this page. These inhibit oxidation.

Anti-inflammatories are used to calm inflamed tissues and swelling.

Adaptogens are tonics thought to help enhance the immune system and the endocrine system, which affects our reactions to stress.

Bitters have been used for hundreds of years as a "tonic" after a meal. They are thought to help improve digestion and absorption of food.

Carminatives relieve cramping and bloating caused by gas that builds up in the intestine.

Demulcents are believed to soothe the mucous membranes and digestive system by coating the tissues and protecting them from further irritation.

Expectorants reduce the viscosity of secretions from or decrease the persistence with which mucus adheres to the respiratory system, allowing them to be expelled more easily.

Cooking for Health: Herbal Culinary Adventures

Culinary herbs have potential healing and preventive properties. These properties are believed to be due in part to phytochemicals. Phytochemicals, sometimes called phytonutrients, are plant-based compounds that give herbs color and are believed to have health-enhancing or medicinal properties. Phytochemicals are substances that plants naturally produce to protect themselves against viruses, bacteria and fungi. Many phytochemicals are antioxidants—natural cell protectors—that include: flavonoids, polyphenols, phytoestrogens, lignans, organosulfurs, phytosterols, saponins and capsaicin.

Antioxidants are classes of compounds including flavonoids and phytoestrogens listed below that are thought to neutralize free radicals, which are molecules produced in our cells and formed from sources such as smoking, pesticides and smog. Over time, free radicals damage DNA and cell structures, which can promote cellular aging and cancer.

Flavonoids are members of the phenolic family that have antioxidant properties. They are thought to protect tissue from free-radical damage that can lead to heart disease and some types of cancers. Many people became familiar with flavonoids (but did not know that's what they were) when resveratrol, found in wine and grape juice, was touted for a healthy heart.

Polyphenols and phenols are part of the largest category of phytochemicals—phenolics—and among the most widely distributed in the plant kingdom. They may protect the body from some diseases by blocking the formation of nitrosamines that are believed to cause some types of cancers. Tea, coffee, cranberries, turmeric, mustard, curry and parsley all contain beneficial phenolic compounds.

Phytoestrogens are compounds from plants that are transformed by the intestines into estrogen-like compounds. Isoflavones (which include genistein and daidzein) make up one of the major groups of compounds classified as phytoestrogens. Found in the largest amounts in soy products and flaxseed, isoflavones are believed to reduce the risk of hormone-sensitive cancers, such as breast and prostate, by substituting weak plant estrogens for human estrogen. However, this belief remains controversial. Studies in humans have shown contradictory results for both reducing the risk of breast cancer and affecting the survival of breast cancer patients. Data that indicates soy has the ability to suppress the spread of existing cancer cells is also contradictory and controversial. Isoflavones may help reduce cholesterol levels and prevent bone loss after menopause.

Organosulfur compounds are responsible for the onion or allium cepa family's distinctive taste and odor. They have been found to boost the immune system, reduce cholesterol production in the liver and assist the liver in neutralizing carcinogens.

Lignans, found in flaxseed, are the fibers that are believed to give flax its cholesterol-reducing properties. Lignans may also act as a bulk-forming laxative.

Phytosterols are compounds found naturally in a wide variety of plants including nuts, seeds, fruits and vegetables. Phytosterols inhibit intestinal absorption of cholesterol by about 50 percent. Some phytosterols are also thought to enhance immunity, reduce inflammation and may reduce the risk of cancer.

Saponins are a type of carbohydrate, found in ginseng and soy, that neutralizes enzymes believed to cause cancer in the intestine. Wound-healing and

Sources of Some Herbal Phytochemicals

Herb	Main Phytochemicals
Flaxseed	Lignans
Garlic, onions, leeks	Organosulfur compounds
Hot peppers	Capsaicin
Licorice	Triterpenoids
Rosemary	Phenolic compounds; Ellagic acid
Cranberries	Ellagic acids
Tea	Polyphenols
Watercress (a member of the cruciferous vegetable family—cabbage family)	Isothiocyanates

immune-boosting properties may also be credited to saponins.

Capsaicin, a purified compound from red peppers, may provide temporary pain relief for arthritis and some neuralgias. It is also considered a digestive stimulant and may inhibit production of cancer-causing substances.

Nearly all of us are familiar with the culinary uses for herbs. Herbs enliven foods and give dishes flavor without salt. At the same time, they provide some essential nutrients and potentially active plant constituents that treat disease and support overall health and wellness. Herbs contain phytochemicals that have many actions in the body, like blocking the uptake of various hormones, including estrogen. They also activate enzymes that help metabolize and get rid of carcinogens. These actions may reduce the risk of developing cancer. Herbs have been found to have higher antioxidant activity than fruits and vegetables.

Although primarily regional in use, herbs have been used for thousands of years to flavor foods. The flavors of herbs and spices define cooking worldwide. Rice and beans are Asian and Mexican ingredients, but it is the herbs or spices added to the dish that define it as one or the other. It is only recently that herbs common to cooking have received attention for their medicinal properties. Fresh from your garden, herbs appear to have a higher level of antioxidants than their dried or processed version. Fresh garlic, for example, is one and one-half times higher in antioxidants than garlic powder. Increasing the use of herbs in cooking provides flavor and a daily dose of phytochemicals that can provide health-promoting and -protecting benefits.

Herbal Use Through the Ages & Cultures

Most ancient cultures have a long history of using plants and their byproducts to treat diseases and promote health. Many people around the world continue to practice herbal medicine because of tradition and, in some cases, because modern medicines are not available. Traditional healers who use herbal medicines rely on experience and word of mouth to understand the plants they use, the plants' safety and strength, how to prepare them and how to combine them with other herbs and therapies.

Although there are numerous cultural influences from ancient civilizations, including Greek, Islamic, Tibetan and Medieval, we will look at the four civilizations we hear about most often: Chinese, Ayurveda (or Indian), Mexican and Native American.

Traditional Chinese Medicine (TCM)

TCM has been used for more than 3,000 years for prevention and treatment of "disharmony" or imbalances in the body—disease concepts that are foreign to Western healthcare. The basic idea is that energy flows through the body along pathways called meridians, or qi. In TCM, disease is recognized as an imbalance in qi and therapies are focused on balancing the qi. To balance the person, practitioners use the principles of the five elements and yin-yang as described below.

TCM vs. Western Medicine

Unlike Western medicine, TCM has changed very little over the centuries. The Chinese have documented more than 7,000 kinds of herbs that possess healing benefits. Written records are found as far back as 3494 B.C.E. Chinese herbal medicine has been in the United States as long as Chinese people have lived here. Exposure to Chinese medicine has been limited until recently because it had been confined to large communities with "Chinatown" neighborhoods. Current herbal therapies are still based on the Chinese recipes, standards of purity and dosages of ancient times. Translation of practices from the ancient language is difficult because the language uses many unfamiliar concepts to describe health and disease. Often there are conflicting views regarding the appropriate uses or specific benefits of many herbs because they are believed to have numerous uses. Studies of TCM herbal therapies using Western methodologies are increasing in number, which should mean a better understanding of uses and safety in the future.

The Five Elements & Yin-Yang

The theory of the five elements is central to TCM. Wood, water, metal, earth and fire are the five elements in TCM. According to the theory, these elements are associated with time of life, time of year and specific organ and bodily systems. Yin-yang is the Chinese theory of opposites; everything in the universe has an opposite with an intricate interaction. To promote good health, yin-yang must be balanced.

Chinese Herbs: Medicinal & Culinary Importance

TCM, the most widely practiced form of herbal medicine in the world, usually combines 10 or more herbs in each formula. The current market of Chinese herbal products is unfortunately fraught with problems. Mixtures of herbs sometimes use animal and/or mineral components that may be offensive or dangerous to the user. Several mixtures have been found to be dangerous because they are contaminated with an herb known to contain aristolochic acid. This herb, which causes rapid kidney damage and

The Five Elements of Traditional Chinese Medicine

Element	Wood	Fire	Earth	Metal	Water
Season	Spring	Summer	Indian Summer	Fall	Winter
Color	Green/ blue	Red	Yellow	White	Black/ dark
Taste	Sour	Bitter	Sweet	Pungent/ spicy	Salty
Emotion	Anger	Joy	Worry	Grief	Fear
Direction	Rising	Floating	Centering	Descending	Sinking
Body Part	Liver, gallbladder, tendons, eyes	Heart, small intestine	Pancreas, spleen, stomach, mouth	Lungs, large intestine, nose, skin	Kidneys, bladder, ears, hair, bones
Characteristic	Hot	Cold	Hot	Hot	Cold

failure, can lead to death. Use of animal organs and parts thought to enhance sexual prowess may be offensive to vegetarians. Some Chinese herbal products have been found to be adulterated with heavy metals, pesticides, pharmaceutical drugs or other potential toxins.

Conflicting results from research has led to marketing of some herbs for opposing uses. For example, ginseng is promoted both as a relaxant and a stimulant. In addition, the quality of some products is questionable. Analyses of ginseng products have shown that up to 25 percent of the products sold contained no ginseng at all, and only 40 percent contained what the label stated.

The taste of an herb and its characteristic or environmental influence, hot or cold, is believed to dictate which part of the body the herb will influence. Chinese herbs are believed to be more effective when used in a formula. Knowledge of an individual herb is necessary, even though each herb has its own medicinal and nutritional qualities. To support the concept of balance, several herbs need to be taken in combination in order to systematically correct the imbalance in the entire body. No one single herb can accomplish this. For example, because ginseng is believed to energize the body and because it has strong side effects when used alone, mixing ginseng with another herb, such as astragalus, balances the side effects. Potency and balance of the herbs is believed to be increased when they are combined in the correct proportions.

Several Chinese herbs are used in cooking. Although traditionally thought of as food, several of the items listed in the box on this page are considered Chinese herbal medicines. Due to the amount used in recipes, these herbs may not always bestow a measurable medicinal benefit. Despite not always having a medicinal benefit, they will undoubtedly enhance the nutritional content and flavor of the dishes they are used in.

Chinese medicine is a system of healthcare, not just herbal medicines. It includes therapies such as acupuncture, massage, meditation, concentration, exercises known as qigong, cupping and moxibustion. The Chinese notion of a diet is not about weight loss. Diet is a part of every therapy and helps to balance the body's energy. Studying yin-yang concepts of using food for balancing the body may be the place to begin to understand the concepts of TCM. Many of the TCM practices, including diet, have important roles in health promotion and are worth considering.

Selected Chinese Herbs with Medicinal & Culinary Properties

- Tea (chai)
- Ginger
- Rhubarb
- Mulberry
- Onions and leeks
- Cinnamon
- Licorice
- Cloves
- Peaches
- Garlic
- Reshi-mushroom
- Turmeric
- Soy
- Chinese cucumber
- Citrus fruits

Ayurveda

Ayurveda is believed to be the oldest healing science, originating in India more than 5,000 years ago, with written information dating back to about 2500 B.C.E. Ayurveda is a Sanskrit word that means the "Knowledge of Life." It is derived from two words: *Ayur*, or life, and *veda*, meaning knowledge. Its healing philosophies encompass diet, exercise, spiritual activities and herbal medicine in a holistic approach. The foundation of Ayurveda is similar to TCM in that it has five elements—earth, water, fire, air and ether—which combine to create your own individual constitutional type. This constitutional type, or dosha, is a combination of characteristics—physical, mental and emotional.

Constitutional Types

Ayurveda identifies three constitutional types (doshas) that are present in everyone and everything. The original Sanskrit words for these types are used because there are no English words to describe them. They are vata, pitta and kapha. Everyone has vata, pitta and kapha, but one usually predominates, one is secondary and the third is the least influential.

Vata is dominated by air and ether and is the energy of movement. Vata is associated with bones, the nervous system and the colon. When out of balance, vatas' nervous systems are usually affected and they suffer from problems with cold and dryness.

Pitta is dominated by fire and water and is the energy of digestion or metabolism. When out of balance, pittas usually have difficulties with their organs related to heat—their gallbladder, liver, spleen, blood and eyes. When pittas are stressed, their detoxifying organ—the liver—is unable to process toxins.

The Constitutional Types & Elements of Ayurveda

Dosha	*Vata*	*Pitta*	*Kapha*
Element	**Air, Ether**	**Fire, Water**	**Earth, Water**
Season	Fall/Winter	Spring/Summer	Winter/Spring
Taste/ Flavors	Sweet, salty, sour	Bland, mild sweet, bitter and/or astringent	Pungent/spicy, bitter and astringent
Emotion	Nervous, anxious	Angry, frustrated competitive	Depressed, sad, sluggish
Body Part	Bones, colon nervous system	Kidneys, gallbladder, ears, hair, liver	Lungs, large intestine, nose, skin
Characteristic	Warm, moistening and lubricating	Cool, slightly dry and slightly heavy	Light, dry and warm

Kapha is dominated by earth and water and is the energy of lubrication and structure. When kaphas are out of balance, they tend to be sluggish, sleep too much and lack zest for life. Physically, kaphas are affected by problems with their lungs and chest.

The Six Tastes

In Ayurveda, the six tastes are essential for balancing meals and life. All of these tastes, according to Ayurvedic principles, should be included in each meal, but not necessarily in equal quantities. Balance is the key. The tastes are distinct: astringent, bitter, pungent, salty, sweet and sour.

In addition to the herbs thought to be beneficial for specific doshas, many Indian herbs are becoming known for their purported ability to reduce the risk of numerous diseases, including cancer and heart disease. Tea, with its polyphenol content, is thought to help prevent cancer. Chiles are thought to be anti-inflammatory, and the mint family is believed to be antispasmodic and to reduce sinusitis. Garlic and members of the allium cepa family are thought to thin blood, lower cholesterol, help to fend off colds and reduce the risk of cancer.

Most of the herbs mentioned here are known for their culinary properties and are well-known flavorings and condiments. Their therapeutic benefits are less well known, although further clinical trials are revealing some potential health benefits. Whether you think about the health or culinary benefits of Indian herbs, they are worth considering for their taste and their potential nutritional, including antioxidant, benefit to your diet.

Selected Ayurvedic Herbs with Medicinal & Culinary Properties, by Dosha

Vata	Pitta	Kapha
Basil	Black pepper (small amounts)	Basil
Bay leaf	Cardamom	Black pepper
Cardamom	Cilantro	Black mustard seeds
Cinnamon	Cinnamon	Chiles
Cloves	Coriander	Coriander
Coriander	Cumin	Cumin
Cranberries	Fennel	Fennel
Cumin	Mint	Fenugreek
Epazote	Parsley	Ginger Horseradish
Fennel	Sage	Sage
Fenugreek	Turmeric	*If a Kapha does not tolerate pungent spices:*
Ginger	*Low-salt diet is suggested, except during summer*	Allspice
Mace		Cardamom
Marjoram		Cinnamon
Mustard seed		Nutmeg
Nutmeg		Sea salt in moderation
Oregano		
Savory		
Seaweed		
Thyme		
Turmeric		

Mexican Herbs

Mexican herbs and foods have become as popular as hamburgers and french fries in America. Mexican herbal remedies have a long history but, unlike Chinese and Ayurvedic herbs, Mexican herbs and healing practices are more

Selected Mexican Culinary Herbs with Potential Medicinal Value

- Annatto
- Star anise
- Chayote (vegetable pear)
- Coriander
- Plantain
- Mustard
- Licorice
- Sage
- Mint
- Garlic
- Mexican sunflower
- Onion
- Guava
- Chamomile
- Prickly pear
- Nettle
- Lemongrass
- Epazote
- Basil
- Cinnamon
- Chile
- Bay leaf
- Horehound
- Marjoram
- Rosemary
- Thyme

empiric, less structured and rely more on family and cultural traditions to provide direction in their use. Reliance on word of mouth and tradition often leads to misinterpretations, misunderstandings and confusion regarding use. Names of herbs may be the same in various regions of Mexico, but the plants that produce these herbs may be quite different, with different and sometimes dangerous consequences.

As the Hispanic population increases in America, more Mexican herbs are being introduced for culinary as well as medicinal purposes. At present, there is little clinical evidence that Mexican herbs offer extraordinary health benefits. Because of the increased incidence of diabetes among people of Mexican heritage and the subsequent popularity of certain herbal remedies for the disease, more clinical trials are being conducted to investigate the potential value of some herbs for treating the disease.

In the Southwest and in parts of the country catering to the Hispanic population, numerous herbal products, both culinary and medicinal, are available for purchase. Much of the success of Mexican herbs may be due to the expectation that the herbs will do what they're supposed to do (the placebo effect), particularly if an elder has recommended or suggested using the herbs. One exception does exist in the red pepper, which is the source of the celebrated pharmaceutical capsaicin. Capsaicin is the compound in red pepper (capsicum annum) that makes it spicy hot and valuable for healing. The herb has been used as a digestive aid and as an ointment for treating muscle and joint pain.

Despite the lack of evidence of the medicinal qualities of Mexican herbs, many do provide significant nutritional value by their antioxidant and flavor contributions. For these reasons, including them as part of a healthy diet is considered prudent.

Herbs in Native American Traditions

Native American people, when faced with illness and disease, discovered a wealth of useful healing agents among plants and animals. The use of these medicinal substances and their toxic potential was passed on primarily by word of mouth for at least 12,000 years. Many Native American healing practices have never been written down, only passed directly from elders in closely guarded communication. Some believed that knowledge of medicinal plants was obtained in dreams or visions. Many important herbal medicines were found by following sick animals to see what they ate. Bears were valued for their long claws that could efficiently dig herbs, a practice that taught herbalists many things about the healing properties of herbs. They soon learned that many herbs had immense power and could even kill the patient.

Traditional healing practices vary from tribe to tribe, but all share a use of herbal medicines and sweat lodges or baths, and believe that all aspects of mind, body and spirit are connected in a circle of health. Native American medicine centers around the medicine man or shaman who uses the medicine wheel to find the soul of the sick person and find spiritual energies for healing. As with Chinese and Ayurvedic practices, the physical, spiritual and emotional person is considered during the healing process. As important as curing the illness, and at times identical to it, is making the person whole by establishing balance, harmony, beauty and meaning.

Historical Background of Native American Traditions

When the first European settlers arrived in North America, they adopted some of the Native American herbs including purple coneflower (echinacea), goldenseal and pleurisy root to treat their sick. Echinacea has seen a surge in use during the past few years, and there is growing evidence that this herb is useful as a wound-healing topical agent and as an immune system enhancer. Saw palmetto, a small palm tree found in the southeastern United States, provided food from the tree's seeds for the Seminole Indians. This may have been the beginning of the understanding of saw palmetto's benefits for the prostate gland. Evening primrose was important to Native Americans as food and medicine, and has recently gained popularity in America and Europe for its purported anti-inflammatory properties. Among Native Americans, its use differed from tribe to tribe—from a food source, to a means of reducing external swelling and inflammation and as a weight-loss aid.

Many valuable drugs of today (for example, atropine and digoxin) came into use through the study of native remedies. Several plant-based drugs (for example, morphine and Taxol) are in use today.

Although there was an overlap in the herbs used by various Native American tribes, there were differences which evolved based on where they were grown, the plant part used and the nature of the plant itself. Because Native American traditions have been passed down by word of mouth, it has been more difficult to form a definition of traditional Native medicine from the non-Native.

Selected Native American Foods & Herbs

- Blackberry
- Cranberry
- Evening primrose
- Onion (wild)
- Raspberry
- Juniper
- Black walnut
- Strawberry (wild)
- Sage
- Chokecherry
- Black cherry

Culinary Practices in Native American Traditions

The use of herbs and spices in Native American cooking seems to be more limited than in other cultures. This may be due in part to limited availability of particular herbs and spices, particularly in northern climates. The diet of Native Americans was predominantly animal flesh accompanied by corn, squash, beans and a few other vegetables. Seasonal foods were available when the weather cooperated. Many plants that were not used as part of a meal were prepared as teas or infusions for their medicinal qualities. Several foods common to regions where Native Americans lived are worth listing because of their medicinal and culinary qualities.

Cranberries were a significant part of the diet during the winter, and provided an ingredient to an essential food called pemmican. Made from crushed berries added to buffalo meat and fat, pemmican was described by Lewis and Clark in their writings. This high calorie, high protein snack was adopted by many explorers and travelers in the West because it lasted many months and could be carried easily.

Meals with healing properties include culinary herbs and spices and a variety of fruits and vegetables with antioxidant, medicinal and preventive compounds. The more variety in our meals, the more likely they are to provide the nutrients that will help reduce the risk of disease and promote optimum health. The minimum recommendations of five fruits and vegetables each day, depending on choices, will meet the minimums necessary for health. By eating up to nine or more servings of fruits and vegetables per day, we can actually control blood pressure and reduce our risk for heart disease, obesity and certain types of cancer.

Herbs in Conventional Medicine

Before medicines were made in the laboratory, plants and herbs were all that

Botanicals as Drugs

Botanical	Drug	Used for
Foxglove	Digoxin	Heart medicine
Periwinkle	Vincristine and vinblastine	Anticancer drugs
Opium poppy	Morphine and codeine	Pain relievers
Belladonna	Atropine	Antispasmodic and cardiac drug
Willow bark	Aspirin	Multipurpose pain reliever, blood thinner
Ephedra plant (also called Mormon Tea)	Ephedrine	Forbear of anti-asthma drugs, appetite suppressant
Senna plant	Senna	Laxative
Yew tree	Taxol	Anticancer drug
Coffee tree (beans)	Caffeine	Stimulant

doctors had to treat their patients. Some herbs from the United States were introduced by Native Americans, while others were brought from Europe by colonists and traders. First published in 1820, the *United States Pharmacopoeia* (USP), included medicinal herbs, and at that time, the USP contained some 207 botanical substances that were considered drugs. The numbers dropped off from 79 in 1936 to only 26 in 1990. The USP is in the process of developing a Dietary Supplement Certification Program (DSCP) intended to inform and safeguard consumers who are using dietary supplements. Products that meet USP's rigorous standards must: contain declared ingredients, contain the amount or strength of ingredient declared, meet requirements for limits on potential contaminants, and comply with FDA's good manufacturing processes. (Visit **www.usp.org** for more information.)

Twenty-five percent or more of current prescription medicines come from herbs. Drugs can be made synthetically in the laboratory by copying the chemical structure of naturally growing plants or by deriving them directly from plants. Each herb may have many active ingredients, but only one may be considered the active component—the one used as a drug. Some herbs are helpful, but some may be harmful or even deadly if not used correctly. One example is digoxin, which comes from a plant called foxglove. Digoxin is a powerful heart medicine, but it is deadly if taken in even small amounts above the therapeutic level (the amount required to produce a desired effect).

Some herbs have lost their appeal to consumers, while others are emerging as favorites. Sales of herbal supplements through conventional channels, including grocery stores, drugstores and natural food stores are on the rise. It is impossible to estimate the number of different herbs and the dollar value of herbs and botanicals raised in thousands, if not millions, of backyards throughout the country.

Americans have been using herbs and herbal preparations in increasing numbers since the mid-1990s, despite continuing advancements in medicine. As the number of prescriptions is growing, so are their costs, leading to one possible explanation for herbs' surge in popularity. As

The Popularity of Herbal Supplements

Various sources offer possible explanations for current popularity of herbal supplements. Here are some speculations.

- Consumers may be losing confidence in conventional medicine.
- A search for a miracle cure when all other efforts have failed.
- The belief that herbal supplements will prevent disease and/or improve health and well-being.
- The belief that herbal supplements are natural and safe.
- People believe they can self-medicate and not seek treatment.
- The average price for dietary supplements has been decreasing, while the cost of prescription medication has been on the rise.
- Some people are searching for a competitive edge in sports.
- For weight control.
- Some may offer the same benefits as more expensive prescription drugs.

the use of these popular herbs increases, so do potential dangers—and potential benefits.

In 2000, supplement sales exceeded $16.8 billion, accounting for 9 percent of the healthcare product sales in the United States. Herbal and botanical supplements represent $4.12 billion, or 25 percent of the total, while sports nutrition products that may also contain herbs were 9 percent of the sales, or $1.59 billion. This was in contrast to pharmaceutical and prescription drug sales of $145 billion during 2000.

One in four Americans, or 23 percent, reported they regularly use herbs, with 15 percent of adults taking garlic, ginseng and/or St. John's wort. Women, particularly women over age 65, are increasing their intake of herbs much more than any other group. A survey conducted in Northern California found that 28.5 percent of women over age 65 were taking herbs, including St. John's wort, ginkgo biloba, echinacea and kava. Menopause is the number one specific condition for which women use dietary supplements (herbal and other).

Worldwide Use of Medicinal Herbs

In countries around the world, herbal medicines are government-approved and sold. In Germany, France, Australia, Mexico, Canada and most of Asia, herbal medicines are sold with medical claims regarding their use. In other countries, sales are allowed, but with limited health claims, based on traditional uses.

European Influence on Herb Use in the United States

With the exception of Great Britain and Ireland, most of Europe has never lost its herbal tradition. France, Germany and other European countries have established standards for herbs with regard to dosage, strength and purity. Most scientific and clinical studies on herb use in the West have come from Germany, where the tradition of herbs as medicine has existed for centuries. German physicians use herbal medicine, with as many as 70 percent prescribing the thousands of products available. The *Commission E Monographs,* recently translated into English, provide information on more than 300 herbs that are, with "reasonable certainty," safe and effective. Members of Commission E include knowledgeable healthcare providers, experts and lay persons. Commission E members evaluate trials, data, scientific literature and more in order to compile the monographs and evaluate the safety and efficacy of herbal medicines.

Because of the widespread use of botanicals, particularly in countries that rely heavily on medicinal plants to meet primary healthcare needs, the World Health Organization (WHO) published *Guidelines for the Assessment of Herbal Medicines* in 1991. These guidelines were developed to help regulatory agencies evaluate the quality, safety and effectiveness of herbal medicines, and have expanded to include information about commonly used medicinal plants in China, the South Pacific, Korea and Viet Nam. A collection of 28 monographs covering the quality control and traditional and clinical uses of selected widely used medicinal plants was published in 1999.

Complementary & Alternative Medicine

Complementary and Alternative Medicine (CAM) is defined as a group of diverse medical and healthcare systems, practices and products that are not presently considered part of conventional medicine. Examples of CAM include Traditional Chinese Medicine, homeopathy, dietary supplements and Ayurveda.

CAM and the use of herbs beyond prescription medicine was not taught in medical schools much before the 1990s, but it is taking an ever-increasing role in medical education today. Medical schools are beginning to understand the need for physician education about CAM, including herbal medicines. Approximately 75 percent, if not more, of schools of medicine are including some form of training in integrative medicine (a blending of holistic approaches with the best of Western medicine) in their core curricula. Numerous centers for integrative medicine are also being established in prominent university medical schools. Many insurance carriers and Health Maintenance Organizations (HMOs) are now covering some forms of alternative treatment, usually because of consumer demand.

There is great demand for CAM as is seen in the rising out-of-pocket spending for CAM since 1990. Between 1990 and 1997, there was a 47 percent increase in visits to alternative practitioners, from 427 million to 629 million, which exceeded the estimated total number of visits made to all conventional primary care physicians in 1997. It was estimated that payments to alternative practitioners increased 45 percent to $21.2 billion. The total estimated out-of-pocket expense for alternative therapies in 1997 (whether or not a practitioner was involved) was $27 billion, comparable to the amount paid out-of-pocket for all physician services in the United States. These figures do not represent just herbal medicines, but also the role alternative therapies are playing in healthcare today.

A 1998 survey of attitudes and practices of 783 primary care physicians in the United States found that they most frequently reported training in biofeedback, relaxation, psychotherapy, behavioral medicine and diet and exercise counseling. These therapies were more likely to be considered valid. The least accepted therapies were Eastern medicine, Native American medicine and electromagnetic applications. Physicians who personally used complementary therapies were much more likely to refer patients to these therapies. The longer the provider had been in practice, the less likely the provider was to use an alternative therapy, either personally or in their practice.

Healthcare providers who are more likely to include some form of CAM, including herbal therapies, in their practice include: doctors of TCM, chiropractors, naturopaths and osteopaths. Some providers with less formal education and training bill themselves as "experts." A title does not always guarantee quality training or experience. There are numerous correspondence schools that are not accredited that grant degrees without ever seeing the student. Some practitioners may have an advanced degree, but in an unrelated field. The practice of CAM is not as regulated as the practice of conventional medicine. You may want to check with local and state health regulatory agencies and consumer affairs departments about a specific practitioner's license, education, accreditation and whether there are any complaints filed against the practitioner.

There is no official certification program for "herbalists" in the United States; there are herbalists who are very knowledgeable about herbs and their use, and about diagnosing health problems. Technically, anyone can call him- or herself an herbalist without any training or experience. The only exception may be in the practice of Oriental medicine, especially TCM, where practitioners have earned a doctorate in Oriental medicine, an O.M.D.

Questions to ask about a particular herb

- Is the herb safe to use for my condition?
- Is there any evidence that the herb may be potentially harmful to me?
- Is the herb harmless, or at best, may it increase my quality of life?
- What are the best treatments in the world today for my condition?
- How long must I take the herb before I see improvement? Natural healing can take time and effort and you must often be committed to the efforts and time involved for the effects to be seen.
- How much money am I willing to spend? Although herbs are less costly than prescription medications, the expense is usually out-of-pocket.
- What do I know about my ability to raise the herb for my own use or, if I am going to purchase it, what do I know about the manufacturer? How can I ensure quality, safety and effectiveness?
- If the practitioner provides the herb, ask about the quality, safety and manufacturing and/or growing practices of the company that supplies it.

Finding an Integrative or Herb-friendly Practitioner

Herbal and complementary medicine is not meant to replace conventional therapies, but can be used in addition to conventional medical therapy. The key is finding a provider you are comfortable with—someone you are willing to share information with about what you are using, what your goals and expectations are, and someone who is open to trying some therapies that may have been considered unconventional in the past. The following topics are helpful when considering any therapy or practitioner.

Become Informed

Learn about your options. Whether you want to be healthier or need help treating an illness, the more credible information you have the better. First, ask your current doctor. If he or she appears uninterested or dismisses your questions, you may want to consider looking for a doctor who is more open. If your provider already includes herbal medicines in their treatments, then ask about the safety and effectiveness of the therapy he or she uses. It is critical that you inform your primary doctor, whether he or she practices CAM, about any alternative (and conventional) treatments or therapies you are using. Some herbal therapies can interfere with other treatments you may be getting.

Don't rely on friends, other patients or book and advertising testimonials as the deciding factor for choosing a therapy. Everyone is different and reacts to herbs and drugs differently. Furthermore, some books and seemingly honest testimonials that extol the virtues of particular "cures" are little more than quick and easy moneymakers for their authors or advertisers. The best information about effectiveness and safety comes from clinical trials and should be sought whenever possible. If the information is questionable in your mind, seek more information or other therapies that have more supportive evidence.

Even after you have chosen a practitioner or have started using a particular herb, supplement or therapy, stay informed! Data change almost daily as new information is learned about herbs and therapies that may impact you.

Places to look for more information

- Libraries, particularly at hospitals or universities.
- Advocacy and health organizations such as the American Heart Association and the American Cancer Society.
- The Internet. CAM on PubMed (www.cancer.gov/occam/pubmed.html) is a wealth of information with bibliographic citations on complementary and alternative medicine. The service is free, but not all articles can be accessed free of charge.
- Support groups.
- Other patients or friends, especially those who have been treated recently.

Find Out About the Practitioner

Get good referrals by asking a variety of people. Contact schools of medicine that have integrative or functional medicine centers and ask them for names of providers in your area. Contact state or local regulatory authorities that oversee practitioners who use herbal therapies or the therapies you are seeking. Check to see if the practitioner must be licensed or certified in your area and, if so, whether he or she has a license or certification from a recognized accredited agency.

Talk with the practitioner's office staff to learn more. They can be an invaluable source about the practitioner's expertise, educational background, additional training and professional organizations he or she belongs to. Determine the success the practitioner has had with a particular herb or therapy you are interested in. Find out about cost for treatments and coverage by insurance or third-party payers. You can also get an idea of how patients are treated by the staff themselves.

Talk with the practitioner. Verify information you have received elsewhere and find out how he or she communicates treatment plans, side effects and potential problems to patients. Talk with them about your condition and goals for treatment, and do not be afraid to give them information about what you already know. Find someone you are comfortable talking with and who is open to your questions.

What About Service?

Find out how much time the physician is able to spend with each patient. When you visit the office or clinic, aside from talking with the staff, look at the physical condition and cleanliness of the location. Can all services be obtained in one place? Does the cost seem excessive for what is provided? Does service delivery follow regulated standards for medical safety and care? For example, does the staff wash their hands between patients, use exam gloves appropriately and clean equipment between patients? These may sound like obvious questions, but they are nonetheless important as they may uncover signs of poor service.

None of this information guarantees that the practitioner you choose will meet your expectations after you have formed a partnership with them. It will at least give you a place to start and questions to consider in hopes that you will find the ideal match. Once you have found someone you can work with, it is important that you partner with your provider, that you follow the treatment guidelines, be honest about the care and success (or failure) of the treatment, communicate openly about questions and concerns and share information about other treatments or herbs you may be taking.

Safe Use of Herbs: Herb Use Through the Life Cycle

Herbs are best used to help support and maintain overall health. Many people look at herbs as miracle cures when all else has failed, but more often than not, herbal medicine's ability to turn a patient around from a terminal illness is rare. Although herbs are considered "natural," they should be given the same respect as prescription medicine. Some herbs are perfectly safe for people to use, no matter their age, while others can be dangerous or even deadly. It is important to understand when an herb may be helpful or harmful.

Some Herbs Used with Infants & Children*

Herb	Form	Condition	Action
Chamomile	Tea	Infant colic	Antispasmodic
Fennel seeds (not oil)	Tea	Infant colic; upper respiratory infections	Antispasmodic Reduces mucus
Lemon Balm	Tea	Infant colic	Antispasmodic
Ginger	Dried or as tea	Upset stomach	Antinausea
Aloe Vera	Gel liquid from the leaf	Burns, itching or topical pain reliever	Soothing, anti-inflammatory, immune-stimulating, anti-microbial

* **Note:** Information here is based on limited historical and folklore use. Always check with the child's primary physician before using herbal medications.

Some Herbs to Avoid During Pregnancy*

Class or Characteristic	Herb	Reason
Bitters	Barberry, celandine, feverfew, goldenseal, mugwort, rue, southernwood, tansy, wormwood	Uterine-stimulating action resulting in bleeding and possible spontaneous abortion
Alkaloids	Autumn crocus, barberry, bloodroot, broom, golden seal, mandrake, ephedra	Wide range of effects; several herbs are also listed as bitters
Essential oils of oil-containing plants	Juniper, nutmeg (fresh in large amounts), pennyroyal	Smooth muscle, uterine-stimulating action
Herbal laxatives	Senna, cascara sagrada, aloe bitter latex	Strong laxatives causing intestinal peristalsis, may affect the uterus in the same manner
Other herbal medicines	Black cohosh	Large amounts may cause nausea, vomiting, dizziness and impaired circulation
	Guggul	May stimulate uterine contractions
	Licorice	May cause fluid retention, high blood pressure
	Turmeric	May stimulate uterine contractions

* **Note:** This is a partial list of herbs that may be contraindicated in pregnancy. For further information on specific herbs, see individual listings in chapters 2 and 3. Always consult your healthcare provider when considering the use of herbs during pregnancy or lacation.

Herbs for Infants & Children

Herbs have been used for centuries for treating children with upset stomach and infants with colic. There have been few clinical trials that have studied the effects of herbal medicines on children, but the absence of known adverse reactions does not necessarily mean safety. Reports to the Poison Control Center of accidental poisoning from herbs have been far fewer than for other pharmaceutical and over-the-counter drugs and with only rare harmful effects, but they do occur. In one year the American Association of Poison Control Centers identified 704 adverse reactions to herbs in children ages 6 to 18. During the same year, there were more than 475,000 reports of adverse reactions to pharmaceuticals in children older than age 6. Of those reports, more than 39,000 were vitamin or vitamin/mineral preparations. To avoid potential problems, it is always wise to seek the advice of a practitioner before beginning herbal therapy in children or infants.

If you decide to give your child an herbal preparation, begin with a small amount and evaluate how well he or she tolerates it. The amount of herb required to treat a child is not the same as for an adult. Dosage is usually based on body weight. A child half the weight of an adult receiving 500 mg of an herb would require 250 mg, or half the dose. Know the side effects that have been reported for herbs beforehand so you know what to do if there is a reaction. Some herbal preparations are to be used on the skin (topically) and not internally. The risk with topical use is less, but the chance for a reaction is still possible, so you should know what those risks might be.

Herbal medicines should not be given to children on an ongoing basis. The potential exists for allergies to develop as a side effect of extended use. For example, children given chamomile for an extended period of time may develop an allergic reaction to ragweed or members of the daisy family. If a rash, stomachache, headache or any other new symptom develops when using an herbal remedy, discontinue using the herb immediately and call the child's healthcare provider.

Stimulant herbs, like caffeine or ephedra, should not be used without a reputable practitioner's guidance and should be kept from children's reach. Other supplements intended for use by adults, especially those with weak estrogenic activity, are not recommended for children.

Herbs During Pregnancy & Lactation

Most references do not recommend the medicinal use of herbs during pregnancy unless under the supervision of a qualified healthcare provider, regardless of safety information. Most drugs will pass from the mother to the baby through the placenta during pregnancy, and this may be true of herbs as well. While nursing, many drugs, and presumably herbs, will pass to the baby in the mother's milk. The effects are unknown because testing of some herbs has not been initiated on humans, and animal testing does not always produce the same effects as might be seen in humans. Herbs used as seasoning in food, such as garlic and ginger, are considered safe when used in recipe amounts. Avoid using additional amounts for flavoring or medicinal purposes.

Studies on the safety of echinacea

during pregnancy reported what appeared to be no increased risk of birth defects or adverse reactions when used as recommended. Echinacea used for upper respiratory tract symptoms was found to be effective in relieving the symptoms in 81 percent of the participants. Forty-eight percent of the women had consulted their healthcare providers, who felt that echinacea posed no significant safety concerns. A conservative, and probably safer, recommendation is for pregnant women to avoid using echinacea because its use during pregnancy and lactation has not been established as safe. Before using echinacea during pregnancy or lactation, first consult your healthcare provider.

Garlic, as a major food and ingredient, has a long history of safe use. Eating garlic as a food during pregnancy is considered safe. Concentrated garlic products may, on the other hand, result in garlic passing into the breast milk, possibly resulting in colic in sensitive infants or it may flavor the breast milk.

Ginger used in pregnancy has no known side effects and may be beneficial in relieving morning sickness. Because ginger has been used as a food for centuries and there have been no negative effects noted with it, it can also be used while nursing. It is usually taken as a tea of boiled fresh gingerroot, sweetened as needed. Consult with your healthcare provider before using ginger during pregnancy and lactation.

There are several groups of herbs that are contraindicated in pregnancy and lactation, whether home-grown or purchased. Although useful remedies for non-pregnant women and adults, these have a chemistry that in some way irritates the placenta or causes muscular contractions in the uterus.

Herbs for Adults

Most people who are considering using herbal therapies for health improvement or for treating illness are interested first in what the therapy can do for them, then how safe it is. These should be considered equally, however. Herbs are drugs, sometimes weak, sometimes strong and sometimes poisonous; they are not risk free. The majority of the herbs you will be able to grow yourself and many that are available in bulk will be safe, even in large amounts. Some herbs may cause allergic reactions, but this is usually rare. Some herbs will interact with drugs or with other herbs. Any particular cautions will be listed when the herb is discussed in Chapter 2 and 3. Herbs that may be purchased as supplements, and the cautions for using them, will be discussed in Chapter 3.

Herbs as We Age

"Of all the self-fulfilling prophecies in our culture, the assumption that aging means decline and poor health is probably the deadliest."

—Marilyn Ferguson
The Aquarian Conspiracy, 1980

Many people approach getting older with the assumption that their health will eventually decline and they will no longer be able to do what they enjoy, or worse, that they will live out their days in bed rather than playing golf, walking or even reading a favorite book. Herbal therapies cannot correct years of neglecting one's body, but for those who have been successful in maintaining a relatively healthy lifestyle, herbs may promote longevity.

In most cases, herbs are safe for those of us who are "over the hill," if we choose wisely and inform our healthcare

Herbs, Aging & Chronic Disease

It is only human nature to look for the fountain of youth as we age. Some people are taken in by worthless and sometimes dangerous promises for a cure because they are desperate for a miracle. In a society where a youthful appearance is paramount, many people are looking for the easy fix to stop or reverse the aging process. Although there may be products that can help sooth the wrinkles, aging of the body is inevitable. A better choice for healthy aging is a healthy diet, regular exercise and stopping smoking.

Many older folks suffer from the debilitating effects of arthritis. There are numerous remedies on the market that promise to reduce pain and make movement easier. Many of these are popular and widely sold, not necessarily because they are effective, but because many symptoms of arthritis come and go.

Young and old alike fall prey to cancer prevention therapies, cures and treatments; however, most, if not all, have little proven value and some may in fact be dangerous. Choosing alternative therapies may keep a person from seeking and receiving effective treatment for their disease.

Unproven herbal and alternative therapies can be costly. In addition they are usually not paid for by insurance. Persons who choose supplements may do so as a substitute for food because of cost and the belief that supplements replace food. This may put a person already at risk, whether elderly or not, at increased risk due to poor nutrition.

If you are seeking cures for aging or a particular disease, you may want to reconsider if the therapies you are using are costly, paid for out of pocket and/or promise any one of the following:

- A quick or painless cure
- A special cure or product that is only available through the mail, Internet or one person or company
- Testimonials of miraculous cures or results from satisfied patients
- The product is effective for all that ails you, or at least a variety of complaints
- A cure that is not yet understood by traditional medicine

Herbs you can grow and enjoy at home that promise to hold back the clock include echinacea, garlic, milk thistle, peppermint, purslane, rosemary and thyme. Some of you may also be able to cultivate ginger and American ginseng at home. Herbs available as supplements include ginkgo biloba, Siberian ginseng, evening primrose, gotu kola, and willow bark.

provider about what we are taking. Herbs can interfere with medication and with other herbs as well. Some herbs that help lower your risk for heart disease—garlic, for example—can decrease blood-clotting time. So if you are taking a blood thinner, using more than one or two fresh garlic cloves (or its equivalent in a dietary supplement) might not be right for you.

Herbal Use in Preventive Care & Illness

Options for disease prevention are limited, primarily due to how a person's lifestyle choices affect health, including obesity, inactivity and heart disease. Through prescription drugs that control, and in some cases prevent, disease, heathcare's focus has begun to lean toward disease prevention. As healthcare costs continue to increase, many consumers are recognizing that self-care—including making lifestyle changes—and preventive medicine can help improve overall health and reduce healthcare costs in the long run. Part of self-care includes measures readily endorsed by conventional doctors, like taking a low-dose aspirin each day to reduce the risk of heart attack and stroke or adding exercise to your daily routine. Other measures, such as herbal therapies, are not as readily accepted, probably because of quality concerns and few scientific studies. As research continues to show promise for herbal therapies, this will change, but only with time and education.

It is already recognized and generally accepted that some vitamins and minerals are protective. Their antioxidant properties help protect the body's cells against damage from free radicals. We are beginning to understand, through research and European and American clinical trials, that many herbal medicines convey much of the same protection as well. Herbs are believed to play a role in the prevention of diseases of the heart and liver. Herbs may also play a role in fighting some types of cancers. They may contribute to a feeling of well-being, ease the ravage of menopause, protect our urinary and respiratory tracts, and reduce the incidence and/or severity of headaches.

Herbal products that have been tested in European clinical trials are products that are formulated and manufactured to high-quality standards to ensure their safety and efficacy. This is not to say that herbs you can raise in your backyard will not provide the same benefits. However, these over-the-counter products have been grown, harvested and compounded under conditions that the home gardener cannot match. If you are looking for specific effects from an herb, then it might be worth it to try one that is specifically formulated for that condition. Then, once you know how it benefits you, consider raising it yourself, if possible.

Herbal Therapy in Illness

Some herbal therapies might one day replace one or more of the traditional drugs used to treat a variety of illnesses. The ability of an herb to cure diseases that drugs have not been able to cure is difficult to prove at this time. Until more well-researched evidence is available, herbs may be useful as a complement to conventional therapies, when safe, rather than as a replacement. Herbs can be

Herbal Solutions

Herb	Commercially Available Product (Importer)	This Herb Is Used to Treat	Can You Grow This Herb Yourself? Is It Available in the Wild?
Bilberry	Bilberry Extract (PhytoParmacia/ Enzymatic Therapy, Solaray)	eye health, capillary strengthening, benefits spider and varicose veins	Possibly. Bilberry is related to the American blueberry
Black cohosh	Remifemin (GlaxoSmithKline)	menopausal discomforts	Yes
Chamomile	Camo Care (Abkit)	used topically for skin inflammations and irritations	Yes
Echinacea	Echiaguard (Nature's Way)	healthy immune system, colds and flu	Yes
Garlic	Kawi (Lichtwer Pharma)	cardiovascular health, cholesterol and blood pressure control, infections	Yes
Ginkgo	Ginkgold (Nature's Way) Ginkoba (Pharmaton) Ginkai (Lichtwer Pharma)	cardiovascular health, improved circulation to brain and extremities	No
Ginseng (Asian)	Ginsana (Pharmaton)	Endurance, overall health and energy, stress and fatigue	American ginseng can be grown and is wild in some parts of North America
Horse chestnut	Venastat (Pharmaton)	varicose veins, venous insufficiency, hemorrhoids	No
Milk thistle	Thisylin (Nature's Way)	liver health and detoxification of harmful chemicals, alcohol, drugs and pollution	No
Saw palmetto	Propalmex (Chattem)	benign prostatic hyperplasia (BPH), prostate health preservation	Yes
St. John's wort	Kira (Lichtwer Pharma)	mild to moderate depression and insomnia, fatigue and anxiety related to depression	Yes
Vitex (Chasteberry tree)	Femaprin (Nature's Way)	premenstrual syndrome (PMS), menopause, reproductive health (women)	Yes

good medicine when used wisely and tailored to meet individual health goals. Unfortunately, many widely exaggerated claims are advertised to consumers. Effective marketers convince consumers through testimonials, money-back guarantees and promises of health and longevity, not to mention healing. They are focusing on the "quick fix" mentality with the least amount of effort and commitment on the consumer's part. Natural healing takes time and commitment including, in many instances, a change in lifestyle. Studies have shown that those who are interested in complementary and alternative medicine, and who practice one or more forms, are often more committed to the efforts necessary for alternative therapies to be successful.

Chapter 4 will give more details about the usefulness of herbal remedies in treating illnesses. Some of the areas that hold promise and are worth mentioning here include:

Heart Disease

Heart disease includes a laundry list of ailments related to the heart and its vessels. High blood pressure, high cholesterol and peripheral artery disease all have serious consequences. Adding a fresh crushed garlic clove to your salad each day may be beneficial to controlling cholesterol levels in your blood. One of the most promising herbal therapies is the Ayurvedic herb guggul, which has been used for hundreds of years for heart health.

Cancer

Although not the number one killer worldwide (that distinction is left to heart disease), cancer is the most feared. The flavonoids found in herbs, fruits and vegetables provide another reason to eat your greens and yellows and reds. Their antioxidant abilities help protect the body from free-radical damage and help strengthen the immune system. Garlic shines once again in cancer protection, as studies have shown that garlic may protect against stomach cancer.

Liver Disease

The liver filters everything we eat, drink and breathe, detoxifying otherwise harmful chemicals that enter our body, including alcohol. It filters toxic products of metabolism from the blood and converts them to substances that the body can get rid of. It also helps process drugs and medications we take so that our body may use them more effectively.

When we have a disease of the liver, like hepatitis or cirrhosis, the liver does not work as effectively. Herbs, which are drugs, may not be broken down by the liver and may build up in toxic amounts in the body. Some herbs have been reported to cause liver-related complications ranging from acute hepatitis and jaundice to cirrhosis and death from liver failure. Herbs may also interfere or interact with drugs that are used to treat certain liver diseases.

Milk thistle is one herb that has promise in treating certain diseases of the liver. Studies are currently being conducted and evaluated to determine its effectiveness and safety in liver disease. If you are considering trying an herbal preparation discuss the preparation you are taking or planning to take with your healthcare practitioner so that potential side effects, drug interactions and results can be more safely and appropriately monitored.

Kidney Disease

The kidneys, much like the liver, act as the body's waste disposal. After the body has taken what it needs from the food, the byproducts that are not useable for growth, repair or energy are sent to the blood. Our kidneys filter out about two quarts of waste products and extra water from about 200 quarts of blood each day. The waste and extra water become fluid that is excreted from the body as urine. If the kidneys do not remove these wastes, they build up in the blood and become toxic to the body.

A person with kidney disease may be enticed to use an herb that acts as a diuretic to help with fluid removal. However, herbs with diuretic action can lead to problems with fluid balance and may worsen existing medical conditions. Herbal medicines that contain potassium may also lead to fluid balance and heart problems. Some herbal medicines can affect blood pressure. People who use prescription blood thinners and anticoagulants should be cautious when using any herbal medicine with anticoagulant properties. These herbs can prolong bleeding time or interact with anticoagulant drugs.

Many older persons with multiple diagnoses, including kidney disease, suffer from constipation. Using herbs with laxative properties may do more harm than good if used regularly. In such cases they can accumulate in the kidney and lead to electrolyte and fluid imbalance.

The kidney transplant patient, or any transplant patient for that matter, is at risk from improper herbal medicine use. Immune system stimulants should not be used by anyone with an autoimmune disease (such as lupus or rheumatoid arthritis), or anyone on immunosuppresants—including transplant patients. And lastly, the effectiveness of the transplant drug cyclosporine can interact with some herbal medicines. Herbs affecting blood pressure should be avoided by kidney transplant patients.

Herbal medicine use has even been shown to cause damage to healthy kidneys. If you are considering adding herbal medicine to your daily regimen and you have a history of kidney disease, discuss your plans with your healthcare practitioner so that drug interactions, effectiveness and safety can be monitored.

Common Cold & Respiratory Infections

Echinacea, along with other immune-enhancing herbs like ginger, has shown promise in shortening the duration and severity of colds. Peppermint, chamomile, lavender, wintergreen, garlic and other aromatic herbs help alleviate nasal congestion. Anise seed can be used as an expectorant. The controversial herb ephedra (ma huang) helps open bronchial passages but is also a stimulant that has been used in diet drugs and is associated with increased health risk. Some unwanted side effects include insomnia, jitters, high blood pressure, and in some cases, death.

Menopause

All women face the inevitable midlife change: menopause. With the decline of natural estrogen in the body, women begin to suffer from symptoms like hot flashes, mood swings, anxiety, dry skin and more. Some herbal therapies hold promise in helping decrease some of the side effects. Black cohosh, soy isoflavones and red clover are among those that are being studied closely at this time.

Migraine Headaches

Although they are usually not life-threatening, migraine headaches can incapacitate a person for days and can cause, in their most severe instances, blurred vision, nausea and vomiting. If used consistently, feverfew may be the answer to a migraine sufferer's prayers. Feverfew is an easy-to-grow herb that is a good example of an effective preventive herbal medicine with a specific use.

Benign Prostatic Hypertrophy (BPH)

As men age, their prostate increases in size. As it grows larger, it makes urination more difficult. Saw palmetto is one herb that has been hailed as effective in treating BPH in much the same way some prescription medicines do. Licorice can help as well, but does have some side effects. Pumpkin seeds may be a benefit for many reasons, including their ability to increase urination and because of their high zinc and amino acid content. As with Saw palmetto, pumpkin seeds may also prevent the conversion of testosterone to dihydrotestosterone (DHT). Excess accumulation of DHT is thought to be related to problems of the prostate gland. As with all diseases, it is important that you get the correct diagnosis before using herbal therapies for prostate symptoms. Prostate cancer can present itself through symptoms similar to BPH.

Vision Loss & Macular Degeneration

More and more people over the age of 65 are discovering they have an irreversible condition known as macular degeneration. Antioxidant herbs, vegetables and fruits have shown up in research as strong candidates for the prevention of this devastating disease. Although the disease may not be cured, further damage can be slowed. Bilberry is loaded with antioxidants that strengthen the capillaries in the retina, which helps slow macular degeneration and possibly play a role in reducing the risk of glaucoma. Grapeseed extract has shown promise, as has the isoflavone genistein in legumes, particularly soybeans, in helping the retina stay healthy. The disease glaucoma, the leading cause of blindness, is treated by many prescription medicines that have herbal origins. This disease is serious and must be treated by a physician. Some herbs, including bilberry, oregano and fruits and vegetables high in vitamin C, are thought to be adjuncts to conventional medicine for glaucoma and macular degeneration.

Who Cares Whether I Am Using an Herbal Medicine?

The conditions and diseases listed above are but a few of those that may benefit from the addition of herbs to conventional therapies. It is very important that as a healthcare consumer you inform your medical care provider of your use of herbal therapies, particularly if they are more than for culinary purposes. Even those herbs you grow and use at home have the potential to interact with drugs that may be prescribed for a particular illness, may increase the risk of bleeding during surgery or may interact with each other. When asked by your provider if you are taking any medications, don't forget that herbs are medicines too. Even though they have not been "prescribed," herbal supplements and other dietary supplements do have an impact on your health and any treatment you may receive.

Do I Need to Tell My Doctor or Healthcare Provider that I Am Taking Herbs?

Our doctors or healthcare providers routinely ask if we are taking any medications or drugs. Often, we either do not think of herbs as drugs or we are too embarrassed, intimidated or afraid to say we are taking them. It is important to inform our healthcare providers that we are taking herbs. If your provider scolds you for taking herbs, maybe it is time to look for another provider. But more important, why should you tell them?

One reason for doctors to know your herb intakes is that some herbs interact with prescriptions and over-the-counter (OTC) drugs. Herb interactions with prescription medications will be discussed in Chapters 3 and 4. Taking herbs and medicines together could cause undesirable—even fatal—reactions.

Additionally, some supplements can have adverse effects during surgery. They may change your blood thickness, heart rate, blood pressure and more, and could adversely affect the outcome of your surgery. It is important to quit taking any herbal supplements at least 2 weeks prior to surgery. This also applies to vitamin supplements; check with your healthcare provider or surgeon.

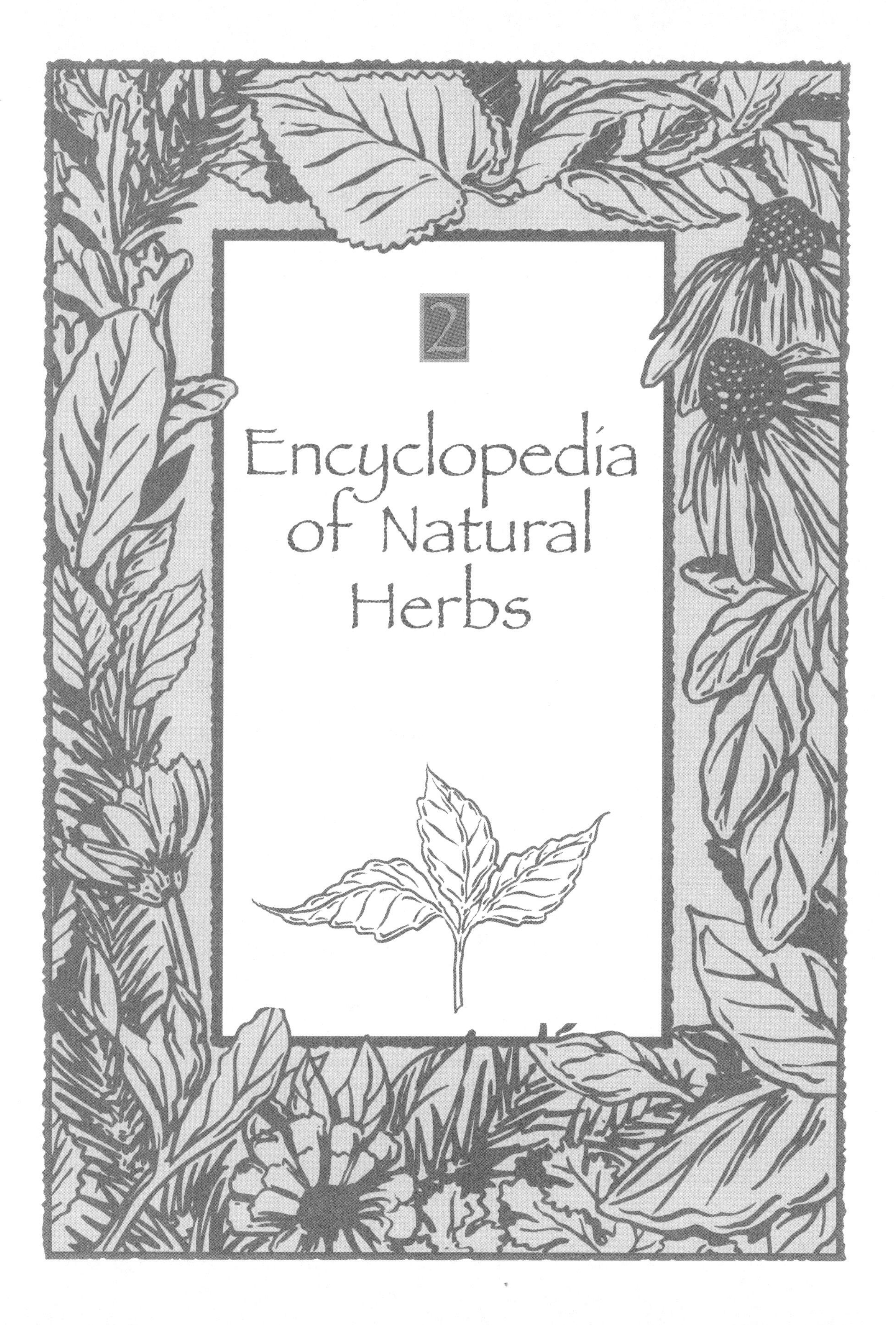
2
Encyclopedia of Natural Herbs

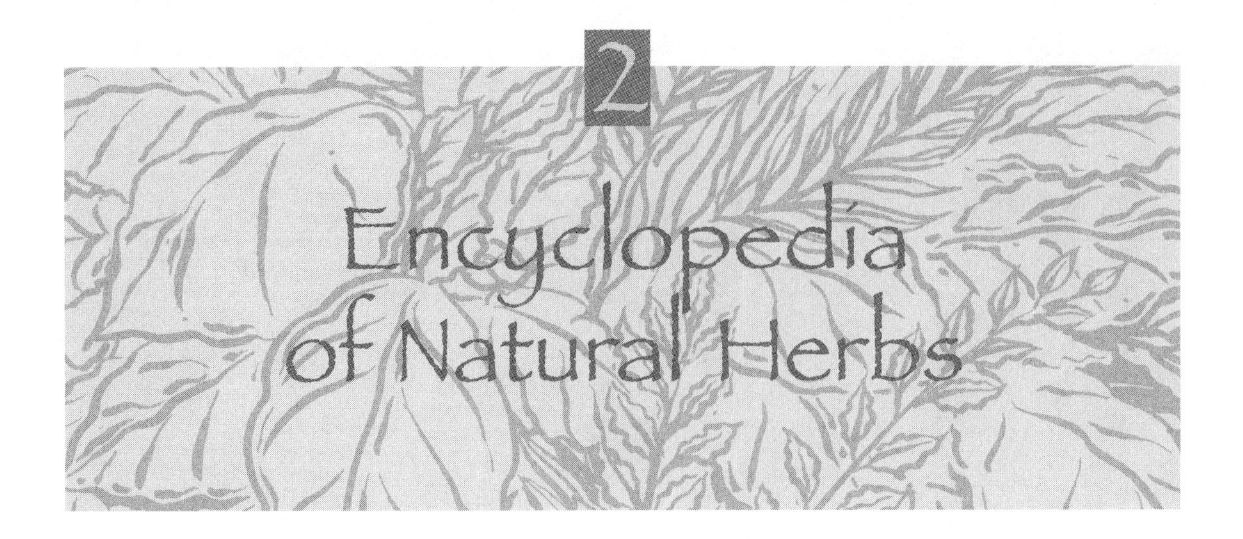

2 Encyclopedia of Natural Herbs

All of the herbs, medicinal and culinary, listed in this chapter can be grown in the home garden, depending on your location and climate. This list is by no means inclusive of all the herbs you might be able to grow. The ones listed here can be purchased through seed catalogs as either seed or plant, and some may be available from your local nursery.

Whether you choose seeds or buy starter plants, it is important that you know what you are buying and that you get what you think you are getting. Remember that all plants are categorized according to family. Plants within a family share some characteristics. Families are further divided into genus and species. Within a family, there may be more than one genus and species. For example, the Apiaceae/Umbelliferae family has several species of the genus Angelica, including *Angelica archangelica* and *Angelica sinesis,* also known as dong quai. These two herbal medicines have differing uses and safety. Within a family, there may also exist a beneficial genus and species, as well as a toxic or poisonous one.

Cautions

Know what you are buying. If you are buying seed, know how to identify the plant as it grows. If you are buying plants from a nursery, ask questions about the plants and again, make sure you know that it is of the family, genus and species you want. If the nursery is unable to answer your questions, go elsewhere.

Be familiar with common and local names of herbs used in different regions of the country and world. Differing species may carry the same name from one part of the country to another—or even within the same region. This occurs because of confusion in translation or interpretation of an herb's use, or its similarity of appearance.

Astragalus is an example of a commonly known herb that has medicinal value but can be toxic. In the genus in which it belongs, Papilionaceae, there are some 2,000 species known in North America. Locoweed, a member of this family, is extremely toxic to livestock.

Creating & Using Your Own Herbal Supplements Safely

The virtues of herbs and plants are gaining acceptance from consumers and healthcare practitioners. More than 25 percent of modern-day prescriptions are derived from plants. Some books, articles and magazine advertisements make us believe that herbal supplements, plants and other dietary supplements are the answer to all of our illnesses. Some supplements may help, some may harm. Here you will learn about herbs and herbal preparations that may be healthful and healing and how to create many of these at home. If you are not yet ready to venture into making your own, then chapter 3 will provide suggestions on herbal supplements you can purchase. No matter which route you choose, it is important to be informed about the use of these plants and how they may help maintain health. That is the purpose of this book.

Buy Your Herbs, Grow Them or Pick Them in the Wild?

Buying herbs in bulk and making your own preparations can be economical and allows you the chance to experiment with and become more familiar with the herbs. Buying herbal preparations from herbalists who mix their own preparations may make you feel that you are getting the best preparation for you, which may or may not be the case.

Growing medicinal and culinary herbs in your backyard provides much pleasure. Whether indoors or out, gardening can be very therapeutic for the mind and body. You will delight in watching your garden grow, get some exercise while cultivating and harvesting and eagerly anticipate trying herbs in a new dish or as a remedy for yourself or your family. When planning what to grow, give it some careful thought and consideration.

It is beyond the scope of this book to provide all the information you need to grow herbs or to pick them in the wild. This book will provide you with a beginning. There are numerous books on gardening and plant identification in bookstores that will provide more details specific to your area and zone.

Buying Herbs in Bulk

Bulk herbs are available at many natural food stores, specialized herb shops and from herbalists. However, bulk herbs can vary considerably in quality and potency. Batches may be mixed, resulting in genetically different products with differences in active compounds and potency. Other considerations include:

- Growing conditions, including geographic location, time of year and stage of maturation at harvest.
- Purity. Do you know whether the herb you are purchasing contains only that herb? Do the herbs undergo any type of testing for purity or quality assurance at the supplier's level? How does the supplier guarantee that what is being sold is what it is labeled as? If the retailer indicates that it or its supplier has done no testing, you might want to look elsewhere.
- How the herbs are handled once harvested. Are they dried immediately or left for days before drying, increasing the potential for mold and fungus?
- Storage. Are herbs stored properly in dark glass containers and not exposed to excess light or air?

- Turnover at the store or in the herbalist's inventory. How often are products purchased and replenished? Are they purchased in amounts that will be sold quickly, allowing for freshness? Are batches mixed when product supplies get low? Are there ways to ensure that the products are genetically the same and that potency, quality and effectiveness are consistent?
- The seller's knowledge. What does the seller know about the supplier? What does the seller know about herb/herb, herb/drug and herb/food interactions? Does the seller "prescribe," recommend, or imply that a particular herb will heal or prevent a disease?

If these questions cannot be confidently answered to your satisfaction, it may be best to go elsewhere, or to purchase only herbs that you do not intend to use for medicinal value.

Growing Your Own Herbs

Numerous herbs can be grown in containers indoors. Those suited for indoors will often grow outside with ease. Some may need more coaxing if they are natural to subtropical climates and you live in the Rocky Mountains, for example. But in the right spot, with the right light and a bit of TLC, almost anything is possible. Culinary herbs provide a welcome bit of fresh color to a dull and drab winter meal and add some beneficial compounds as well. A garden of various medicinal herbs complemented by a kitchen windowsill garden full of culinary herbs offers a virtual powerhouse that tastes good and is good for you.

Herbs can be grown from seeds, pits, cuttings, suckers, greenhouse-grown plants and division from a clump of herbs. The method you choose may depend in part on your gardening experience, what you want to grow, and where you will grow your herbs.

Once you have chosen a site, it is important to plan what you want to grow. If you don't plan, you may end up with large plants shading smaller ones or you may forget what you have planted where. Although herbs do not need the heavy application of manure that may be beneficial for vegetable gardens, they do require feeding and mulching that is suitable for the herb. Bulky organic fertilizers will feed and mulch herbs. Synthetic fertilizers, herbicides and pesticides are not recommended for herbs, as they introduce risk of contamination. Natural fertilizers are important to the health of the plants and will help ensure you get the beneficial compounds you want.

Weeding, deadheading (removing faded flowers) and pruning give you the chance to get to know the characteristics of your herbs. Care of herbs, while growing and during harvesting and storage, will influence their potential effectiveness.

Herbs can be successfully grown in containers, hence their popularity in the kitchen. They can be placed on a sunny windowsill so bits can be snipped for flavoring meals or for soothing cuts and burns. Depending on your climate, some herbs may be grown in pots and left out all year long, while others must be brought in to survive. Regular watering and a biweekly feeding with an organic liquid fertilizer are necessary to keep herbs healthy. If a plant has outgrown its pot, it will begin to fade, have weak growth and be susceptible to pests. It is best to repot plants before this happens. As with garden-grown herbs, the quality of the resulting herb will depend on the care and feeding it receives.

Wildcrafting

Gathering plants in the wild, also known as wildcrafting, has grown in popularity, particularly because some botanicals cannot be grown quickly enough commercially or in home gardens. Also, many people feel that these wild plants provide a more natural—thus preferred—product, and the process of gathering is therapeutic in itself. This poses several problems:

- Many plants in North America and the world are threatened because of overharvesting.
- There is a risk of unintentional contaminants, including pesticides, herbicides and heavy metals.
- Positive identification may be difficult without accurate information, including detailed pictures.
- Ingredients and strength can differ considerably depending on location and growing conditions.

Preparing Your Own Herbal Supplements

Once you have decided what form of herbs you will be using—purchased in bulk, home-grown or wildcrafted—it is time to decide the most effective way to use them. They can be used as foods, seasonings, herbal medicines or teas. Some ways may be more effective than others, but no matter how you choose to use them, you will benefit from their potential healing properties.

There are numerous types of herbal remedies. Which you use will depend on the herb and the desired results. The best way to preserve the strength of an herb is to make it into a tincture or extract, if the particular herb is suited for it. Other methods of preservation and use include traditional drying, decoctions, compresses, poultices and infusions.

Do not confuse the term *extract* used here with the term *standardized extract.* In other words, "extract" does not equal "standardized extract." Standardized herbal extracts have been processed to ensure that they contain minimum levels of one or more of the active ingredients. The active ingredients are what give the herbal preparation its healing properties. These standardized herbal extracts are usually sold in capsule or tablet form. An extract in this instance is similar to the extracts used for flavorings in cooking. Tinctures are also extracts and are most commonly made by steeping a quantity of herb in alcohol. The alcohol will extract the water and oil-soluble compounds from the herb. Extracts are more often purchased than made at home. Extracts are measured to a pharmaceutical grade to ensure the herb's strength. Some herbs do lend themselves to a homemade extract and are described where appropriate.

The following are some of the most common ways of preparing herbs for use at home. Since the same methods of preservation or preparation may not be appropriate for every herb, additional information, including standard quantities and doses, will be given with each herb discussed.

Drying Herbs

Drying is an easy way to preserve your harvest, but it needs to be done with care. When herbs are gathered, drying conditions, the time it takes to reach the correct level of dryness and proper storage will affect the therapeutic effectiveness of the herb. When dry, herbs should be stored in airtight, preferably dark glass containers, where they may be kept for 12 to 18 months. Each part of the plant should be treated differently, as each has different qualities that you should try to preserve.

Leaves & Stems. You can dry large leaves individually, but leave smaller leaves on the stem. If the aerial part (growing into the air, as opposed to roots that grow underground) of the plant is to be included, harvest it with the stem and leaves. Tie the herbs in small bunches, with no more than eight leaves or stems to a bunch, and hang them upside down to dry. When dry and brittle to the touch, crush them for immediate use or store them in an airtight dark glass container. Stems may be dried much like small leaves bunched together and hung upside down to dry. When thoroughly dry, break into small pieces and store in a glass container.

Seeds. Harvest seeds just before ripe, keeping the head and a small part of the stalk attached. Tie into small bunches and hang them upside down over a towel or wax paper to catch seeds as they fall out. Seeds should be dry in about 2 weeks.

Roots & Rhizomes. Harvest roots and rhizomes when the aerial part of the plant has died and before the ground freezes (sometime in autumn, depending on the herb). Wash thoroughly to remove any soil, then chop into small pieces before they have the chance to dry and become hard to cut. Spread the pieces on a tray lined with paper towels and dry for 2 to 6 hours in a cooling oven. (Heat oven to 200°F, turn off, then place tray with roots in the oven to dry with door ajar about 1 inch to let moisture escape.) Drying time depends on the size of the root pieces. Transfer to a cooling rack and place in a warm sunny room out of direct sunlight to complete drying. Roots and rhizomes should be dry and brittle and stored in airtight dark glass containers.

Fruit. Dry fruit in a dehydrator or on trays. Turn fleshy fruits often to make sure they dry completely. If it's not dried thoroughly, fruit will mold.

Bark. To dry tree and shrub bark effectively, remove small amounts of bark in the fall when sap is flowing to lessen damage to the plant. Lightly dust the bark to remove moss, fungus or insects. Break bark into 2x2-inch pieces and lay out on racks to dry. Never remove all of the bark from the tree as it may die.

Bulbs. Dig garlic and other bulbs when the aerial part has wilted. To store bulbs, hang them or place them in a container that allows for sufficient air circulation.

Flowers. Flowers can be very fragile; they require careful handling. Pick small flowers before maturity, early in the morning but after dew has evaporated. Cut the stems from the flower heads and dry out of the sun on a tray lined with paper towels. When thoroughly dry, store in an airtight dark glass container. As an exception, lavender should be dried upside down on the stem with a small bag lightly tied over the flowers. If you choose to use them fresh, harvest when they have just bloomed.

Fluid Herbal Extracts

Begin with a weighed portion of powdered dry or finely cut fresh herb. Fill a large glass jar (canning jars work well) approximately two-thirds full with the herb. Fill the jar with vodka, cap tightly and allow the extract to steep; each day, shake the jar gently for a few seconds until contents are mixed. After two weeks, strain the extract through several layers of cheesecloth and squeeze to remove all of the liquid from the herbs. Weigh the finished extract to obtain an approximate ratio of herb to extract. If 100 grams of the herb are extracted and produces about 100 grams of extract, the extract ratio is 1:1. For other proportions such as 1:5, 100 grams of the herb is extracted to produce 500 grams of extract. Larger volumes of extract require larger volumes of alcohol to herb. Store the finished extract in an airtight glass container, preferably one that is dark. Vodka is one of the best solvents because it is colorless and odorless and, at 70 percent alcohol, extracts the desired compounds.

For a fluid extract that is reliable—one that is more certain to meet your needs—purchase a commercially prepared fluid extract prepared according to pharmaceutical grades, providing a concentrated preserved extract.

Herbal Vinegars

Although their use is a bit more limited, herbal vinegars can make a delicious alternative to alcohol-based tinctures. They are most suited for salads and cooking. Herbal vinegars can be made using the same ratios as for tinctures by simply steeping the herbs in vinegar instead of alcohol.

Herbal Infusions

Similar to teas, herbal infusions can be made with water or oil. This method is used mostly for the flowers and leafy parts of herbs and should be made fresh each time you want to use it. Fresh or dried herbs are placed in a glass or pottery pot with a tight-fitting lid. Bring water to a boil and remove from heat; pour over herbs and steep for 5 to 10 minutes. Standard quantities are 75 grams (2.5 ounces) of fresh or 30 grams (1 ounce) of dried herb to 500 mL (17 ounces) of water. Strain while pouring into a cup or mug and enjoy. Any herb that is suitable for tea may be made into an infusion.

Infused oils can be used for massage oils, creams and ointments. They can be made by gently heating olive or vegetable oil and herb in a heavy glass bowl (or double boiler) over boiling water for 2 to 4 hours. Strain by pouring through cheesecloth, and carefully squeeze out all of the oil from the herb. Be careful, as the liquid will be hot. Pour into an airtight bottle and store up to one year. For more potent oils, make smaller batches more frequently. For cold-infused oils, pack a large jar tightly with herbs and cover completely with oil. Seal well and place in a sunny place for two to three weeks. Strain the same way as hot infused oils.

Herbal Teas

Also referred to as tisanes, teas are infusions made from herbs. All of the usable portion of the plant may be used for teas, but generally they are made with leaves, flowers and sometimes fruit. They are a weaker solution than an infusion and are usually steeped for 5 to 10 minutes.

Herbal Decoctions

Decoctions are extracts from roots, bark and/or berries. Creating a decoction involves simmering the herbs for up to 1 hour until the liquid is reduced by one-third, then straining. Decoctions should be made fresh each day and in amounts recommended for the desired result.

Standard quantities are 60 grams (2 ounces) of fresh or 30 grams (1 ounce) of dried herb to 500 mL (17 ounces) of water.

Herbal Tinctures

Tinctures are similar to fluid extracts and decoctions. Use an alcohol-water mix, generally a strength of 750 mL alcohol (preferably vodka) to 250 mL water, with proportion of one part herb to four or five parts solution, depending on the herb, and steep for at least 12 hours. Each herb that is appropriate for use as a tincture will have its own proportion indicated under the heading "Making the Remedy & Dosage."

Herbal Compresses

To make an herbal compress, soak a cloth in a hot herbal extract. Apply the compress to the affected area. Herbal compresses are popular for treating muscle strains and sprains and for healing wounds.

Herbal Poultices

Poultices are time-tested remedies effective for drawing out infections. The whole herb is used, rather than just the extract, and is applied directly to the affected area. Fresh herbs can be boiled, or chopped in a food processor for a few seconds, then squeezed of excess moisture. Dried herbs may also be used for poultices. Prepare the skin with a light film of oil, apply the poultice, then cover the area with gauze to hold it in place.

Herbal Salves or Ointments

Salves or ointments can be made from herbs, but the process tends to be messy because they are made with beeswax, petroleum jelly, paraffin wax, animal fat or vegetable fat. The wax or fat is melted in a double boiler over boiling water. Then the herbs are added and heated until crisp, about 2 hours or more. The mixture is strained through cheesecloth, then poured quickly into clean, dark glass jars. Wear rubber gloves to protect your hands from the hot mixture.

Dried Herb Capsules

Capsules can be made from the powders of dried herbs. They are useful for those herbs that are foul-tasting and are convenient to carry with you. Capsules, either gelatin-based or vegetarian, are available in most natural food stores. You may make your own powder for the capsules, but potency and effectiveness may differ from powders and capsules available commercially. Most capsules hold approximately 200 to 250 mg of a powdered extract. This translates into a dose of approximately 2 to 3 capsules per day, depending on the herb. An equivalent amount of powder is about 1 teaspoon.

Children, immune-compromised individuals and the elderly often need smaller doses. If you are in doubt whether a preparation should be used, ask your physician before using it.

Note: Measuring herbs for preparations, their dosages and liquid measurements are listed in metric and when possible, U.S. measurements. Because metric measurements allow for more precise measure, they provide more exact doses. For the best results a metric scale and liquid measures are recommended.

Starting from Scratch

Anyone with an herb garden will want to include several medicinal and culinary herbs. The following list is a suggestion of herbs to begin with. They are easy to grow and easy to prepare for use. More detail about the specific herbs and their uses will be provided under their individual listings.

Calendula, for sore throats or inflammations in the mouth and for minor skin irritations and injuries.

Catnip, as an insect repellent or tea. Any feline friends you might have also appreciate catnip!

Chamomile, for digestive problems, insomnia and, externally, for wounds, sunburn and hemorrhoids.

Echinacea, for its immune-stimulating potential.

Garlic, as a possible anti-hypertensive, anti-cholesterol and anti-diabetic compound. Also thought to be useful for infections and colds.

Lemon balm, for its possible antiviral, anti-bacterial and insect repellant uses.

Parsley, which is known for its breath-freshening effects and for its potential benefits for persons suffering from bladder infections and kidney stones.

Peppermint, for a wonderful tea that purportedly eases gastrointestinal (GI) spasms and nausea, as well as head and chest congestion.

Rosemary, as a digestive aid, for promoting menstrual flow, for loss of appetite, gallbladder and liver complaints and for blood pressure irregularities.

Sage, a common culinary herb that is thought to be an effective treatment for mouth ulcers, gingivitis and sore throats.

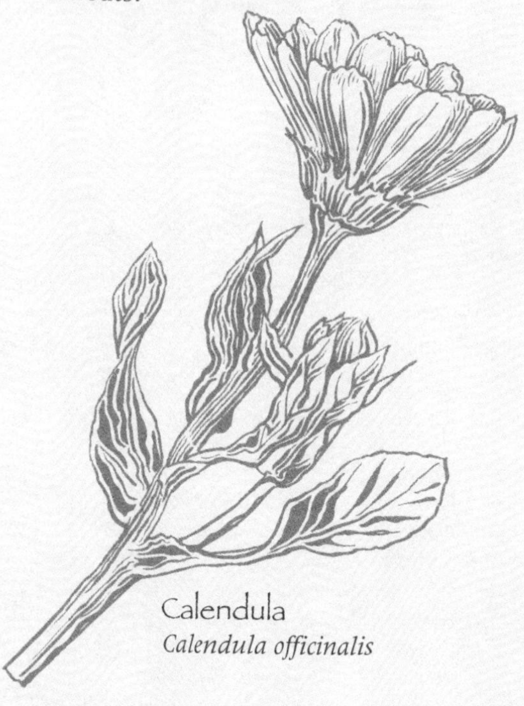

Calendula
Calendula officinalis

How To Use This Chapter

For quick reference and ease of use, this encyclopedia outlines each medicinal and culinary herb in the same fashion. You can turn right to the information you need regarding a particular herb, or skim-and-search the pages efficiently. Here is a summary of the information you'll find with each herb.

Common Names
These are the names the herb is called or known by. Many herbs have more than one name and some have names that are similar to each other, which makes identification tricky.

Family
This is the plant family to which the herb belongs. It is part of the botanical name. Sometimes family members have similar properties… for example, members of the Asteraceae/Compositae family. Several plants from this family are used to fight infections, but if you are allergic to one member of the family, you may also be allergic to others.

Genus & Species
These are parts of the botanical name that further identify the herb.

Description
This describes the herb's appearance. A description is helpful if you are growing the herb, or looking for it in the wild.

Historical Use
This information is based on numerous references that describe how the herb was used in ancient cultures, folklore, traditional medical practices, and present-day herbal medicine. Information in this section is not meant to recommend how to use the herb.

Parts to Use
This describes which parts of the herb are commonly used.

What It Does
Although this section might repeat some information from "Historical Use," the purpose here is a bit different. What It Does describes what the herb is thought to help, based on traditional and current use as well as documented evidence. When possible, only human information has been included; however, some information may be based on animal data, *in vitro* (laboratory) data or word of mouth/tradition. This information does not intend to recommend or prescribe but rather to overview the conditions the herb is used for.

What It Might Help Treat
Based on traditional use and results that have been seen when it is used, information here is not necessarily research based. This section also includes speculative information on what the herb might treat based on ongoing or planned research, the final results of which are not reported at this time.

Medicinal Herbs

Dandelion

Profile

Common Names: Common dandelion, blowball, dandelion herb, wild endive
Family: Asteraceae/Compositae (daisy and marigold are also in the family)
Genus & Species: *Taraxacum officinale*
Description: Does dandelion need a description? Dandelion is a perennial with a taproot that seems to go on forever. When cut, the stem excretes white latex. The leaves are saw-toothed and the plant usually produces one bright yellow flower followed by a fine tuft that contains the fruits or seeds of the plant.
Historical Use: This poor herb is scorned. It is considered a nuisance, a pest and a weed. But many of us do not realize that dandelion has a rich medicinal history. Chinese and Ayurvedic physicians have used the herb to treat colds, respiratory tract ailments, dental problems, obesity, ulcers and numerous other conditions. It has been linked to the health of the liver, to its use as a diuretic and as a tonic used by Early American colonists. Lydia Pinkham's Vegetable Compound in the 1800s contained dandelion.
Parts to Use: Whole plant, above-ground parts.

What It Does

The FDA believes that dandelion is a weed and has no therapeutic uses. In Germany, the Commission E recognizes dandelion as a diuretic that may reduce bloating in women with PMS, and endorses its roots and leaves for bile stimulation.

78 *Herbs for Health and Healing*

What It Might Help Treat

- Gallstones
- Premenstrual syndrome (PMS) and associated fluid retention
- High blood pressure
- Loss of appetite

Research Insights

There is possible anti-tumor activity as demonstrated in animals. The Japanese use dandelion in treating breast cancer. In animals, dandelion has been shown to have an anti-inflammatory activity, and also lowers their blood sugar.

How It Is Used

Fresh, as an infusion, decoction or tincture.

Growing
Anyone with a patch of grass in their yard knows that dandelions will grow just about anywhere, no matter what the conditions are.

Harvesting
When to harvest depends on intended use:
- Leaves are picked in the spring before the plants flower. Picked fresh, leaves may be used in salads.
- Dig roots in the fall or in the spring.
- Flowers are picked for wine-making in the spring; leaves and stems are removed.

Preserving
- Leaves picked in spring may be juiced or dried.
- Roots can be pressed for juice, dried or roasted for a coffee substitute. Dried roots and leaves should be kept in a sealed dark glass container out of direct sunlight.

Dandelion
Taraxacum officinale

Research Insights
If there is research data regarding the usefulness of this herb, it is listed here. The same information might also be listed under What It Does.

How It Is Used
This section tells you how to grow the herb, the climate in which the herb grows best, preparation for its use, and information on preserving the herb. Also listed here are the most popular types of herbal remedies associated with the herb. Tips on how to make typical home remedies and doses are provided.

Best Herbal Remedy Forms

Information here describes the form that the herbal remedy is best suited for: tea, tincture, dried or powdered… how the herb is best used to get the maximum effect.

Making the Remedy & Dosage

Making the remedy varies from practitioner to practitioner. There are as many recipes for making tinctures and teas as there are for making chicken soup! This section outlines the most common recipes with the simplest preparation techniques.

Best Herbal Remedy Forms

Tea or decoction, fresh in salads or cooked, and tincture.

Making the Remedy & Dosage

- **Decoction** is made by using 30 grams of dried root (or 60 grams of fresh) to 750 mL of water, simmered and reduced to about 500 mL. Drink up to 3 cups a day.
- **Tinctures,** 1:5. Use 1 to 2 teaspoons of tincture in a small amount of water preferably up to 3 times each day.
- **Tea** made of leaves is a less effective preparation, but is still effective as a digestive stimulant. Use 30 grams of dried (or 25 grams of fresh) dandelion leaves steeped in 1 cup of hot, not boiling, water for 10 minutes, then strained. Take up to 3 cups a day.
- For dandelion root **tea**, use 3 to 8 grams of dried root in 1 cup of hot, not boiling, water. Drink up to 3 times a day.
- **Dried leaves and roots** may be used for any of the above preparations.
- **Juice** made of fresh leaves is given as 1 to 2 teaspoons a day.

Safety & Effectiveness

When taken as a food or medicinally as directed, dandelion is considered safe. Dandelion may be effective for stimulating bile flow, loss of appetite and diuresis. There is insufficient research to conclusively support other uses for the plant.

Interactions

Drugs. Use of dandelion with diuretics and drugs used to control blood sugar may interfere with drug therapy. Use of dandelion with the drug lithium, may cause lithium toxicity because of sodium loss caused by dandelion.

Dandelion may interfere with drugs used to decrease stomach acid.

Other Herbs. Theoretically, dandelion may have additive effects when taken with other herbs that have diuretic properties. When used with herbs that lower blood sugar, dandelion may have an additive effect, thus lowering blood sugar even more.

Foods. No known interactions.

Vitamins or Minerals. No known interactions.

Effects In Laboratory Tests

No known adverse effects.

Adverse Reactions

- Low blood sugar in persons with diabetes. Blood sugar levels should be monitored closely.
- Dandelion taken orally can cause increased stomach acid.
- Persons allergic to members of the Asteraceae/Compositae family, including daisies, ragweed, chamomile and marigolds, may be sensitive to dandelion.

Who Should Not Use Dandelion

- People with active gallbladder disease should consult their primary care physician before using dandelion.
- People with bowel or bile duct obstruction should not use dandelion.

Comments

Dandelion is one of the best culinary sources of vitamin A, surpassing that of carrots.

Medicinal Herbs

Encyclopedia of Natural Herbs 79

Effects In Laboratory Tests

Some herbs affect blood and urine tests. For example, many herbs lower blood sugar. So if you are taking drugs for diabetes, be careful about herbs that affect your blood sugar as the drug and herb may work against each other and result in inaccurate test results.

Adverse Reactions

These are negative reactions that can occur when an herb is used—maybe an allergic reaction or a potential toxicity. Many known adverse reactions are included here, but the list is not all-inclusive because information changes so quickly. If you have questions regarding a specific herb, ask your healthcare provider.

Who Should Not Use the Herb

Certain conditions should not be treated with herbs. Those that are known are listed here.

Comments

You'll find interesting background and cautions about an herb here.

Interactions

Here you'll find information on what drugs, foods and herbs the particular herb may interact with, and what the effect might be. Many herbs are listed with no interactions or adverse reaction; interpret this cautiously. This does not imply that the herb is 100 percent safe; it just means there is no published information.

Safety & Effectiveness

This section addresses the most important information that is known about the safety and the effectiveness of the herb. This section includes the most up-to-date, comprehensive information known about the herb. As with drugs and food, the information about safety and effectiveness can change from day to day.

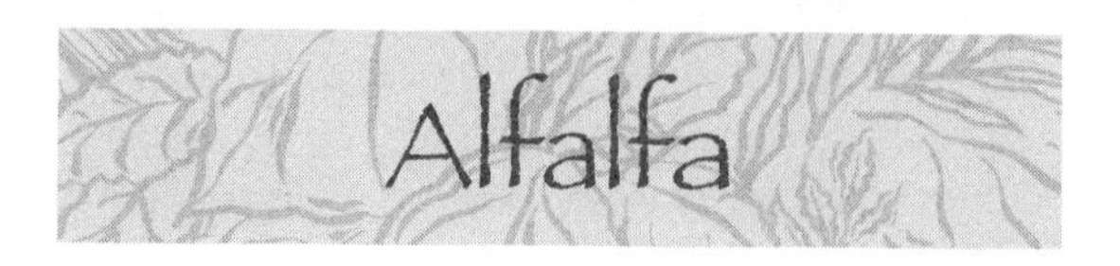

Profile

Common Names: Buffalo grass, Chilean clover
Family: Leguminosae (this family also includes soybeans)
Genus & Species: *Medicago sativa*
Description: Bushy perennial with blue-green leaves and light mauve to purple and sometimes yellow flowers.
Historical Use: Primarily known as a crop for livestock, alfalfa is rich in vitamins, especially beta-carotene and vitamin K, and minerals.
Parts to Use: Whole plant, leaves and seeds. Seeds, when sprouted, are a popular addition to salads.

What It Does

Taken internally, it might be helpful for urinary tract conditions, including prostate and bladder problems. In people with diabetes, it may help lower blood sugar. People with asthma, arthritis and indigestion may experience relief when using alfalfa.

What It Might Help Treat

- Elevated cholesterol
- Fungi
- Menopausal symptoms

Research Insights

Alfalfa contains saponins that may decrease the body's absorption of cholesterol. It may lower blood sugar and contains several isoflavones, which appear to have weak estrogen-like properties.

How It Is Used

- Fresh young leaves can be used in teas or cooking.
- Seeds may be sprouted for use in cooking.
- Dried, in capsule form.
- Dried alfalfa can be used in making tea.

Growing

- Relatively easy from seed sown in spring or autumn. May self-propagate if allowed to go to seed.
- Benefits from fertilizing with manure.

Harvesting

Cut plants before they flower.

Preserving

Dry by hanging small, loose bunches upside down in a dry area away from strong sunlight. When dry and brittle, crumble and store in an airtight dark glass container. You may separate the stems from the leaves if desired.

Best Herbal Remedy Forms

As teas for internal use, tincture and dried for use in capsules.

Making the Remedy & Dosage

- 5 to 10 grams **powdered** in capsule form, 3 times a day.
- 5 to 10 grams dried herbs steeped and strained as a **tea**, 3 times a day.
- As a 1:1 **extract**, 5 to 10 mL (1 to 2 teaspoons) 3 times a day.

Safety & Effectiveness

Alfalfa is relatively safe in recommended doses. It may be effective for lowering cholesterol, but there is no reliable research about other medicinal uses. Alfalfa is an excellent source of antioxidants, including vitamins and minerals.

Interactions

Drugs. Alfalfa may interfere with anticoagulant medications, hormone therapy and oral contraceptives. May cause sensitivity to sunlight in some people using the tranquilizer Thorazine.

Other Herbs or Dietary Supplements. Using multiple herbs with alfalfa, which is rich in vitamin K, can increase the risk of clotting in people using anticoagulants.

Foods. No known interactions.

Effects In Laboratory Tests

Might lower blood cholesterol levels and test results in persons with type II hyperlipoproteinemia. May lower blood sugar test results, particularly in people taking diabetic medication.

Adverse Reactions

- Ground seeds may worsen Systemic Lupus Erythematosis or bring the disease out of remission.
- May lower blood sugar; monitor blood sugar regularly.
- Theoretically, because of its weak estrogen properties, it may affect estrogen-sensitive diseases.

Who Should Not Use Alfalfa

Pregnant and lactating women should not use alfalfa in supplemental form because of its possible estrogenic activity.

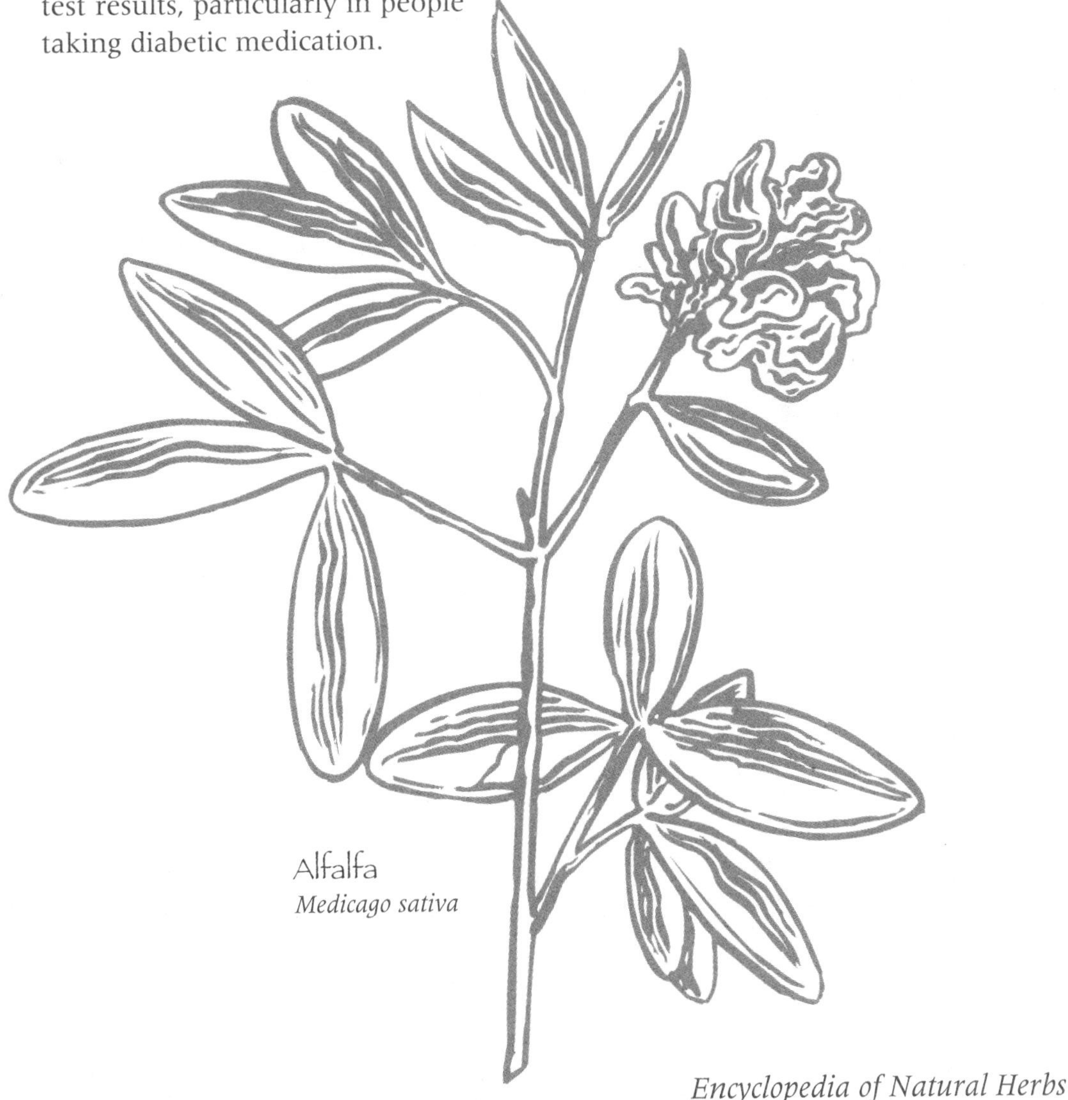

Alfalfa
Medicago sativa

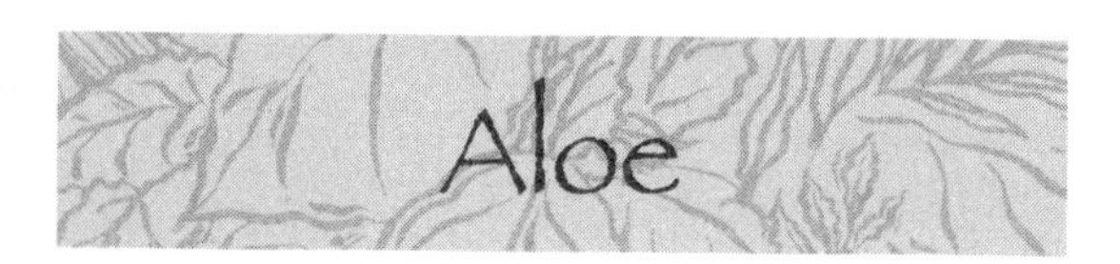

Profile

Common Names: Aloe vera, burn plant, miracle plant, plant of immortality, lily of the desert
Family: Liliaeae
Genus & Species: *Aloe vera, Aloe barbadensis, Aloe perfoliata, Aloe arborescens natalenis, Aloe ferox, Aloe africana, Aloe spicata, Aloe perryi, Aloe capensis* and approximately 500 other species
Description: There are more than 360 members of the aloe family and many of them look alike. They vary in size from 2 to 3 feet tall (a typical houseplant) to as much as 60 feet tall (grown naturally in Africa). Aloes have thick, spiky, spiny leaves that are about 99 percent water.
Historical Use: One of the oldest medicinal plants known, aloe is mentioned as far back as 1552 B.C.E. It has been used for ailments from healing wounds and cuts to constipation. Because of its bitter taste, it has been used on children's fingernails to stop nail biting and thumb sucking.
Parts to Use: Leaves and gel (the thick fluid from the leaf's center).

What It Does

Taken internally, it acts as a laxative. Externally, it is well known for wound healing, reducing inflammation, treating minor burns and other skin conditions.

What It Might Help Treat

- Diabetes
- Virus infection
- Stomach ulcers

Research Insights

Current information on the effectiveness of aloe juice/gel does not fully support the use of aloe for other than its laxative and wound-healing properties. Further study is being conducted on aloe's role in blood sugar, triglyceride and lipid control in diabetes. Aloe is also being considered for its ability to prevent and heal gastric ulcers and for preventing the replication of viruses, including HIV, herpes simplex and its relative, canker sores.

How It Is Used

Growing

Aloe can be cultivated in the subtropical regions of the United States and Mexico but is more commonly found in the wild in northern Africa, the Near East, Asia and the southern Mediterranean. An excellent houseplant, aloe may grow several feet tall given the right conditions.

Harvesting

Pick or cut desired number of leaves directly from plant at any time.

Preserving

Cut leaves, drain gel and use fresh. Gently boil larger quantities of sap down to a thick paste and store in dark glass jars. Dry leaves.

Best Herbal Remedy Forms

Fresh from the plant as a gel, tincture, ointment or powdered dried herb.

Making the Remedy & Dosage

- Aloe gel can be applied directly to the skin for wounds or burns. If you gather more than you need, store it in a dark glass container.

Aloe
Aloe vera

- Use 2 to 6 teaspoons (up to 30 mL) of aloe **gel** in water or fruit juice 3 times a day for constipation. Do not let it become contaminated with the white milky latex beneath the plant's skin as it may cause severe intestinal cramping and loose stools.
- For an **ointment,** gather a large amount of gel from several leaves and boil until reduced and thick. Apply cooled ointment directly to affected area.
- For a **tincture**, place equal amounts of leaves and vodka in a clean glass jar. Cover tightly and steep for 2 weeks, shaking occasionally. Use 3 to 15 mL (about 1½ to 7 teaspoons) in 8 ounces of water for constipation taken in the evening as needed.
- **Powdered** leaf juice is available in gelatin capsules. Follow directions on label for use.

Safety & Effectiveness

Aloe gels and dried leaves may be safe and effective for constipation when used as directed. Aloe may be effective when applied to the skin, although some allergic reactions have been reported. It may enhance healing and possibly reduce pain and inflammation of wounds and burns.

Interactions

Drugs. Aloe taken internally can lead to potassium deficiency if used with some diuretics, licorice and corticosteroids. The actions of cardiac glycosides and antiarrythmic drugs can be enhanced if used with aloe.
Other Herbs. Using aloe with other stimulant laxative herbs, licorice or horsetail may increase the risk of potassium depletion. Herbs that contain cardiac glycoside can be toxic if used with excessive amounts or continuous use of aloe.
Foods. No reactions with foods have been reported.
Vitamins or Minerals. No known interactions.

Effects In Laboratory Tests

Continuous or excessive use may result in potassium depletion. Dried aloe juice may interfere with urine testing that relies on color changes, and may reduce blood glucose.

Adverse Reactions

- No adverse reactions except rare mild allergies have been noted in topical use. Some cases of delayed wound healing when used on wounds from cesarean sections or laparotomies.
- For internal use, aloe contaminated with aloe latex may cause severe diarrhea, cramping and uterine contractions.
- Long-term use of aloe as a laxative can cause dependency, requiring increased doses to maintain effectiveness.
- Occasional abdominal cramping.

Who Should Not Use Aloe

- Pregnant women should not use aloe internally, but may use it topically.
- Aloe should not be used internally for children under 12 years of age.
- Do not use internally if you have stomach pain of unknown origin.
- Persons with ulcerative colitis, Crohn's disease or intestinal obstruction should not use aloe internally.

Comments

- Do not confuse with *Agave Americana*, or American Aloe, which is not a true aloe.
- Aloe of the Bible, a fragrant wood used for incense, is unrelated to medicinal aloe.

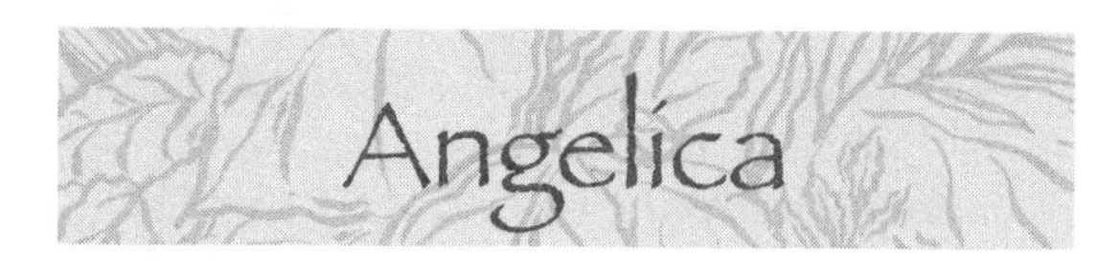

Profile

Common Names: Wild Celery, Root of the Holy Ghost, Wild Angelica, Dong Quai (China)
Family: Umbelliferae (carrots, parsley, celery, fennel and dill also belong to this family)
Genus & Species: *Angelica archangelica, Angelica atropurpurea, Angelica sinensis* (Dong Quai)
Description: Angelica grows anywhere from 20 inches to almost 9 feet tall. The flowers are greenish white and shaped somewhat like an umbrella. The leaves are very large, from 20 to 35 inches long.
Historical Use: Angelica was one of the most popular herbal medicines in Europe during the 15th century and is recorded in Chinese medicine as early as 200 C.E. Angelica has been connected to the Archangel Michael and the Feast of the Annunciation and was believed to protect against evil and cure all disease.
Parts to Use: Seed, whole plant and root.

What It Does

Angelica leaves and seeds are used as a diuretic and to stimulate perspiration. The root is thought to stimulate the appetite, promote menstrual flow, stimulate the uterus, act as an expectorant and a topical anti-inflammatory. Angelica is also used in candied products for decorating cakes and pastries.

Angelica
Angelica archangelica

What It Might Help Treat

Fruit

- Fevers and colds
- Urinary tract infections
- Feeling of fullness, heartburn, bloating and nausea after eating
- Loss of appetite

Leaves (these are unproven uses, but are found in historical documents)

- Diuretic
- To stimulate perspiration

Root

- Complaints of fullness, heartburn, bloating and nausea after eating
- Loss of appetite

Research Insights

There is insufficient reliable information available about the effectiveness of angelica root, fruit or seeds for uses except in combination with other herbs as a topical cream to prevent premature ejaculation.

How It Is Used

Growing

Angelica archangelica is relatively hardy and can be grown from seed sown in autumn or spring. It prefers moist, rich soil in sun or partial shade. Plants will self-seed if not harvested.

Harvesting

Leaves are gathered before the plant flowers, stalks are cut in early summer, seeds are harvested as they ripen and roots are dug in autumn before the ground freezes.

Preserving

All parts of the plant are dried for medicinal use. For culinary use, the foliage may be eaten like celery. The stalks can be combined with rhubarb for stewing and jams. The flower buds, before opening, can be eaten raw or cooked. The essential oil from the root gives the liqueur Benedictine its characteristic flavor.

Best Herbal Remedy Forms

As a fluid extract, tincture, or tea made from dried leaves and seeds. Dried root used as a decoction, as a powdered supplement in capsule form or as an extract or tincture.

Making the Remedy & Dosage

- **Extract,** 1:1. Use 1 to 3 teaspoons a day.
- **Tincture,** 1:5. Use 1 teaspoon up to twice a day.
- **Tea or Infusion,** add 1 teaspoon of powdered seeds or leaves to 1 cup of boiling water and drink twice a day.
- **Dried Root,** the typical dose is 4.5 grams a day in capsule form. **Note:** Do not store angelica root preparations in plastic. The essential oil will react with the plastic.

Safety & Effectiveness

Angelica preparations, when used topically, can increase photosensitivity, so excess exposure to sunshine is not recommended. Large amounts of angelica root can cause poisoning when taken internally.

German Commission E has approved angelica for use in treating fevers, colds, infections, gastrointestinal complaints related to eating and for loss of appetite. It may be effective when used topically for pain, inflammation and psoriasis. In a topical multiple herb preparation it has been used to treat premature ejaculation.

Interactions

Drugs. Angelica contains coumarins, compounds used to thin the blood. Use with prescription blood thinners may increase the risk of bleeding. Because of its proposed use for post-meal gastrointestinal complaints, Angelica might interfere with antacids, sucralfate (Carafate), H-2 antagonists (e.g., Pepcid), or proton pump inhibitors (e.g., Prilosec).
Other Herbs. Simultaneous use of herbs that have coumarin compounds or affect the viscosity (thickness) of the blood could possibly increase the risk of bleeding in some people.
Foods. No adverse reactions or interactions have been noted.
Vitamins or Minerals. None reported.

Effects In Laboratory Tests

None reported.

Adverse Reactions

- No significant side effects have been noted when angelica is used in the recommended therapeutic doses.
- Sensitivity to sunlight may occur when angelica preparations are used topically or if you come in contact with the plant juices while harvesting.

Who Should Not Use Angelica

- Pregnant women
- Nursing women

Comments

Dong quai, or *Angelica sinensis,* will be discussed in Chapter 3.

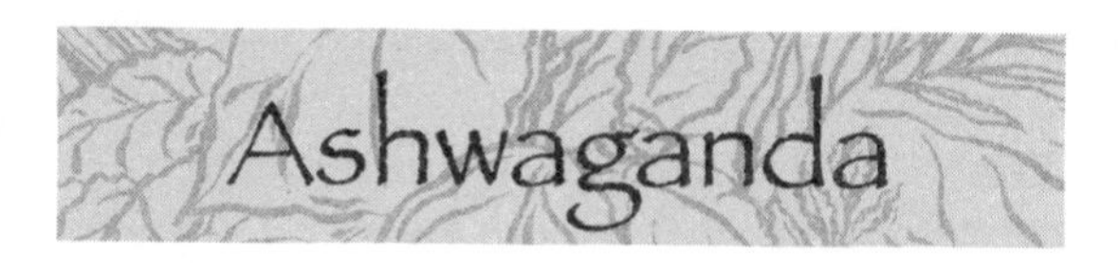

Profile

Common Names: Winter cherry, Indian ginseng, Ashwagandha
Family: Solanaceae (the nightshade family)
Genus & Species: *Withania somnifera*
Description: Ashwaganda is an evergreen shrub with oval leaves and greenish yellow flowers that are followed by orange-red berries.
Historical Use: Ashwaganda has been used in Ayurvedic, Chinese and Middle Eastern Medicine. The plants are toxic to livestock except in specific veterinary medicines.
Parts to Use: Roots, leaves and fruits.

What It Does

According to Ayurvedic practitioners, ashwaganda can help treat male impotency and erectile problems. Ayurvedic medicine also promotes ashwaganda for balancing life forces and for its anti-stress effects. May also affect the reproductive and nervous systems. Currently, there is insufficient substantiated information available about the effectiveness of ashwaganda.

What It Might Help Treat

- May be an immunosuppressant.
- May help treat inflammatory conditions.
- Can be used as a poultice for swelling caused by stings, wounds, burns and snake or scorpion bites.
- Ashwaganda is thought to be an adaptogen that rejuvenates and boosts strength, stamina and vigor, as well as sexual energy.

Research Insights

As documented in animal studies, in combination with other anti-inflammatory herbal medicines it may have an anti-inflammatory activity. Although the plants are toxic to livestock, who do ignore them, Ashwaganda is used to treat mastitis in lactating cows.

How It Is Used

As a tea, tincture or in capsule form as an ingredient in various Ayurvedic formulas.

Growing

Ashwaganda is indigenous to the Mediterranean, Middle East, India and Sri Lanka. Although not traditionally grown in the home garden, it may be tolerant in Zones 8 to 11. Most Ashwaganda preparations are available commercially.

Harvesting

Roots are harvested in the fall when above-ground parts have wilted.

Preserving

Dry the root only.

Best Herbal Remedy Forms

Powdered root for tea or capsules.

Making the Remedy & Dosage

- **Extract or tincture,** commercially purchased. Follow label directions.
- **Tea or infusion,** prepare 1 to 2 teaspoons chopped roots in 1 cup hot (not boiling) water for 15 minutes; cool. Drink 1 cup 3 times a day.
- **Dried whole ashwaganda,** typical dose is in capsule form, containing 1 to 2 grams herb each day.

Safety & Effectiveness

There is insufficient information regarding the safety and effectiveness of ashwaganda.

Interactions

Drugs. Used with amphetamines, ashwaganda may increase the stimulant properties of the drug. Theoretically, use of ashwaganda can increase the effectiveness or strength of barbiturates and sedatives.
Other Herbs. Theoretically, use of ashwaganda may increase the effectiveness and adverse effects of herbs with sedative properties.
Foods. No known interactions.
Vitamins or Minerals. No known interactions.

Effects In Laboratory Tests

No known interactions or adverse effects.

Adverse Reactions

- None have been reported. However, because of the theoretical adverse reactions, refer to Who Should Not Use.

Who Should Not Use Ashwaganda

- Pregnant women, as it may cause excessive bleeding and abortion.
- Nursing women, as there is insufficient data regarding its safety.

Comments

Avoid confusing ashwaganda with winter cherry (*Physalis alkekengi).*

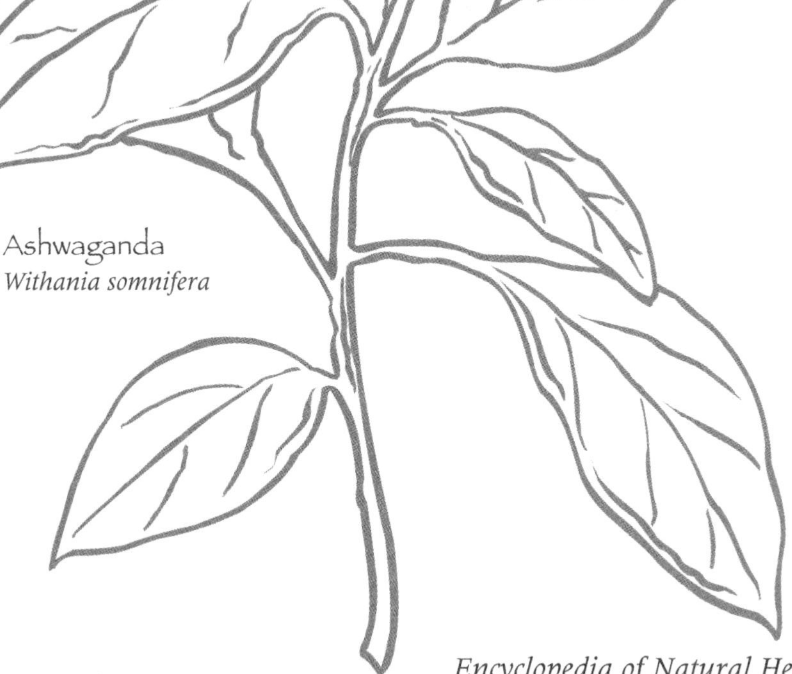

Ashwaganda
Withania somnifera

Astragalus

Profile

Common Name: Milk vetch
Family: Leguminosae (the family that includes alfalfa, soybeans and other legumes)
Genus & Species: *Astragalus membranaceus*
Description: Astragalus is a perennial with light green leaves and yellow pea-like flowers. In the fall, it has papery pods with small, kidney-shaped seeds.
Historical Use: Astragalus has been used in Traditional Chinese Medicine for thousands of years as a tonic equal in effectiveness to ginseng. Astragalus is believed to "tonify the Spleen, Blood and Qi," and is used for "wasting and thirsting syndrome."
Parts to Use: Roots.

What It Does

Astragalus is believed to be an antiviral and antibacterial herb and may have antioxidant properties. It may also provide some relief from inflammation and edema (swelling), and may be helpful in treating disorders of circulation and blood pressure.

What It Might Help Treat

- The common cold and upper respiratory tract infections
- May be used as adjunctive therapy, in combination with glossy privet (*Ligustrum lucidum*), for breast and lung cancer
- Angina
- Relieve symptoms of congestive heart failure
- Hepatitis

Research Insights

Research has shown that the root and its extracts are powerful stimulators of the immune system.

In laboratory animals, astragalus has been shown to have a protective effect on the livers of animals exposed to chemotherapy drugs.

How It Is Used

Dried root powder.

Growing

Native to eastern Asia, astragalus is not usually grown in North America. Some herb gardening references do offer information regarding zone and growing conditions, indicating that with the right conditions, cultivation might be possible.

Harvesting

Roots are dug in the fall and dried for decoctions, powders and tinctures.

Preserving

Dry the root only.

Best Herbal Remedy Forms

Tincture, tea or dried root for capsules.

Making the Remedy & Dosage

- **Tincture,** use purchased, commercially prepared, 1:5. Take 15 to 30 drops, twice a day,
- **Tea,** mix 120 grams of whole root powder with 1 liter of water; drink ½ to 1 liter a day.
- **Decoction,** simmer 4 to 5 sticks of root in 4 cups of water for 1 hour. Drink 1 cup, 2 times each day.

- **Dried,** may be made into a powder for capsules of 400 to 500 mg; take up to 8 to 14 (400- to 500-mg) capsules of astragalus powder daily.
- **Culinary,** may be used in soups or other cooked foods, including rice, as desired. Astragalus tastes mildly sweet.

Safety & Effectiveness

Toxicity of astragalus is considered low when used topically. Astragalus may be effective when used for the common cold and mild upper respiratory infections. It may be effective for relief of angina symptoms.

Interactions

Drugs. Interactions with drugs are primarily theoretical, based on the function or action of the herb. May contribute to antiviral effects when used in combination with antiviral medications. May interfere with drugs that suppress the immune system, such as drugs taken to prevent transplant rejection.

Other Herbs. No interactions have been noted.

Foods. No interactions have been noted.

Vitamins or Minerals. No interactions have been noted.

Effects In Laboratory Tests

None known.

Adverse Reactions

Toxicity is considered to be very low.

Who Should Not Use Astragalus

- Pregnant and nursing women, because of insufficient information regarding the effects of astragalus.
- May not be appropriate for persons with high fevers or those who are acutely ill.

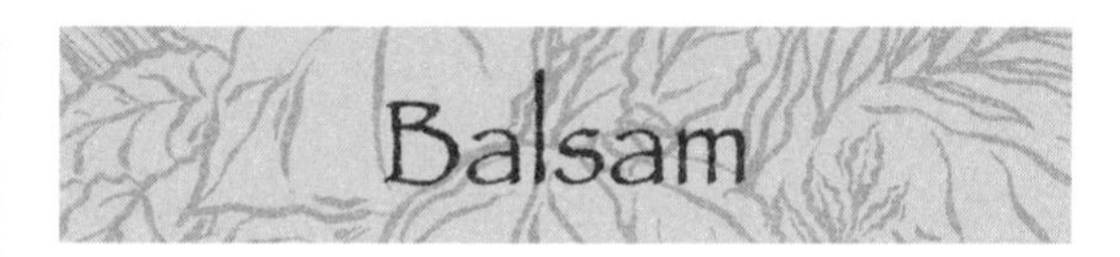

Profile

Common Names: Balsam fir, Canada balsam
Family: Pinaceae
Genus & Species: *Abies balsamea*
Historical Use: Canada balsam has been used for burns, sores, cuts, angina, cancer, mucous membrane inflammation, colds, coughs, warts, wounds, urinary tract complaints and for pain relief. The resin is used as flavoring in foods and beverages and for mounting microscopic slides. The oil is used in dentistry as well as for fragrance and cosmetic use.
Description: There are between 40 and 50 species of evergreen trees, found mostly in mountainous regions. Most are very large and not suitable for the home garden. They prefer the colder zones.
Parts to Use: Bark, twigs and needles (leaves).

What It Does

It acts as an expectorant and respiratory system stimulant.

What It Might Help Treat

- Chest infections (respiratory, colds)
- Wounds and burns

Research Insights

There appears to be no research on balsam and its medicinal uses despite its long history of use.

How It Is Used

Fresh shoots, dried leaves (needles), bark and resin. Shoots, leaves and bark are used for tea. Resin is used commonly in dentistry and as an ingredient in foods and beverages.

Growing

Balsam prefers cooler climates and can be found growing in the wild in central and eastern Canada and in the northeastern United States. The balsam fir is somewhat smaller than its cousins and may be suitable for use in home landscaping.

Harvesting

- Shoot tips may be picked fresh in the spring and used for teas.
- Bark and leaves may be picked fresh and used as needed. Leaves are best picked fresh in the spring. Bark may be harvested at any time, but to minimize damage to the tree, the best time is autumn.
- Leaves for drying should be picked in spring. Take care not to remove entire limbs as this may cause permanent damage.
- Sap and resin may be collected in the fall; however, use caution and respect for the tree so as not to damage or kill it. Collect the resin or sap by drilling a small hole in the tree and catching the resin in a bucket.

Preserving

- Dry the root only.
- Never remove all of the bark from the tree. Do not remove an entire band encircling the tree, either. Both practices can kill the tree. Cut bark into small pieces and spread on a tray to dry.
- Leaves—use standard leaf drying instructions.

- Resins can be stored directly in a clean, sterile, dark glass jar until ready for use.
- Leaves may be spread to dry on a fine mesh screen. When they are brittle to the touch, store in dark glass away from sunlight.

Best Herbal Remedy Forms

Tincture or tea.

Making the Remedy & Dosage

- **Tincture,** 1:5. Take 5 to 20 drops of tincture in a small amount of water up to 3 times daily.
- **Tea,** steep 2 to 6 tablespoons of leaves and bark in 1 cup boiling water to make a weak tea of Canada balsam. Take up to 3 times daily.

Safety & Effectiveness

Balsam is considered safe when needles and twigs are used appropriately in food or topically as directed. There is insufficient documented information on the effectiveness of balsam for medicinal purposes.

Interactions

Balsam is considered safe if used in the appropriate dosages. There are no known drug, herb or food interactions, nor does it have an effect on laboratory tests.

Effects In Laboratory Tests

No interactions or effects on laboratory tests have been observed.

Adverse Reactions

No adverse reactions have been reported.

Who Should Not Use Balsam

Because insufficient data is available regarding use during pregnancy, pregnant women should avoid using balsam as an herbal supplement.

Comments

Hemlock spruce is also referred to as Canada balsam, but it belongs to a different family altogether: the Coniferae family. Hemlock spruce is used for many of the same conditions as Canada balsam, but a useful part of hemlock spruce is the oil obtained by steam distillation from the needles, branch tips or branches, a process best left to experts! Hemlock spruce may worsen whooping cough and asthma, should not be used in cardiac insufficiency (patients whose hearts do not pump efficiently) or on open skin lesions. Hemlock spruce should not be confused with the toxic water hemlock. The typical dose is 4 drops of oil on a lump of sugar taken 3 times a day for respiratory ailments. As an inhalant, add 2 grams of oil to hot water and inhale 2 to 3 times each day. For sprains and strains, a topical preparation of 1 to 5 parts Hemlock spruce oil to 1 to 5 parts petroleum jelly may be rubbed into affected areas.

Balsam
Abies balsamea

Bergamot

Profile

Common Name: Bergamot orange
Family: Rutaceae
Genus & Species: *Citrus bergamia*
Description: There are some 16 species of the small evergreen trees and shrubs that make up this genus. The tree has white fragrant flowers during spring and summer, followed by an aromatic fruit with a yellow rind.
Historical Use: Orange flower water from bergamot has been used for colic in babies. Bergamot oil is used on the skin to treat loss of pigmentation and as an insecticide for body lice.
Parts to Use: Flowers, ripe fruit, peel and oil.

What It Does

It can be used topically for skin conditions. In aromatherapy, bergamot oil may soothe anxiety. Bergamot oil is used as a citrus-flavoring agent in many commercially prepared foods.

What It Might Help Treat

- Psoriasis
- Loss of skin pigmentation (vitiligo)
- Anxiety

Research Insights

When used with long-wave UV light, it may be effective for treating psoriasis. Bergamot may be effective as a topical preparation for mycosis fungoides, which is a rare chronic lymphatomous skin malignancy. For this condition, it should be used only under the care of a physician. There is insufficient reliable research regarding bergamot and any other uses.

How It Is Used

Purchased essential oil. Dried or fresh for culinary use.

Growing

In tropical climates, *citrus bergamia* can be grown as part of the home's landscape. It appears to be hardy to 7°F for a short period of time.

Harvesting

Harvest flowers right after they have opened or the ripe fruit when it separates easily from the stem. The oil is obtained from the skin of the ripe fruit.

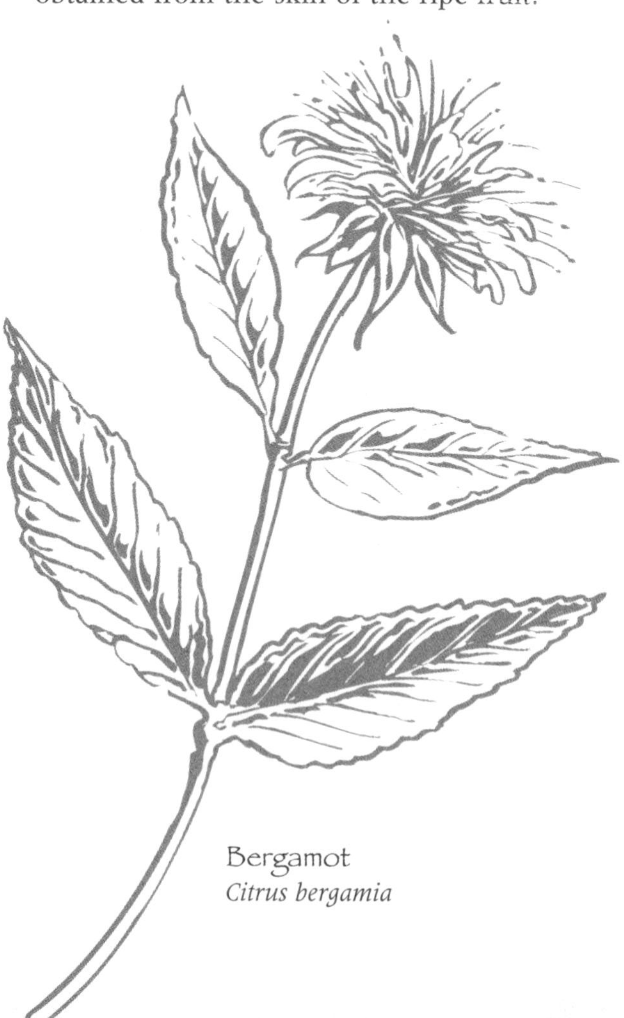

Bergamot
Citrus bergamia

Preserving

Flowers and fruit are best used when fresh. The oil may be preserved in a dark glass container.

Best Herbal Remedy Forms

Aromatherapy and some topical applications.

Making the Remedy & Dosage

- **Tinctures and salves,** it is best to purchase already prepared essential oil that may be used for inhalants and in preparation of tinctures and salves. Bergamot oil is cold-pressed from the peel.
- For an **inhalant**, add 3 to 5 drops of the essential oil to 1 quart (4 cups) steaming water.
- **Culinary,** dried (or fresh) zest of the peel can be used to flavor teas and dishes that call for orange peel.

Safety & Effectiveness

It is generally safe when consumed in amounts used in food. Bergamot may be effective for treating psoriasis, vitiligo and some fungus when used (medically and topically) with long wave UV light.

Interactions

Drugs. Using bergamot oil topically while taking drugs that increase photosensitivity may compound the risk of side effects from either or both drugs.
Other Herbs. No interactions have been noted. However, if used with herbs that increase photosensitivity, the risk of side effects may be compounded.
Foods. No interactions have been noted.
Vitamins or minerals. No interactions have been noted.

Effects In Laboratory Tests

None known.

Adverse Reactions

- The oil may act as a photosensitizer when used topically. Photosensitivity reaches its peak approximately 2 hours after contact.
- Frequent exposure to the peel or oil can result in skin reactions, such as rash, hyperpigmentation and blisters.

Who Should Not Use Bergamot

- The oil should not be used for children because it may cause intestinal colic, seizures and possibly death.
- When used topically, bergamot is considered safe for pregnant women. There is not enough information about its use internally to recommend it during pregnancy or lactation.
- Individuals who are sensitive to the sun should avoid using topical oil of bergamot while exposed to the sun.

Comments

- Do not confuse bergamot with bee balm (*Monarda didyma*), which is sometimes referred to as bergamot. Bee balm belongs to the Lamiaceae family and is found in the prairies, dry scrub and woodland. Bee balm is called bergamot because its scent is similar to that of *Citrus bergamia*.
- Bee balm is a brightly colored plant that attracts bees, butterflies and hummingbirds.
- The whole bee balm plant, including leaves and flowers, is used as an aromatic, stimulant and expectorant herb thought to benefit digestion.
- Culinary uses of bee balm include flavoring tea and adding the flowers to salads.

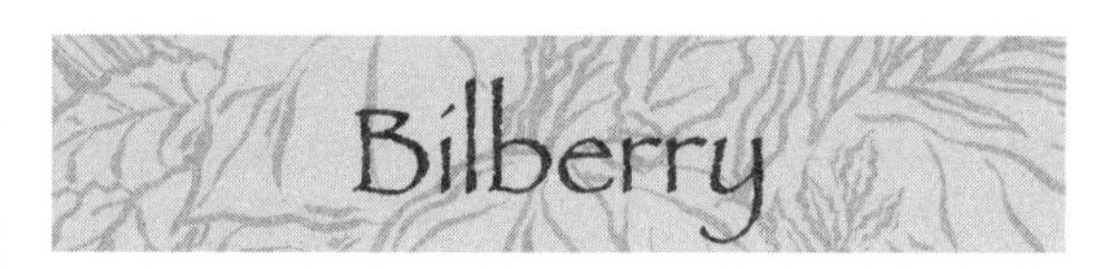

Profile

Common Names: Blueberry, dwarf bilberry, huckleberry, whortleberry and wine berry
Family: Ericaceae
Genus & Species: *Vaccinium myrtillus*
Description: Bilberry is a deciduous shrub with glossy, oval leaves and bell-shaped flowers that become blue-black fruits in summer.
Historical Use: Bilberries belong to a large genus that has approximately 450 species. The most important members of this family include bilberries, cranberries (Vaccinium macrocarpon) and blueberries (Vaccinium corymbosum). Medicinal use began in the 12th century when women used bilberry fruit to relieve symptoms of menstruation. The berries are considered tonics, astringents and antiseptics when used both internally and externally. Europeans have used it for respiratory and GI conditions. In the 18th century, it was often used as a mouthwash. It has long been considered a nutritious food, with its high vitamin C content.
Parts to Use: Leaves and fruits.

What It Does

Bilberries contain powerful antioxidants called anthocyanosides, which prevent free-radical damage to cells.

What It Might Help Treat

- Vision problems
- Heart disease
- Inflammation of the mucous membranes of the mouth and throat

Research Insights

Bilberry may help relieve diarrhea and irritation of the mouth and throat mucosa. On the other hand, excessive quantities of fruit may be an effective laxative.

Bilberry improves blood flow and the structure and permeability of blood vessels. It may improve retinal lesions as a result of diabetic or hypertensive retinopathy.

It's a powerful antioxidant, may have antiplatelet activity, may be effective for spider and varicose veins and also may lower blood triglyceride levels.

How It Is Used

Fresh bilberries may be used for constipation or to relieve diarrhea. May be taken internally in capsule form, as a decoction or an extract. May also be applied topically.

Growing

Cultivated primarily in Europe, on hillsides. In the United States, they are large and sweet, more like the blueberry.

Harvesting

Leaves are picked in spring. Fruits are picked in late summer.

Preserving

- Leaves are picked in the spring and dried for teas and decocting.
- Fruits may be used fresh, dried or juiced.

Best Herbal Remedy Forms

- Fresh, juiced or dried berries.
- Leaves dried for teas and decoctions.
- Commerically available purchased supplements.

Making the Remedy & Dosage

- **Dried ripe berries**, 20 to 60 grams a day for constipation. May also provide some benefits for the eyes as well. Take with at least 8 ounces of water.
- Make a **tea** from 1 to 2 teaspoons of dried leaves. Steep leaves in 1 cup hot, not boiling, water for about 15 minutes and enjoy up to 4 times a day.
- Dried berries may be used for a **tea** by adding 30 grams of herb to 500 mL of hot, not boiling, water steeping for 5 to 10 minutes and straining. This is an excellent non-caffeinated tea substitute.
- **Juice** made from the berry, taken with out sweetening, may help relieve chronic diarrhea. Take 2-4 ounces. If diarrhea persists, seek medical attention. Diarrhea may be a symptom of a more serious condition.
- Mix equal amounts of witch hazel and bilberry juice to make a **lotion** for skin inflammation and sunburn.
- Take 160 mg of a commercially prepared **extract** twice a day for retinopathy.

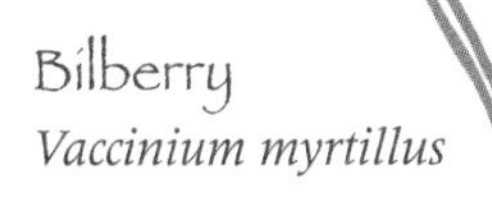

Bilberry
Vaccinium myrtillus

Safety & Effectiveness

Bilberry is considered safe when taken in recommended dosages. High or prolonged doses of bilberry leaves (1.5g/kg/day) may be toxic or lethal.

Interactions

Drugs.

- Drugs used for diabetes may require adjusting as bilberry leaf extract may lower blood sugar. Bilberries are not known to have the same effect.
- People taking drugs to treat alcohol abuse may have an adverse reaction if the herbal preparation contains alcohol.

Herbs. No known interactions with other herbs.

Foods. No known interactions with foods.

Effects In Laboratory Tests

Use of bilberry leaf has been shown to lower blood sugar and triglyceride levels.

Adverse Reactions

Intoxication has been reported in animals that have consumed the leaves. No adverse reactions have been observed in humans using bilberries.

Who Should Not Use Bilberry

Because of potential toxicity for pregnant women, the leaves should not be used. When the fruit and dried fruit are used as a food, bilberries are considered safe to consume.

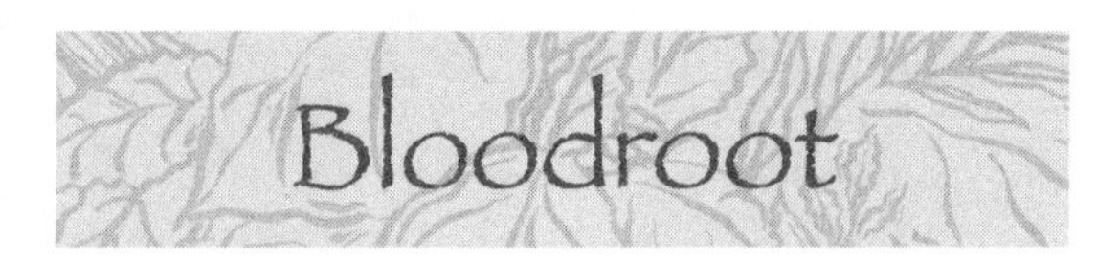

Profile

Common Names: Sanguinaria, Indian red paint, bloodroot, snakebite
Family: Papaveraceae
Genus & Species: *Sanguinaria canadensis*
Description: It is a perennial with kidney-shaped, scalloped gray-green leaves and the rhizome responsible for its name. Its flowers are tiny, white to pink-tinged and appear in the spring as the leaves appear.
Historical Use: Bloodroot was used by Native Americans to dye the skin and induce vomiting for therapeutic reasons. It was also used to treat sore throats, ringworm and rheumatism and to act as a stimulating expectorant, despite its toxic nature. It is now used as a dental plaque inhibitor. Its name comes from the red color of its roots.
Parts to Use: Rhizomes.

What It Does

It reduces dental plaque and treats cancers of the ear and nose.

What It Might Help Treat

- Wounds and minor abrasions
- Heart conditions

Research Insights

There is insufficient reliable information regarding its effectiveness for other uses.

How It Is Used

Dried rhizomes are used for numerous topical preparations as well as some internal uses, but should be used with caution.

Growing

It is relatively easy to grow from seed, cuttings or divisions of the rhizomes. It is a common plant in the wild and in home gardens in the eastern United States.

Harvesting

Dig rhizomes in the fall; handle them carefully, as they are brittle.

Preserving

Rhizomes may be dried. (Rhizomes are similar to roots. They are a stem which grows underground, horizontally. They branch at intervals and bear roots and leafy shoots.)

Best Herbal Remedy Forms

Dried herb, liquid extract or tincture.

Making the Remedy & Dosage

- **Liquid extract,** 1:1. Take 1 to 5 drops in a small amount of water, 3 times a day.
- **Tincture,** 1:5. Take 5 to 40 drops in a small amount of water, 3 times a day.
- **Dried roots and plants** may be made into capsules and taken in doses of 60 to 500 mg, 3 times a day.

Safety & Effectiveness

Considered safe and effective for dental purposes and when used orally and appropriately short-term.

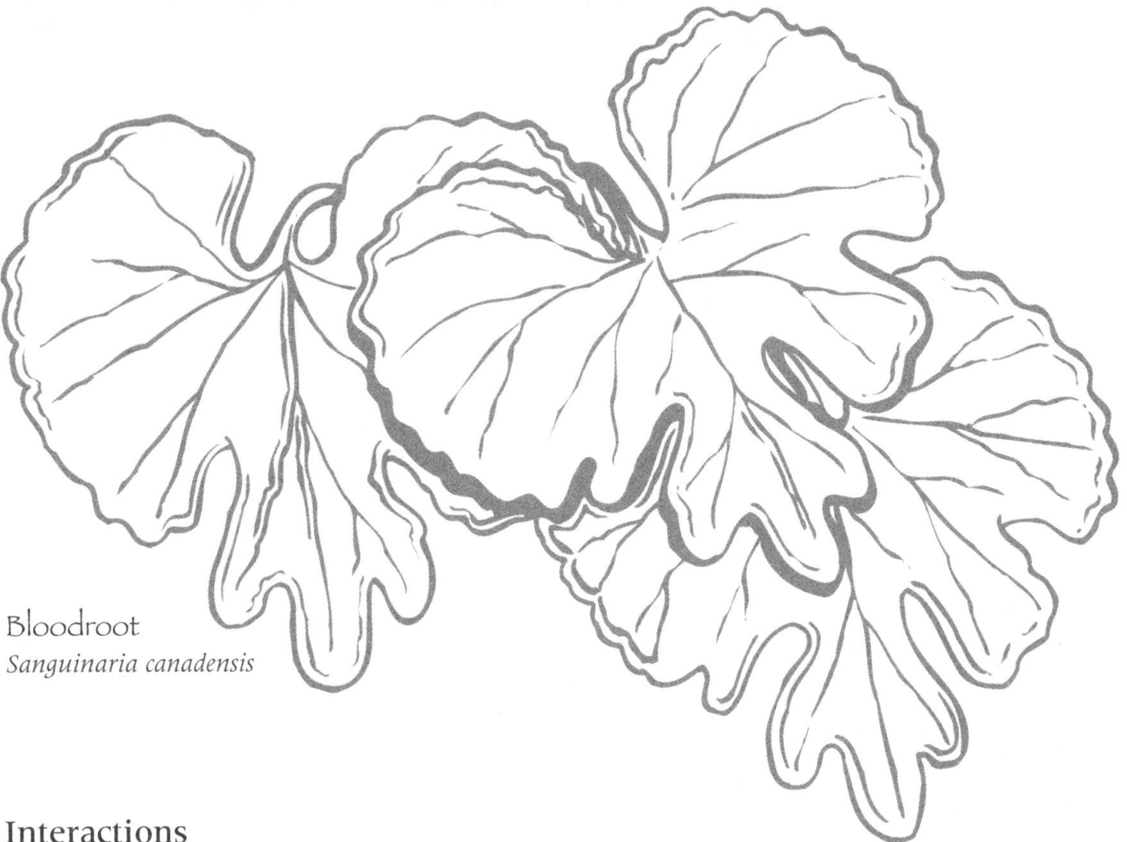

Bloodroot
Sanguinaria canadensis

Interactions

Drugs. No known interactions.
Other herbs. No known interactions.
Foods. No known interactions.
Vitamins or Minerals. No known interactions.

Effects in Laboratory Tests

None known.

Adverse reactions

- When taken internally, bloodroot can cause GI upset, nausea, vomiting or CNS (central nervous system) depression.
- High doses can result in low blood pressure, shock, coma and glaucoma. It can also irritate the skin upon contact.

Who Should Not Use Bloodroot

- People with GI irritation including ulcers, irritable bowel and chronic diarrhea.
- People with glaucoma.
- Pregnant and nursing women because of its potential for GI side effects.

Butcher's Broom

Profile

Common Names: Jew's myrtle, box holly
Family: Liliaceae
Genus & Species: *Ruscus aculeatus*
Description: It is a small, clumping shrub with erect shoots and small oval leaves. There are tiny green flowers in the late winter and spring, followed by small red fruits on the female plants in the summer.
Historical Use: Butcher's broom was known in the first century C.E. as a remedy for kidney stones. In some cultures, the young shoots were eaten as food, similar to asparagus. Its common name comes from its traditional use in bundles to clean floors of butcher's shops.
Parts to Use: Whole plant, young shoots, roots.

What It Does

Butcher's broom acts as a laxative, a diuretic and a vasoconstrictor.

What It Might Help Treat

Butcher's broom might help relieve:

- the burning and itching of hemorrhoids.
- the symptoms of chronic venous insufficiency, including varicose veins, peripheral vascular disease and associated leg heaviness, pain, itching and swelling.
- constipation.
- inflammation.

Research Insights

Research corroborates that when taken internally, butcher's broom may relieve the symptoms of hemorrhoids and may effectively treat the symptoms of chronic venous insufficiency.

How It Is Used

The typical dose is measured by the amount of active plant constituents—ruscogenin—available per dose. As this amount is unknown in home-cultivated plants, purchasing the herb ready-to-use is advised if you want to be sure of the dose. Otherwise, a tea or tincture for topical application may be made.

Growing

Butcher's broom is native to Europe, North Africa and the Azores. It may be cultivated in areas of the United States that are within a similar hardiness zone, usually in areas that are no colder than 10°F during the coldest part of the year.

Harvesting

Harvest young shoots in early spring for eating. Cut whole plants in late spring. Dig roots in the fall.

Preserving

Whole plant and roots may be dried. See standard instructions.

Best Herbal Remedy Forms

- Topical applications
- Teas, decoctions
- Capsules

Making the Remedy & Dosage

- **Decoction** is made with 30 grams of dried herb (5 teaspoons), or 60 grams of fresh, to 750 mL of water, reduced by simmering to 500 mL. Strain and drink hot or cold.
- **Ointment** is made with petroleum jelly and dried herb and is available commercially.
- **Tincture,** purchased commercially, is made with alcohol. May be taken in doses of 20 to 40 drops 2 to 3 times a day.
- **Tea** is made by steeping 1 teaspoon of dried root in one cup of hot, not boiling, water. Strain after 10 minutes and drink hot or cold. Drink up to 3 cups per day.
- **Dried roots** and plants may be made into a capsule; take 2 to 3 capsules containing 500 mg of herb, with water, 2 or 3 times a day.

Safety & Effectiveness

Considered safe when used appropriately, especially if taken orally. May be effective in relieving the burning and itching of hemorrhoids and for relief of venous insufficiency.

Interactions

Drugs. No interactions are known to occur. Theoretically, however, there could be some adverse reactions (compounding effects) if taken with drugs that are vasodilators.

Other Herbs. No interactions are known to occur. Theoretically, however, there could be some adverse reactions (compounding effects) if taken with other herbs that are vasodilators.

Foods. No interactions are known to occur.

Vitamins or Minerals. No interactions are known to occur.

Effects in Laboratory Tests

None known.

Adverse Reactions

When taken internally, can cause GI upset.

Who Should Not Use Butcher's Broom

Avoid using during pregnancy and lactation, as there is insufficient research regarding its safety.

Comments

Do not confuse with Scotch or Spanish broom.

Calendula

Profile

Common Names: Pot marigold, garden marigold
Family: Asteraceae/Compositae; other family members include daisies, ragweed and chrysanthemums.
Genus & Species: *Calendula officinalis*
Description: Calendula is a small, bushy annual with flowers that can grow to 3 inches across. Its leaves are lance-shaped, growing from branched stems.
Historical Use: Calendula has been known for thousands of years as "pot marigold." Originating in Mediterranean countries, it is often confused with the Tagetes species of marigold that is more commonly planted in the United States. It has been referred to as the "poor man's saffron" because of the yellow hue it gives to dishes it is prepared in. Medicinally, calendula has been used to induce menses, produce sweat during fevers and to cure jaundice. It has been noted for its antiseptic and anti-inflammatory properties and used to speed the healing of wounds, sores, burns, bruises and cuts.
Parts to Use: Whole flower heads, petals.

What It Does

It acts as an anti-inflammatory. Also helps heal leg wounds and ulcers.

What It Might Help Treat

Gastric and duodenal ulcers

Research Insights

- External applications in conjunction with other herbs may reduce pain.
- In vitro studies show antibacterial, antifungal, antiviral and antiparasitic properties.

How It Is Used

Dried flowers are used for preparations that treat inflammation both internally and externally.

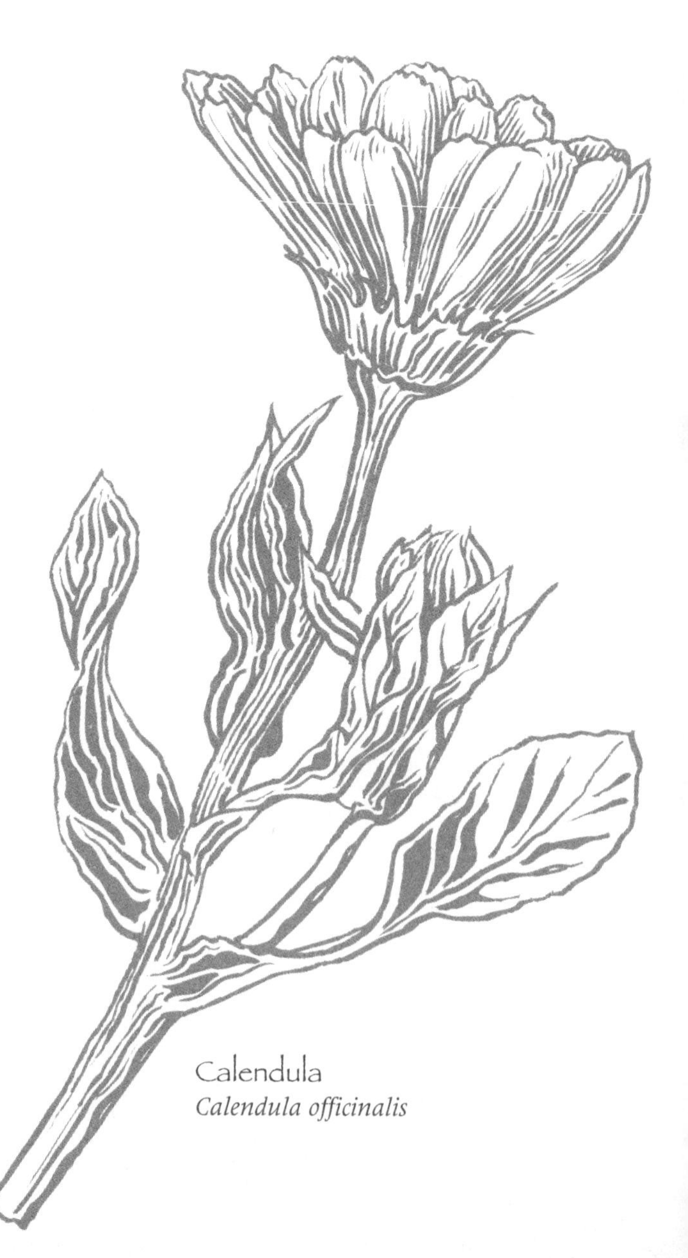

Calendula
Calendula officinalis

Growing

Calendula is a hardy plant that adapts well to the home garden. Sow seeds in the spring or fall in well-drained soil in full sun. Remove dead flowers to prolong flowering.

Harvesting

Cut flowers when just barely dry and used fresh or dried.

Preserving

Dry flower heads in a well-ventilated shady area.

Best Herbal Remedy Forms

In cooking, tea, liquid extract, tincture or ointment.

Making the Remedy & Dosage

- **Tea,** made using 1 to 2 grams of dried flowers in 150 mL of boiling water, left to steep for 5 to 10 minutes. Strain. Drink 3 times a day. Tea also may be used as a mouthwash or gargle.
- **Liquid extract,** 1:1. Take in 1/4- to 1/2-teaspoon doses in a small amount of water, 3 times a day.
- **Ointment,** made with 100 grams petroleum jelly or other suitable cream and 2 to 5 grams of the herb.
- **Tincture,** 1:5. Take 1/2 to 1 teaspoon in a small amount of water, 3 times a day.
- **Compresses,** made with the tea and applied to the affected area with a clean cloth.

Safety & Effectiveness

Considered safe and effective for inflammations in the mouth and for poorly healing leg ulcers.

Interactions

Drugs. May cause additive adverse effects with sedative drugs.
Other Herbs. Herbs with sedative properties may have an additive and adverse effect.
Foods. No interactions are known to occur.
Vitamins or Minerals. No interactions are known to occur.

Effects In Laboratory Tests

None known.

Adverse Reactions

Allergic reactions develop in persons sensitive to the Asteraceae/Compositae family.

Who Should Not Use Calendula

Persons sensitive to other Asteraceae/ Compositae family members including daisies and marigolds.

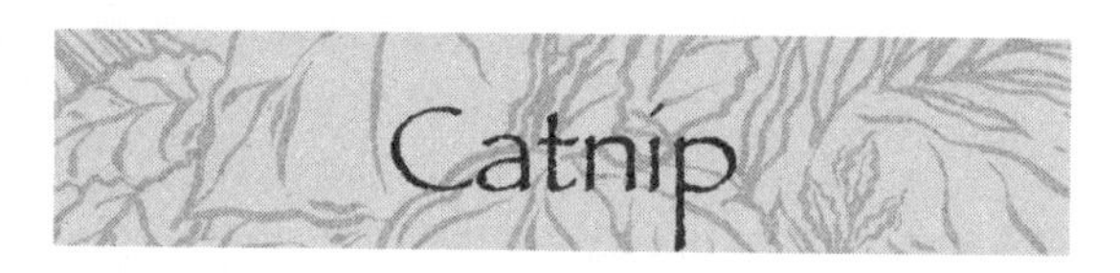

Profile

Common Name: Catmint
Family: Labiatae/Lamiaceae (the mint family)
Genus & Species: *Nepeta cataria*
Description: Catnip looks very similar to other members of the mint family with a square stem, fuzzy leaves and flowers with twin lips. It is greenish gray in color and grows up to 3 feet tall.
Historical Use: Catnip has been used in China and Europe for more than 2,000 years. Its history includes treatment for smallpox, colic and toothache; it also has been used as a tranquilizer and digestive aid. The settlers introduced it to North America and its use (and the plant itself) quickly spread to Native Americans.
Parts to Use: Whole plant and leaves.

What It Does

Catnip soothes or calms the smooth muscles. Also has antispasmodic properties.

What It Might Help Treat

- Digestive ailments, including indigestion, colic, cramping and gas.
- To initiate menstruation.
- As a tonic for anxiety, upper respiratory infections and headaches.
- Insomnia.

Research Insights

Because of its smooth muscle-calming effect, it may have a relaxing and tranquilizing effect on the stomach, intestines and uterus. The same chemicals that make catnip intoxicating to cats are responsible for its sedative effect in humans, supporting its traditional use as a mild tranquilizer and sedative.

How It Is Used

Orally or topically, depending on the ailment it is intended to treat.

Growing

Catnip grows easily from seed or transplants under almost any conditions.

Harvesting

Pick leaves and flowers in late summer when plants are in bloom.

Preserving

Dry catnip in bunches and hang them upside down in a well-ventilated area, shaded from direct sunlight. Or, separate leaves and flowers and spread to dry. It is dry when brittle to the touch. Store in sealed dark glass containers in a cool, dry, shaded area.

Best Herbal Remedy Forms

As a tea, infusion or as a poultice for cuts and scrapes while in the garden.

Making the Remedy & Dosage

- **Tea,** made using 2 teaspoons of dried herb per cup of boiling water. Steep 10 minutes, strain and drink hot or cold. (Do not boil the herb itself as it destroys the healing oil.)
- **Dried,** in capsule form, with approximately 380 mg of herb per capsule. Take 2 capsules, 3 times each day.
- **For a poultice,** pick a few fresh leaves, crush and apply directly to the wound. May be held in place using a light bandage or cloth.

Safety & Effectiveness

Although extensive supporting research data is unavailable, historical use and some recent studies have confirmed that catnip may be effective in treating problems that affect the smooth muscles, particularly of the GI tract and nerves. Catnip is considered safe when used as recommended.

Interactions

Drugs. Sedatives and barbiturates used with catnip may cause additive effects and adverse side effects.
Other Herbs. Herbs with potential sedative and barbiturate properties used along with catnip may compound each other and result in adverse side effects.
Foods. No known interactions.
Vitamins or Minerals. No known interactions.

Effects in Laboratory Tests

No known adverse reactions.

Adverse Reactions

In excessive amounts, catnip may cause headache and vomiting.

Who Should Not Use Catnip

- Because catnip is thought to stimulate menstruation, it should not be used when there is excessive uterine bleeding or pelvic disease.
- Pregnant and lactating women should not use catnip because of its theoretical uterine stimulating properties.

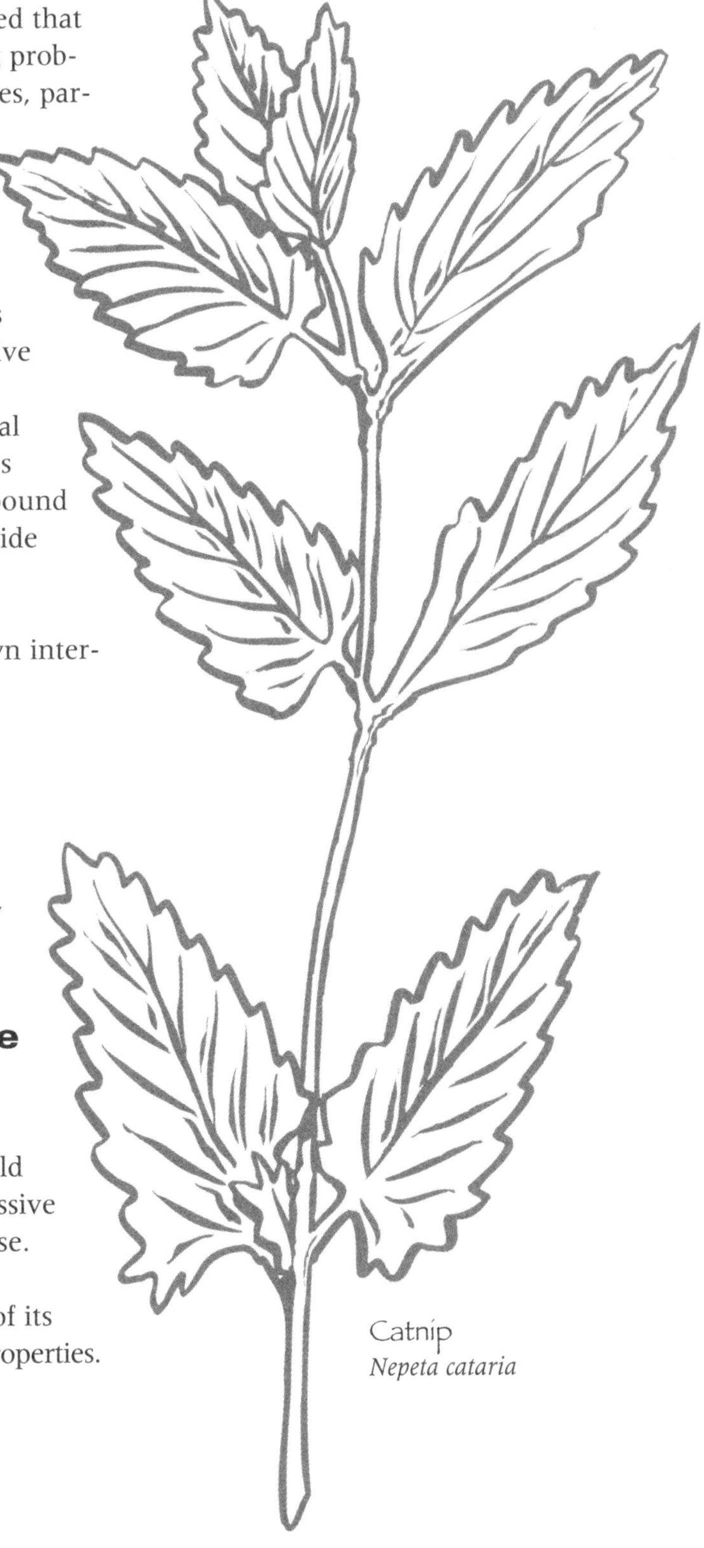

Catnip
Nepeta cataria

Chamomile

Profile

Common Names: Chamomile, ground apple, matricaria
Family: Asteraceae/Compositae (daisies, dandelions and marigolds also belong to this family)
Genus & Species: *Matricaria recutita* (German and Hungarian) or *Anthemis nobilis* (English and Roman)
Description: *Matricaria recutita* (German and Hungarian) is an annual that reaches about 3 feet in height, with multi-branched stems and daisy-like flowers. *Anthemis nobilis* (English and Roman) is a clump-forming perennial with upright single stems, finely divided leaves, and bright golden-yellow daisy-like flowers.
Historical Use: Although two different herbs, botanically unrelated, these two types of chamomile have similar properties and applications. Immigrants from Germany and Britain introduced both types into North America, but German chamomile is most frequently grown here today. During the 1800s, chamomile was used for poultices, wound-healing, digestive complaints, menstrual problems and problems associated with pregnancy and childbirth. Today, chamomile is used as a beverage (tea) more than as an herbal remedy. Found in many herbal cosmetics, Chamomile is still used to give luster to blond hair. Chamomile is listed as an official drug in the pharmacopoeias of 26 countries and is approved for external and some internal use by Germany's Commission E.
Parts to Use:
Flowers.

Chamomile
Matricaria recutita

What It Does

It acts as an antispasmodic, particularly for the smooth muscles of the GI tract. Chamomile has mild sedative effects. It acts as an anti-inflammatory.

Roman chamomile has been used as a hair tint and conditioner. German chamomile's essential oil and extracts are used in foods and beverages for flavoring and in cosmetics, soaps and mouthwashes.

What It Might Help Treat

- Digestive upsets, particularly indigestion, nausea, vomiting, morning sickness, gas.
- Inflammation of the mouth and mucous membranes.
- Anxiety and stress.
- Skin irritations, inflammations and infections.
- Relief of menstrual cramps.

Research Insights

Note: Most research has focused on German chamomile.

Chamomile may help prevent stomach ulcers and speed ulcer healing. It may stimulate the immune system. In animal research, it has been shown to relieve arthritis-related joint inflammation. Chamomile may have an effect similar to tranquilizers and anti-anxiety drugs.

Chamomile oil and the herb have anti-inflammatory properties. Chamomile is endorsed by the German Commission E for treating wounds.

How It Is Used

Tea, liquid extract, tincture and as purchased standardized extracts.

Growing

This hardy annual can be grown from

seed or from plants. If left to bloom and die without being picked, it may re-seed itself. Roman chamomile is a perennial whose clumps may be divided in spring.

Harvesting

Harvest when flowers are just fully open.

Preserving

Use fresh, but may be frozen or dried. When dried, flowers lose their volatile oil, so fresh or frozen is preferable.

Best Herbal Remedy Forms

Teas, extract, tincture or powdered in capsule form.

Making the Remedy & Dosage

Extract 1:1; use 1 to 4 mL (a scant 1/4 to 1 teaspoon), 3 times a day. For mucositus resulting from chemo or radiation therapy, use a rinse made with 10 to 15 drops German chamomile liquid extract in 100 mL warm water, 3 times a day. This may relieve inflammation in the mouth and throat.
Tincture of 1:5. Take 10 to 40 drops, 3 times a day.
Tea, steep 3 grams of dried flowers (about 1 teaspoon) in 150 mL hot, not boiling, water for 5 to 10 minutes and then strain. Take 3 to 4 times each day.
Mouthwash or gargle made with freshly prepared tea and used to treat inflammations of the mouth.
Dried flowers, 2 to 8 grams, 3 times a day, taken in capsule form.
Poultices, steep 4 teaspoons dried flowers in 1 1/2 cups hot, not boiling, water for 10 minutes; strain and apply herb to affected area.

Safety & Effectiveness

Chamomile is recognized by the German Commission E and is on the list of herbs that are generally recognized as safe (GRAS) by the U.S. Food and Drug Administration (FDA).

German chamomile may be effective when used orally for GI complaints, including spasms, GI tract inflammation, inflamed mucous membranes, menstrual cramps and for insomnia. Topically, it may be effective for hemorrhoids, leg ulcers, inflammations of the skin and irritated mucous membranes, mouth and gums.

Interactions

Drugs. May interfere with psychotropic and hypnotic drugs, sedatives, anti-arthritic pain relievers and anticoagulants (blood thinners).
Other Herbs. May interfere with herbs that have sedative properties and anticoagulant or antiplatelet activity.
Foods. No known interactions.
Vitamins or Minerals. No known interactions.

Effects In Laboratory Tests

No known interactions.

Adverse Reactions

- May aggravate asthma.
- People sensitive to other members of the Asteraceae/Compositae family, including daisies and ragweed, may have an allergic reaction to chamomile.
- Large amounts of Roman chamomile taken internally may result in vomiting.
- Topical use of Roman chamomile has been shown to cause allergic skin reactions.

Who Should Not Use Chamomile

Although used for conditions associated with pregnancy and premature labor, women who are pregnant or who are trying to conceive should avoid chamomile in medicinal amounts.

Chaste Tree

Profile

Common Names: Chasteberry, Vitex, Monk's Pepper
Family: Verbenaceae
Genus & Species: *Vitex agnus-castus*
Description: Chaste tree is a deciduous shrub that bears small, tubular, lilac-scented flowers followed by tiny red-black fruits.
Historical Use: This native Mediterranean plant began its history during Hippocrates' time as a treatment for injuries and inflammations. Later, it became known for treatment of menstrual and menopausal complaints and for problems with nursing. In the Middle Ages, the flowers were scattered before the feet of persons entering convents and monasteries to prepare them for their vows of chastity. The fruits of the tree were used to suppress sexual urges in monks, hence the name Monk's Pepper. The dried berries have been used as a substitute for black pepper.
Parts to Use: Fruit.

What It Does

Chaste tree may regulate hormonal function. It may promote the flow of milk in nursing mothers. May relieve spasms and pain during menstruation.

What It Might Help Treat

- Breast tenderness.
- Premenstrual syndrome (PMS).
- Menstrual irregularity and disorders when used long term.

Research Insights

It may be beneficial in treating acne. Chasteberry influences the balance of female sex hormones, reducing estrogen and increasing progesterone levels.

In Germany, a proprietary preparation has been used for ovarian insufficiency and dysfunctional uterine bleeding. Uncontrolled studies have shown the benefit in treating uterine fibroids and infertility as a result of inadequate progesterone levels.

How It Is Used

Orally in tincture, extract, tea or capsule form.

Growing

Although a native of the Mediterranean, Chasteberry was introduced to North America by European colonists. Today, it can be found along streams and riverbanks throughout the southeastern part of the United States and from Florida through the South as far west as Texas and Oklahoma.

Harvesting

Fruits are picked in the fall and used fresh or dried.

Preserving

Dry the root only.

Best Herbal Remedy Forms

Extracts and tinctures are the most often recommended and believed to be the most effective. Capsules of dried fruit may also be used.

Making the Remedy & Dosage

- **Extracts** are available commercially and are measured by pharmaceutical grades. They may be made at home; however, the strength of the mixture may not produce the desired results. The dose in the clinical studies was 40 drops of standardized extract taken once a day.
- **Tinctures** are similar to extracts and can be made at home using dried berries; however, most studies using Chasteberry extract have used 100 mL of an aqueous-alcoholic solution that has been standardized to contain the equivalent of 9 grams of berries. Take 40 drops of tincture up to 3 times each day.
- **Teas or infusions** may be made with tinctures or extracts added to water or by steeping 1 to 2 teaspoons of berries in hot, not boiling, water for 10 minutes. Strain and drink.
- **Dried berries** may be made into a powder that can be taken orally. The recommended dose of commercially available capsules is 175 mg once a day or as recommended.

Safety & Effectiveness

Chasteberry is believed to be safe and effective when used as recommended.

Interactions

Drugs. Chasteberry may interfere, theoretically, with antipsychotic medications, medications that inhibit gastric reflux, oral contraceptives and hormone replacement therapy.
Other Herbs. No known interactions.
Foods. No known interactions.
Vitamins or Minerals. No known interactions.

Effects In Laboratory Tests

No known interactions.

Adverse Reactions

- Side effects rarely have been reported, but can include GI reactions, skin irritation, headaches, dry mouth and increased menstrual flow.
- Complaints of allergic reactions, also minor, are usually resolved when herb use is discontinued.

Who Should Not Use Chasteberry

- Women on birth control pills should not use Vitex as it may counteract birth control pills' effectiveness.
- Pregnant women should not use Vitex because it can have uterine-stimulating properties.
- Do not use during lactation. Not enough is known about its safety, despite the fact that it has been shown to increase milk production without interfering with the quality of the milk.

Comments

Chasteberry does not act immediately; results will take at least two menstrual cycles—longer if menstrual problems have been long-standing.

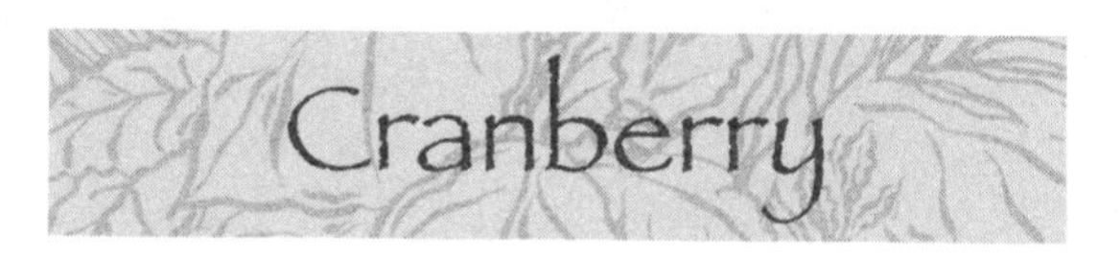

Profile

Common Name: American cranberry
Family: Ericaceae (the same family as bilberry, blueberry and mountain cranberry or Uva-Ursi)
Genus & Species: *Vaccinium macrocarpon* or *Oxycoccus quadripetalus*
Description: Everyone knows what cranberries look like—at least in the grocery store. In the wild, cranberry bushes are small evergreen shrubs that prefer very damp feet. Late spring to late summer pink or purple flowers adorn the shrub, followed by bright red fruits in the fall. They can be found in the wild in parts of the northern United States.
Historical Use: Cranberries have been a staple on the Thanksgiving Day table long before it was known as a healing herb. New England sailors discovered by accident a benefit from their high vitamin C content—they prevented scurvy when taken at sea.
Parts to Use: Fruits or berries.

What It Does

Cranberry helps maintain or improve urinary tract health. It also prevents scurvy, which is no longer a health risk in developed countries.

What It Might Help Treat

- Mild urinary tract infections.
- Prevent bacteria from sticking to the walls of the urinary tract.
- Deodorizes urine in persons who are incontinent.
- May help prevent diseases of the eye, including cataracts, macular degeneration and diabetic retinopathy.

Research Insights

Regular use of cranberry juice cocktail reduced the frequency of urinary tract infections and pus in the urine in elderly women who consumed at least 300 mL a day. It prevented urinary tract infections in nursing home residents who drank 4 to 6 ounces of cranberry juice cocktail a day. The proanthocyanidins (the antioxidant pigments) in cranberries prevent bacteria from sticking to the walls of the urinary tract.

Unpublished research has reported that the antioxidants in cranberries and cranberry juice reduced breast cancer tumors, tumor development and reduced the spread of tumors in mice. Cranberry juice also appeared to inhibit the oxidation of LDL "bad" cholesterol.

How It Is Used

Whole berries, sauce, juice or dried.

Growing

Cranberries are not suitable for the home garden; they require wet, acidic soil. Fresh cranberries are most plentiful in the fall, but their byproducts (canned sauce, juice and dried berries) are available year-round.

Harvesting

Harvest in the fall before the first freeze.

Preserving

Fresh cranberries can be frozen for future use or dried in a home dehydrator. Cranberry juice can be made at home; many traditional cookbooks have a recipe for making juice under the section on preserving.

Best Herbal Remedy Forms

Fresh, dried fruits, in commerically prepared cranberry extract capsules, or juice.

Making the Remedy & Dosage

- Standardized **extract** of cranberry solids available commercially in capsule form. Up to 300 to 400 mg of concentrated capsules, twice a day, has been used effectively in some studies.
- **Fresh or frozen cranberries,** 1½ ounces, can be used instead of 3 ounces of cranberry juice used in recipes that provide at least 1½ ounces of fruit per serving. It is not known how effective dried cranberries may be at preventing recurring urinary tract infections, but adding a few tablespoons to your morning cereal may be a tasty way to experiment. Do not substitute berries or capsules for antibiotics if you have an infection; cranberries are helpful in preventing recurring infections.
- **Cranberry juice cocktail** containing at least 33 percent pure juice or made from purchased natural concentrate in the proportion of ⅓ cup juice to ⅔ cup water. Approximately 1,500 grams (about 3 pounds) of fresh cranberries will produce 1 liter of pure juice.
- **Dried** at home or purchased dried, cranberries are similar to raisins and can be used in cooking or as a snack.

Safety & Effectiveness

Cranberries and their juice are considered safe for adults who are not taking other medicines that may affect the urinary tract or kidneys. Urinary tract infections should not be self-treated. If you have symptoms, notify your primary care provider immediately.

When taken orally to prevent urinary tract infections, approximately 3 to 16 ounces of cranberry juice (or its equivalent) each day appears to do the job. Other forms of cranberry have not been studied enough to know their effectiveness. Using cranberry for other therapeutic uses is still under investigation.

Interactions

Drugs. May decrease the effectiveness of drugs called proton pump inhibitors used for excess stomach acid and as anti-ulcer therapy.
Other Herbs. No known interactions.
Foods. No known interactions.
Vitamins or Minerals. No known interactions.

Effects in Laboratory Tests

No known adverse reactions.

Adverse Reactions

- Persons with diabetes should avoid cranberry juice products sweetened with sugar, as they may increase blood sugar levels when used in amounts considered effective. They may use, with caution, cranberry juice cocktail products that have been sweetened with artificial sweeteners.
- Drinking more than 3 liters of cranberry juice may result in diarrhea and GI upset.
- Because of its acidity, cranberry juice may increase the absorption of dietary vitamin B12 in people with atrophic gastritis or hypochlorhydria.

Cranberry
Vaccinium macrocarpon

Who Should Not Use Cranberries

Women who are pregnant or lactating should avoid using in amounts that exceed what might be consumed in foods because there is not enough reliable information regarding excess amounts.

Dandelion

Profile

Common Names: Common dandelion, blowball, dandelion herb, wild endive
Family: Asteraceae/Compositae (daisy and marigold are also in the family)
Genus & Species: *Taraxacum officinale*
Description: Does dandelion need a description? Dandelion is a perennial with a taproot that seems to go on forever. When cut, the stem excretes white latex. The leaves are saw-toothed and the plant usually produces one bright yellow flower followed by a fine tuft that contains the fruits or seeds of the plant.
Historical Use: This poor herb is scorned. It is considered a nuisance, a pest and a weed. But many of us do not realize that dandelion has a rich medicinal history. Chinese and Ayurvedic physicians have used the herb to treat colds, respiratory tract ailments, dental problems, obesity, ulcers and numerous other conditions. It has been linked to the health of the liver, to its use as a diuretic and as a tonic used by Early American colonists. Lydia Pinkham's Vegetable Compound in the 1800s contained dandelion.
Parts to Use: Whole plant, above-ground parts.

What It Does

The FDA believes that dandelion is a weed and has no therapeutic uses. In Germany, the Commission E recognizes dandelion as a diuretic that may reduce bloating in women with PMS, and endorses its roots and leaves for bile stimulation.

What It Might Help Treat

- Gallstones
- Premenstrual syndrome (PMS) and associated fluid retention
- High blood pressure
- Loss of appetite

Research Insights

There is possible anti-tumor activity as demonstrated in animals. The Japanese use dandelion in treating breast cancer. In animals, dandelion has been shown to have an anti-inflammatory activity, and also lowers their blood sugar.

How It Is Used

Fresh, as an infusion, decoction or tincture.

Growing

Anyone with a patch of grass in their yard knows that dandelions will grow just about anywhere, no matter what the conditions are.

Harvesting

When to harvest depends on intended use:
- Leaves are picked in the spring before the plants flower. Picked fresh, leaves may be used in salads.
- Dig roots in the fall or in the spring.
- Flowers are picked for wine-making in the spring; leaves and stems are removed.

Preserving

- Leaves picked in spring may be juiced or dried.
- Roots can be pressed for juice, dried or roasted for a coffee substitute. Dried roots and leaves should be kept in a sealed dark glass container out of direct sunlight.

Dandelion
Taraxacum officinale

Best Herbal Remedy Forms

Tea or decoction, fresh in salads or cooked, and tincture.

Making the Remedy & Dosage

- **Decoction** is made by using 30 grams of dried root (or 60 grams of fresh) to 750 mL of water, simmered and reduced to about 500 mL. Drink up to 3 cups a day.
- **Tinctures,** 1:5. Use 1 to 2 teaspoons of tincture in a small amount of water preferably up to 3 times each day.
- **Tea** made of leaves is a less effective preparation, but is still effective as a digestive stimulant. Use 30 grams of dried (or 25 grams of fresh) dandelion leaves steeped in 1 cup of hot, not boiling, water for 10 minutes, then strained. Take up to 3 cups a day.
- For dandelion root **tea**, use 3 to 8 grams of dried root in 1 cup of hot, not boiling, water. Drink up to 3 times a day.
- **Dried leaves and roots** may be used for any of the above preparations.
- **Juice** made of fresh leaves is given as 1 to 2 teaspoons a day.

Safety & Effectiveness

When taken as a food or medicinally as directed, dandelion is considered safe. Dandelion may be effective for stimulating bile flow, loss of appetite and diuresis. There is insufficient research to conclusively support other uses for the plant.

Interactions

Drugs. Use of dandelion with diuretics and drugs used to control blood sugar may interfere with drug therapy.
Use of dandelion with the drug lithium, may cause lithium toxicity because of sodium loss caused by dandelion.
Dandelion may interfere with drugs used to decrease stomach acid.
Other Herbs. Theoretically, dandelion may have additive effects when taken with other herbs that have diuretic properties.
When used with herbs that lower blood sugar, dandelion may have an additive effect, thus lowering blood sugar even more.
Foods. No known interactions.
Vitamins or Minerals. No known interactions.

Effects In Laboratory Tests

No known adverse effects.

Adverse Reactions

- Low blood sugar in persons with diabetes. Blood sugar levels should be monitored closely.
- Dandelion taken orally can cause increased stomach acid.
- Persons allergic to members of the Asteraceae/Compositae family, including daisies, ragweed, chamomile and marigolds, may be sensitive to dandelion.

Who Should Not Use Dandelion

- People with active gallbladder disease should consult their primary care physician before using dandelion.
- People with bowel or bile duct obstruction should not use dandelion.

Comments

Dandelion is one of the best culinary sources of vitamin A, surpassing that of carrots.

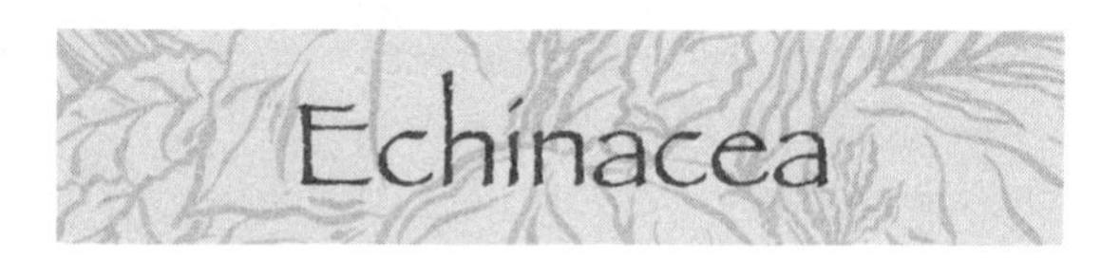

Echinacea

Profile

Common Name: Purple coneflower
Family: Asteraceae/Compositae (marigolds, dandelions and daisies belong to this family)
Genus & Species: *Echinacea angustifolia* and *Echinacea purpurea*
Description: Echinacea is considered an American wildflower. Its purple cone-shaped flower is what gives it the common name "Purple Coneflower," although there is also a white variety of the flower. It is a perennial with a single flower produced on a stem with bristly hairs and slender leaves. Echinacea can grow up to 5 feet tall. Its roots are black.
Historical Use: Echinacea, a native of the Great Plains, was an important medicinal plant for Native Americans of the region. It was used for wounds and bites of all types, for sore gums and teeth and to treat colds and other infectious diseases. It was used by settlers, but was not recognized as an effective remedy until the late 1800s. It was then that pharmacist John Uri Lloyd noticed a patented medicine called "Meyer's Blood Purifier" was being offered by Nebraska physician H. C. F. Meyer. Dr. Meyer claimed it was an "absolute cure" for almost all disorders. It was not introduced in Europe until around 1900. Since the 1930s, echinacea has been widely grown, used and studied, and has become accepted as an herbal medicine by the German Commission E and other European pharmacopoeias.
Parts to Use: Primarily roots, flowers and leaves.

Echinacea
Echinacea purpurea

What It Does

It promotes natural resistance to infections and, when used topically, aids in wound-healing.

What It Might Help Treat

- Treatment of the common cold and flu symptoms.
- May reduce the symptoms and duration of colds when taken at the first sign of symptoms.
- Above-ground parts may provide supportive therapy for lower urinary tract infections and yeast infections.
- May enhance the immune system and rids the body of invading organisms.
- May help the body respond to and fight against cancer.
- As supportive therapy for candida-caused vaginal infections.

Research Insights

When taken internally, root extracts appear to provide supportive therapy for flu-like infections. Extracts of the herb (above-ground part) or combinations of the herb and root, when taken orally, may shorten the duration of the common cold.

Oral extracts of the herb may be effective as supportive therapy for treatment of urinary tract infections. Topical preparations may promote healing of skin wounds and ulcers.

How It Is Used

Fresh juice, tincture, decoction or commercially available preparations.

Growing

Echinacea grows well in almost any condition. It will grow from seed, transplants or root cuttings taken in the fall. The roots require about 4 years to grow large enough to use.

Harvesting

Pick flowers when in full bloom. Fresh juice may be made from leaves. Above-ground parts may be picked and dried, but are thought to be less effective than the root. Dig roots in the fall.

Preserving

Dry the root only.

Best Herbal Remedy Forms

Decoctions, tinctures, dried and powdered roots, capsules and commercial preparations.

Making the Remedy & Dosage

- **Juice** from fresh, pressed leaves, 6 to 9 mL (1 to 2 teaspoons) in divided doses each day. *The German Commission E Monographs* recommend that continuous use of echinacea be limited to 8 weeks, allowing several weeks before resuming use.
- **Tinctures** are available commercially, but may be made at home in a 1:5 proportion. Take 15 to 20 drops in a small amount of water up to 5 times a day.
- **Decoctions** made of 30 grams of dried root to 750 mL of water, reduced by simmering to 500 mL, may be taken in 2-teaspoon doses every 1 to 2 hours during the acute phases of a respiratory infection.
- **Dried root** can be finely ground and used as a dust for skin conditions. In capsule form, 500 to 1000 mg, 3 times a day at the onset of the infection.

Safety & Effectiveness

When used orally and as directed for a limited period of time, echinacea may be safe. Using longer than 8 weeks may depress immunity.

Echinacea may be effective when used at the onset of symptoms for the common cold, urinary tract and kidney infections and for poorly healing skin wounds and infections.

Interactions

Drugs. Echinacea may interfere with the effectiveness of immunosuppressant drugs.
Other Herbs. No known interactions.
Foods. No known interactions.
Vitamins or Minerals. No known interactions.

Effects In Laboratory Tests

No known adverse reactions.

Adverse Reactions

- Persons with a genetic predisposition to allergic conditions and those allergic to members of the Asteraceae/Compositae family including daisies and chrysanthemums should avoid echinacea.
- People with asthma may also react negatively to echinacea because the herb may contain pollens that are similar to environmental and household allergens.

Who Should Not Use Echinacea

- People with progressive systemic diseases, including tuberculosis, multiple sclerosis, collagen disorders and those with immune disorders such as AIDS, HIV infection and autoimmune disorders should be careful when taking echinacea. Although the effect of echinacea is to stimulate healthy cells to destroy microorganisms and cellular debris, theoretically this process may also stimulate the overall immune system.
- Some research suggests its use in pregnancy and lactation may pose no risk for birth defects. However, you should discuss its use with your healthcare provider before using.

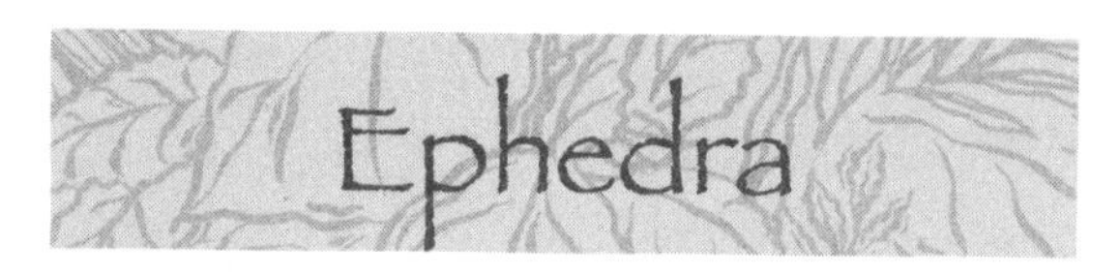

Profile

Common Names: Ma huang, Mormon tea, Yellow astringent, Teamster's tea
Family: Ephedraceae
Genus & Species: *Ephedra sinica, E. vulgaris, E. nevadensis, E. distachya, E. antisypilitica* (Mormon tea)
Description: Ephedra is a dwarf evergreen shrub. The stems and branches are jointed with small scale-like leaves and tiny yellow flowers.
Historical Use: Ephedra has a long history of use for its decongestant and stimulant effects on the respiratory system. Improper use has resulted in serious complications and even death.

Native Americans used an indigenous plant of the same family, *Ephedra antisypilitica*, for many conditions. Mormons were introduced to *E. antisypilitica* in the 1840s and adopted it as a coffee and tea substitute, thus its common name "Mormon tea."
Parts to Use: Stems.

What It Does

Ephedra contains the alkaloid ephedrine, which is responsible for its decongestant and metabolic stimulation properties.

What It Might Help Treat

- Short-term treatment of respiratory diseases.
- Combined with other herbal products as a weight-loss aid.
- In Chinese medicine, ephedra is used for colds, flu, fever, chills, headache, edema, as a diuretic and for joint and bone pain.

Research Insights

Ephedrine, the active constituent of ephedra, dilates the small tubes in the lung that allow for air exchange, thus making breathing easier. Ephedrine increases the metabolic rate and may also suppress the appetite.

How It Is Used

Tea, decoction, tincture or commercially prepared preparations. Voluntary recalls of products with more than 8 mg/dose of ephedra have been called for in the United States and Canada.

Growing

Ephedra grows in climates similar to South Europe and subtropical America.

Harvesting

Collect stems at any time.

Preserving

Drying (the root only).

Best Herbal Remedy Forms

Tea, decoction or tincture.

Making the Remedy & Dosage

- **Decoction,** simmer 30 grams dried herb in 750 mL water and reduce to 500 mL. Take 1 to 3 mL (20 to 60 drops), 3 times a day.
- **Tincture,** 1:4. Take 6 to 8 mL (½ to 1½ teaspoons) in a small amount of water, 3 times a day.
- **Tea,** steep 1 to 4 grams of herb in 150 mL of water for 10 minutes. Strain and drink up to 3 cups a day.

Safety & Effectiveness

When used as directed for less than 7 days, in doses of 8 mg or less and not exceeding 24 mg in a 24-hour period, it may be safe, depending on the health of the person taking it.

When taken for short periods of time, it may be effective for treating upper respiratory tract diseases. The amount usually recommended for these conditions exceeds the safe limit. As a single herb treatment for weight loss, it is considered ineffective.

Interactions

Drugs

- If taken with the antidepressant amitriptyline or drugs to treat migraine headaches, there is a risk of high blood pressure.
- Used with corticosteroids, ephedra may decrease steroids' effectiveness.
- Ephedra may increase blood sugar and may interfere with diabetes drug therapy.
- Used with the cardiac drug digoxin, ephedra may cause arrhythmias.
- Simultaneous use with bronchodilators may increase the stimulatory effects of both drugs.
- Urinary acidifiers increase the excretion of ephedra; urinary alkalinizers reduce excretion.

Other Herbs

- Coffee, cola nut and caffeine-containing herbs may increase the risk of stimulatory adverse effects.
- If taken with foxglove (digitalis), the combination may cause high blood pressure.

Foods. Caffeinated coffee and tea, with ephedra, may increase the stimulatory effects of the herb and beverages.

Vitamins or Minerals. No known interactions.

Effects In Laboratory Tests

Ephedra can result in a urine test positive for the drug ephedrine, a banned substance with the International Olympic Organizing Committee. Ephedra might increase blood glucose level readings. Ephedra may also result in a false positive urine test for amphetamines or methamphetamines.

Adverse reactions

The list of adverse reactions is long. It includes dizziness, anxiety, irritability, insomnia, headache, anorexia tachycardia, arrhythmias, high blood pressure, heart failure and death.

Who Should Not Use Ephedra

- Pregnant or lactating women.
- Children under the age of 6 years.
- People with cardiovascular disease.
- People with diabetes.
- People suffering from anorexia or bulimia.
- Those with genitourinary tract conditions, including BPH, kidney stones and urinary retention.
- People with thyroid disease, myasthenia gravis or essential tremors.
- People suffering from anxiety.

Comments

Variances in the active constituents in over-the-counter products containing ephedra have been observed. This increases the risk of obtaining too little, too much and, in some cases, none of the herb.

Evening Primrose

Profile

Common Names: Evening star, EPO
Family: Onagraceae (the flower fuchsia belongs to this family)
Genus & Species: *Oenothera biennis*
Description: Evening primrose is an annual, or biennial, that is 3 to 5 feet tall with yellow bowl-shaped flowers that open in the evening throughout the summer and fall. Downy pods that contain tiny seeds follow the flowers.
Historical Use: The herb was first used as a food and medicine for Native Americans. The knowledge of the herb was passed on to colonists, who used it as food and as a poultice for wounds. The Shakers made a tea from the seeds to treat digestive upsets and coat sore throats. It was not until the 1980s that evening primrose was noticed as more than a pretty flower and a minor medicinal herb. Then its oil was found to contain an essential fatty acid, gamma-linolenic acid (GLA), which plays many important roles in the body.
Parts to Use: Leaves, stem bark, oil and flowers.

What It Does

Evening primrose oil (EPO), which is the most widely used and researched part of this plant, contains gamma linolenic acid (GLA)—an essential fatty acid which, when broken down in the body, is converted to prostaglandin PGEI. PGEI is one of many prostaglandins that has anti-inflammatory activity in the body, dilutes blood vessels and may prevent abnormal blood clotting.

What It Might Help Treat

- Nerve damage associated with type 1 and 2 diabetes
- Breast pain
- PMS
- Chronic eczema
- Arthritis
- High cholesterol

Research Insights

The strongest case for EPO is for using it to relieve diabetic neuropathy that results in nerve damage in the legs, arms, hands and feet. It is most promising because it does not have the side effects of some prescription drugs.
Women suffering from mastalgia or breast pain appear to experience relief when given EPO.

How It Is Used

The oil contains the most beneficial compounds known at this time. The whole plant can be used for culinary purposes as salad greens or cooked, and undoubtedly provides some nutritional benefit.

Growing

Evening primrose can be grown throughout the United States. It is grown from seed sown in the fall.

Harvesting

Leaves, stems, flowers and immature seed pods may be collected in the summer and used fresh. The seeds are collected when ripe.

Preserving

The evening primrose plant is best used fresh. The oil is best when purchased commercially.

Best Herbal Remedy Forms

Fresh use of the whole plant. As greens, cooked or in salads. Commercially purchased capsules provide the most consistent dose of evening primose oil (EPO).

Making the Remedy & Dosage

- For diabetic neuropathy—8 to 12 **capsules** containing 500 mg of EPO a day with a total of 320 to 480 mg of total GLA.
- For breast pain, 6 to 8 (500-mg) **capsules** of EPO a day.
- For PMS, 4 to 8 (500-mg) **capsules** of EPO a day.
- For rheumatoid arthritis, 1 to 6 (500-mg) **capsules** a day.
- For wounds, apply **leaves** directly.
- **Roots** may be boiled and eaten as a vegetable.

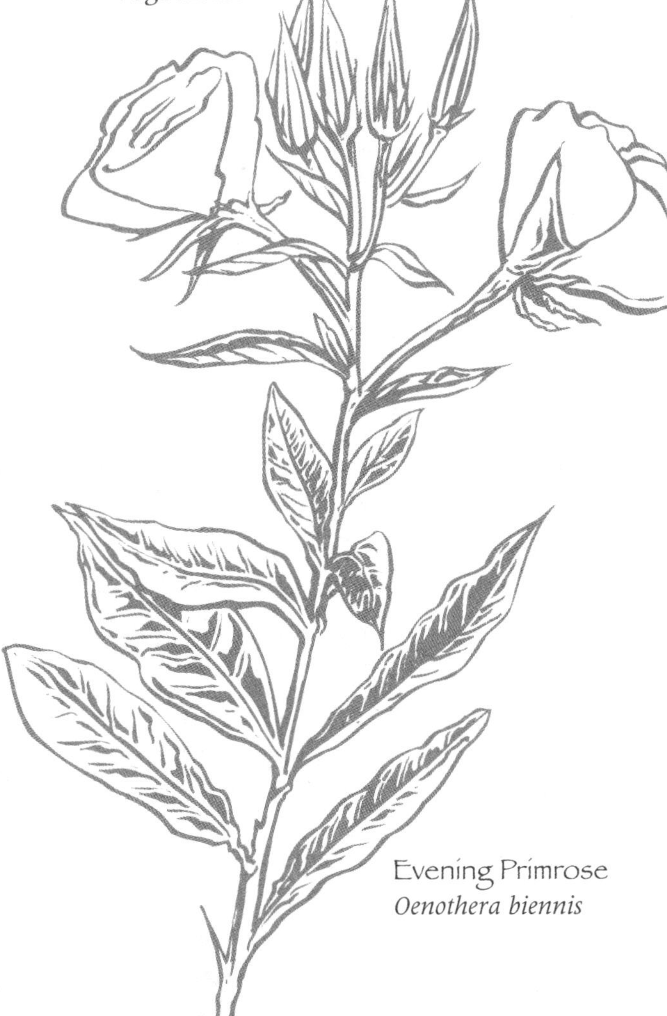
Evening Primrose
Oenothera biennis

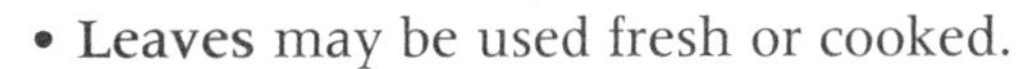

- **Leaves** may be used fresh or cooked.
- **Seeds** have been used as a substitute for poppy seeds in baking.

Safety & Effectiveness

When used as directed, EPO is considered safe and effective for breast pain, possibly for symptoms of rheumatoid arthritis and for use in relieving the symptoms of diabetic neuropathy.

Interactions

Drugs. Interactions with drugs used to treat schizophrenia have been reported in persons taking them along with EPO.
Other Herbs. No known interactions.
Foods. No known interactions.
Vitamins or Minerals. No known interactions.

Effects In Laboratory Tests

No known adverse reactions.

Adverse Reactions

- GI upset in some cases.
- Loose stools when taken in excess.
- Seizures when taken with prescription drugs for schizophrenia.

Who Should Not Use Evening Primrose

- People with seizure disorders, particularly if they are being treated with prescription medications.
- People being treated for schizophrenia.
- Pregnant women should not use EPO as it may increase the risk of some delivery-related complications.
- Women who are lactating might be able to use EPO safely, as the essential fatty acids in EPO are naturally present in significant amounts in breast milk. Consult with your physician before using.

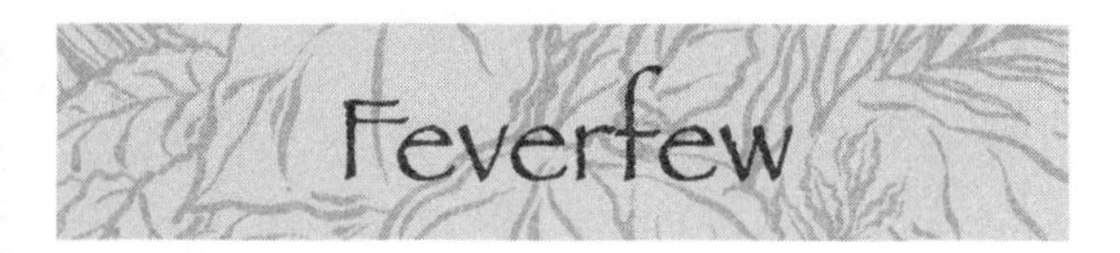

Feverfew

Profile

Common Name: Feverfew
Family: Asteraceae or Compositae. Other members include daisies, dandelions and marigolds.
Genus & Species: *Tanacetum parthenium*
Description: Feverfew is a perennial that grows up to 3 feet tall and will self-seed. Although the daisy-like flowers with yellow centers are pretty, they do not attract bees, and the plant's strong odor may be offensive to some.
Historical Use: Feverfew has been used for migraine headache prevention, fever, non-migraine headaches, digestive upset and menstrual pain.
Parts to Use: Leaves, preferably fresh.

What It Does

Feverfew has been shown to be effective when used as a prophylaxis for migraine headaches. Feverfew may reduce the frequency of migraine headaches considerably. Migraine headaches that do occur appear to have fewer severe symptoms of pain, nausea, vomiting and sensitivity to light and noise.

What It Might Help Treat

- Rheumatoid arthritis
- Non-migraine headaches
- Inflammation
- Intestinal upset that involves the smooth muscles of the stomach

Research Insights

Research methodology has been flawed in a number of the studies conducted on feverfew. It has been shown to be beneficial for preventing migraine headaches in most of the randomized clinical trials, but efficacy has not been established beyond a reasonable doubt. For other uses, effectiveness has not been established.

How It Is Used

As fresh or dried leaves.

Growing

Feverfew is easy to grow and, if left to its own devices, will self-seed and spread, often to unwanted and unlikely places in the garden.

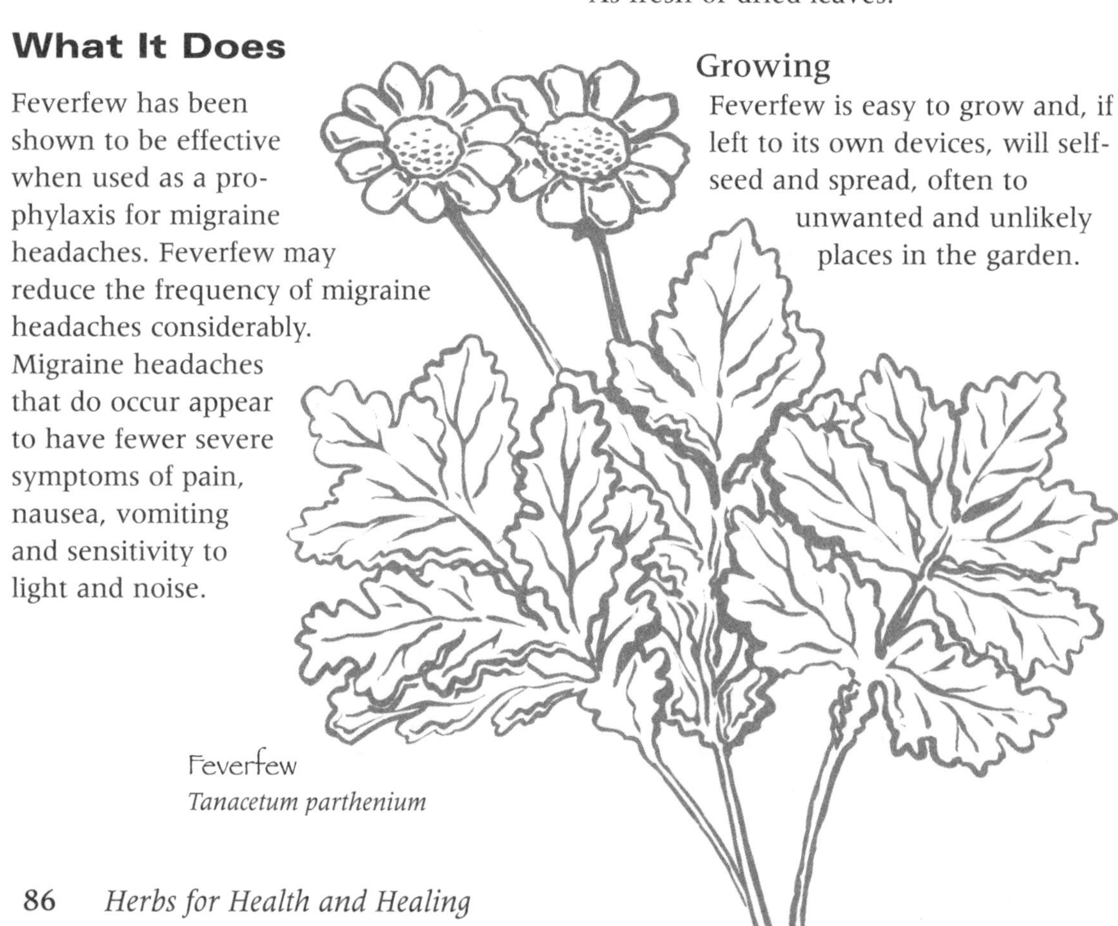

Feverfew
Tanacetum parthenium

The first planting is most successful when made from root cuttings or nursery stock.

Harvesting
When leaves are mature, just before flowering, pick leaves to be used fresh or for drying.

Preserving
May be used fresh or dried.

Best Herbal Remedy Forms
- Fresh leaves
- Tea made from dried herb
- Capsules

Making the Remedy & Dosage
- **Fresh leaf** dosage is 2 to 2½ leaves a day, with or after food.
- **Tea** using ½ to 1 teaspoon of dried herb per cup of hot, not boiling, water.
- **Dried or freeze-dried leaf** is taken at 50 to 125 mg a day, with or after food.

Safety & Effectiveness

When used as recommended and for short term, up to 4 months, feverfew appears to be safe, and for some people, an effective treatment for migraine headaches.

Interactions

Drugs. Because it may affect blood clotting, feverfew might increase the risk of bleeding when used with anticoagulant or antiplatelet drugs. The effectiveness of non-steroidal anti-inflammatory drugs (NSAIDs) may decrease the effect of feverfew.
Other Herbs. Feverfew may inhibit the ability of the blood to clot in laboratory animals. This has not been demonstrated in humans, however. In theory, use of feverfew and herbs that affect blood clotting could increase the risk of bleeding in some people.
Foods. No known interactions.
Vitamins or Minerals. No known interactions. However, persons taking supplemental vitamin E should consult a healthcare provider before taking feverfew.

Effects In Laboratory Tests
No known adverse reactions.

Adverse Reactions
- Feverfew can cause abdominal pain, indigestion, diarrhea, gas, nausea and vomiting.
- The traditional method of using feverfew—chewing fresh leaves—can result in mouth sores, inflamed tongue and mucous membranes, swelling of the lips and occasional loss of taste.
- An allergic reaction is highly likely in individuals sensitive to the Asteraceae/Compositae family, including ragweed, chrysanthemums, marigolds and daisies.

Who Should Not Use Feverfew

- Pregnant women should not use feverfew as it may cause uterine contractions.
- Nursing women should not use feverfew because there is insufficient reliable safety information.
- Children under 2 years of age.

Comments

For children over 2 and adults over 65 years of age, begin with low-dose preparations and increase gradually as needed.

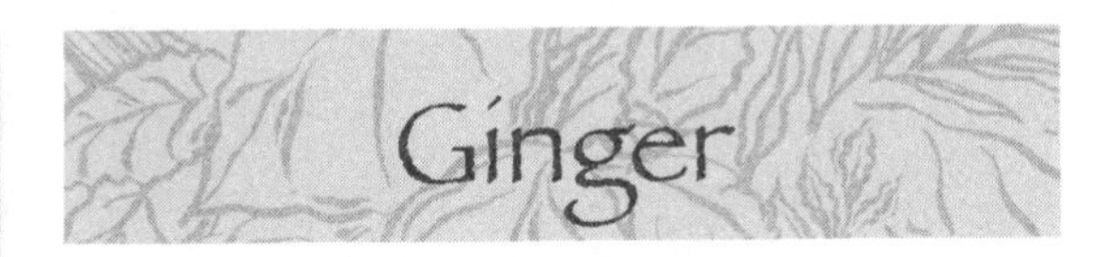

Profile

Common Name: Gingerroot
Family: Zingiberaceae (Other members include turmeric and cardamom.)
Genus & Species: *Zingiber officinale*
Description: Ginger is a tropical perennial that grows from a tuber. The plant itself has thin, pointed leaves and a single large yellow and purple flower.
Historical Use: Ginger has a long history of use documented in ancient Greek, Roman and Sanskrit medical literature. It continues to be an important botanical in Asian medicine, where it has been used for thousands of years to treat GI complaints, arthritis, heart disease and as a "warming" herb. In Germany, it is approved in the *Commission E Monograph* as a component in anti-emetic stomach medicines. In the United States, ginger has been used singularly as a preparation for nausea, flu-like symptoms, GI upset and motion sickness.
Parts to Use: Root or tuber.

What It Does

Ginger appears to provide relief for motion sickness, morning sickness, upset stomach, gas, chemotherapy-induced nausea and loss of appetite. It is used as a flavoring for beverages and foods. Ginger is aromatic and is used for fragrance in soaps and cosmetics.

What It Might Help Treat

It may provide relief in rheumatoid arthritis and osteoarthritis.

Research Insights

Seasickness symptoms may be effectively relieved with ginger preparations. Motion sickness may be lessened when ginger is taken up to 4 hours prior to travel. Some preliminary evidence indicates that ginger may lower blood sugar. Ginger may cause low or high blood pressure. It may help to lower blood cholesterol. Ginger may decrease blood clotting, increasing the risk for bleeding.

How It Is Used

Fresh, dried, teas or tinctures.

Growing

It grows outside in Hawaii, Florida, southern California, New Mexico, Arizona and Texas from young fresh roots that have eyes similar to potatoes. The best place to get ginger to grow is through a nursery. Ginger may also be grown inside in deep pots.

Harvesting

After the plant has grown for about a year, dig the roots, remove some of the tubers and replant the rest.

Preserving

Dry the root only. Because of its moisture content, gingerroot may be difficult to dry thoroughly, so prepared powdered gingerroot may be preferred.

Best Herbal Remedy Forms

Fresh root, commercially prepared extracts or commercially prepared candied ginger.

Making the Remedy & Dosage

- **Decoctions and teas** may be made by adding 1 to 2 slices of fresh gingerroot

to 8 ounces of water and simmering for 10 minutes.
- **Tinctures,** 1:5. Use 1 to 2 teaspoons tincture in water, 3 times a day.
- **Dried,** powdered dose is 0.2 to 1 gram of dried gingerroot taken in capsule form or in a small amount of water up to 3 times daily.

Safety & Effectiveness

When used as recommended, gingerroot is effective for motion sickness, seasickness and to prevent nausea and vomiting.

Interactions

Drugs
- Claims that ginger increases stomach acid mean it might interfere with acid-inhibiting drugs.
- Excessive amounts of ginger may increase clotting time.
- May enhance the effects of barbiturates.
- Ginger may increase or decrease blood pressure and may therefore interfere with blood pressure drugs.
- May interfere with cardiac drugs.
- May interfere with drugs to treat diabetes because of its potential to lower blood sugar.

Other Herbs. Used with herbs that have anticoagulant or antiplatelet activity, ginger may result in increased blood clotting time.

Foods. No known interactions.

Vitamins or Minerals. No known interactions.

Effects In Laboratory Tests

No known interactions; however, due to ginger's potential for lowering blood sugar, it may result in a false-negative reading.

Adverse Reactions

- Skin rash or eruptions in sensitive individuals.
- Large doses may result in central nervous system depression and cardiac arrhythmias.

Who Should Not Use Gingerroot

- Pregnant and lactating women should not take amounts greater than normally in foods. Although ginger has been used in studies on morning sickness, it should be used with caution and under the supervision of a healthcare professional.
- People with gallstones should avoid ginger, as it may worsen symptoms.
- People with diabetes should regularly monitor their blood sugar if taking ginger because of its blood sugar–lowering ability.

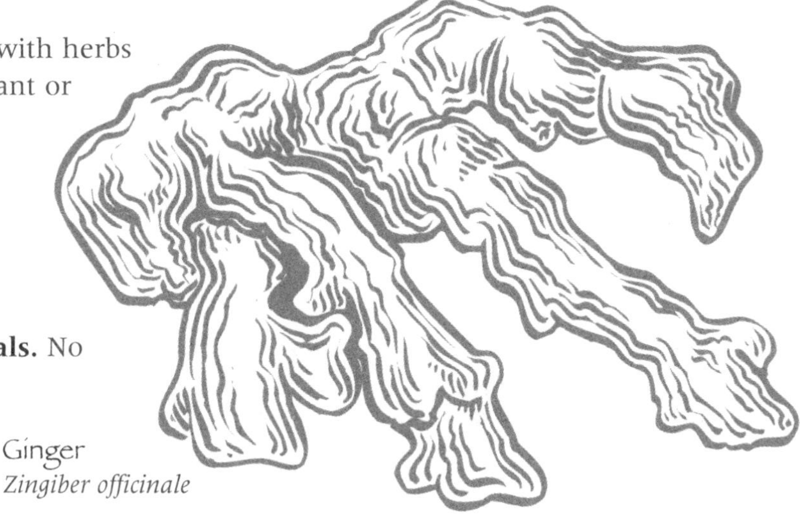

Ginger
Zingiber officinale

Goldenseal

Profile

Common Names: Yellow root, Indian turmeric, Indian dye, jaundice root, eye balm, golden root and more.
Family: Ranunculaceae; other family members are buttercup and peony.
Genus & Species: *Hydrastis canadensis*
Description: Goldenseal is a perennial plant with yellow rhizome and roots. Its leaves are palm-shaped and deeply grooved. Its flowers are tiny in clusters, with green-white stamens, followed by a red fruit.
Historical Use: Native Americans in the northeastern United States used the juice of the goldenseal as a dye. The herb was used medicinally as an eyewash, for skin wounds, sore throat, GI complaints and for recovery after childbirth. Cherokee Indians combined goldenseal with bear fat to make an insect repellant. In the 1800s, it was found to be beneficial as an antiseptic, for hemorrhoids, pinkeye, boils, wounds, colds and women's problems associated with menstruation and the reproductive tract. Goldenseal has been collected in the wild to the point of near-extinction.
Parts to Use: Rhizomes.

What It Does

It may be beneficial in treating diarrhea resulting from Escherichia coli, amoebic dysentery and cholera. Goldenseal is an antiseptic and also an anti-inflammatory agent when used topically.

What It Might Help Treat

Possible treatment for cancer and/or complement to cancer therapy.

Research Insights

May be beneficial in treating diarrhea associated with amoebic dysentery and Giardia.

How It Is Used

Dried in capsule form, tea, liquid extract or tincture.

Growing

Goldenseal is difficult to grow. It may be raised from seeds and plants. It takes 5 years for the roots to become mature enough for use.

Harvesting

Harvest the rhizomes in the fall of the fifth year.

Preserving

Clean the roots, dry in well-ventilated area until brittle.

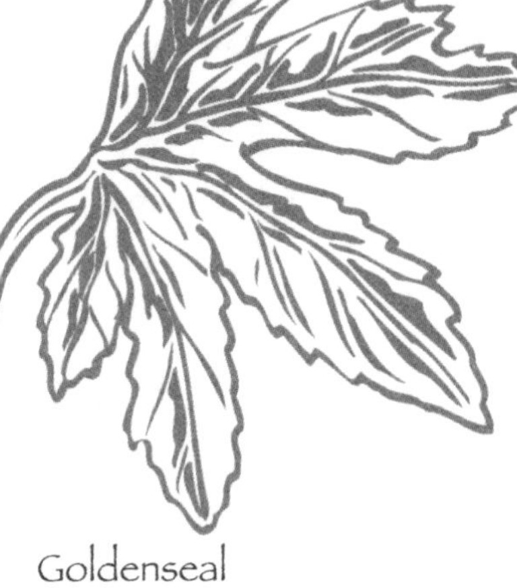

Goldenseal
Hydrastis canadensis

Best Herbal Remedy Forms

Tea, powder or capsule.

Making the Remedy & Dosage

- Make a **dried powder** by thoroughly drying the root and pulverizing it, preferably with a mortar and pestle. Store the powder in an airtight, opaque glass container. Take ½ to 1 gram, divided into 3 doses.
- **Teas** may be prepared using ½ to 1 gram of dried root to 150 mL of boiling water, steeped for 5 minutes and strained.
- **Tincture,** 1:10. Take 40 to 80 drops (2 to 4 mL) in a small amount of water, 3 times daily.
- **Capsules** containing 500 to 600 mg of powdered root, up to 4 times a day.

Safety & Effectiveness

Goldenseal is safe when used as recommended for a period not exceeding 1 week. Contrary to past belief, goldenseal does not mask the presence of illegal drugs during urinalysis.

Interactions

Drugs.

- May interfere with acid-inhibiting drugs (antacids).
- May interfere with blood pressure medications and control.
- May increase sleep time when used with barbiturates.
- May inhibit anticoagulant effects of heparin.
- May interfere with drugs that are bound to protein, such as phenylbutazone.
- May cause additive effects of sedative drugs.

Other Herbs. May enhance therapeutic properties of sedative herbs.
Foods. No interactions have been reported.
Vitamins or Minerals. May decrease B-vitamin absorption.

Effects In Laboratory Tests

May increase bilirubin levels.

Adverse Reactions

- Prolonged use can cause GI disorders, constipation, hallucinations and occasionally delirium.
- Overdose causes nausea, vomiting, nervousness, depression, irregular heart rate, low blood pressure, seizures, paralysis and even death.

Who Should Not Use Goldenseal

- People with diagnosed heart disease should not use without consulting a healthcare practitioner.
- People with infectious or inflammatory GI conditions.
- People with elevated bilirubin and newborn infants.
- People with high blood pressure.

Comments

Because of the high cost of raising goldenseal and its scarcity in the wild, there is a long-standing problem with adulteration and contamination. It has been combined with bloodroot which, when dried, has the same yellow color. Bloodroot is a powerful laxative and has numerous side effects. If you have purchased goldenseal and you begin having symptoms of vomiting, diarrhea, dizziness or intense thirst, stop taking it immediately.

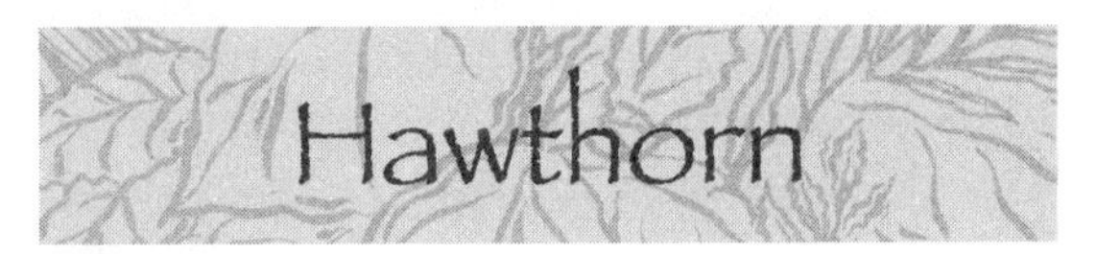

Hawthorn

Profile

Common Names: Hawthorne, May blossom and May flower
Family: Rosaceae. Other family members include rose, peach, almond, apple and strawberry.
Genus & Species: *Crataegus oxyacantha*
Description: Hawthorn is a small tree that loses its leaves in the fall. Its wood is very hard. It possesses sharp thorns and, when it blooms, it has clusters of white, unpleasantly aromatic flowers, followed by bright red fruits that look like small apples.
Historical Use: Hawthorn is believed to have been used in Neolithic times, possibly as food. It has a long history of use. In Greek and Roman times, hawthorn was rich in symbolism linked to fertility, hope and marriage. This changed when Christianity arrived and Christ's crown of thorns was supposedly made of hawthorn, thus making it a symbol of bad luck. As time passed, hawthorn became known as a medicinal herb, primarily for congestive heart failure, angina, high blood pressure and cardiac arrhythmias.
Parts to Use: Flowers, leaves and fruits.

What It Does

Hawthorn is believed to open the coronary arteries and dilate blood vessels throughout the body. It may be effective in treating congestive heart failure (CHF). Leaf and flower extracts have been shown to improve blood ejected during ventricular contractions and exercise tolerance, and to reduce symptoms of breathlessness, fatigue and/or heart palpitations. The greatest benefit is usually seen after 6 to 8 weeks of therapy.

What It Might Help Treat

- High cholesterol.
- Angina.
- Bacterial infections, when applied topically. Hawthorn leaf may be used as a poultice for boils, sores and ulcers.
- Hawthorn fruit can be prepared as a wash or compress for sores, itching and frostbite.

Research Insights

Hawthorn leaf and flowers may be used in combination with conventional cardiovascular medications to help relieve some side effects, such as nausea and indigestion. May improve cardiac insufficiency by promoting vasodilation, coronary blood flow and increasing heart rate and the heart's ability to contract. May act as a sedative and antispasmodic. Hawthorn is an excellent source of antioxidant flavonoids.

How It Is Used

Dried leaves and flowers.

Growing

Hawthorn is well adapted to many conditions in North America and may be easily grown.

Harvesting

Flowering sprigs are collected in the spring. Fruits are gathered when ripe.

Preserving

Flowers and leaves are dried. Dry the root only. Fruits may be used raw, cooked or dried whole.

Best Herbal Remedy Forms

Infusions, decoctions, tinctures and tablets or capsules.

Making the Remedy & Dosage

- **Decoctions** can be made with 30 grams dried (or 60 grams fresh) flowers and leaves to 500 mL of water, simmered for 15 minutes. Take ½ cup (120 mL) up to twice a day.
- **Tinctures**, 1:5. Take 5 mL (20 drops), or 1 teaspoon, in the morning and at bedtime in a small amount of water.
- **Tea** can be made using 2 teaspoons of crushed leaves or fruits to 1 cup of hot, not boiling, water steeped for 20 minutes. Take 2 cups a day.
- **Dried herb** may be used in any of the above preparations.
- **Poultice,** made with enough herb to cover the wound and chopped in a food processor or boiled in a small amount of water for 5 minutes, then applied.

Safety & Effectiveness

Hawthorn is believed to be safe when used short term and in recommended doses. Hawthorn leaf and flower is believed to be effective for some cardiac irregularities when used as a purchased standardized extract.

Interactions

Drugs.

- May cause additive effects to medications used as vasodilators.
- May interfere with conventional drug therapy for CHF, high blood pressure, angina and irregular heart rhythms.

Other Herbs.

- Hawthorn is contraindicated when other cardiac glycoside-containing herbs are being used.
- Use caution when taking other herbs that may affect the heart, including Panax ginseng, parsley, scotch broom flower, ginger and fenugreek, to name a few.

Foods. No known interactions.

Vitamins or Minerals. No known interactions.

Effects in Laboratory Tests

No known adverse reactions.

Adverse Reactions

- Hawthorn is generally well-tolerated with the only side effects reported being mild GI upset, dizziness and headaches in a small percent of those in clinical trials.
- Using hawthorn with conventional cardiovascular drug therapies may interfere with the treatment of heart disease.

Who Should Not Use Hawthorn

- Pregnant women, because of potential uterine-stimulating activity.
- Lactating women, because there is insufficient information about its safety.
- Hawthorn should not be used for acute or chronic heart conditions without the advice of a healthcare professional.

Comments

People with heart disease should use hawthorn only after consulting with their healthcare provider.

Hawthorn
Crataegus oxyacantha

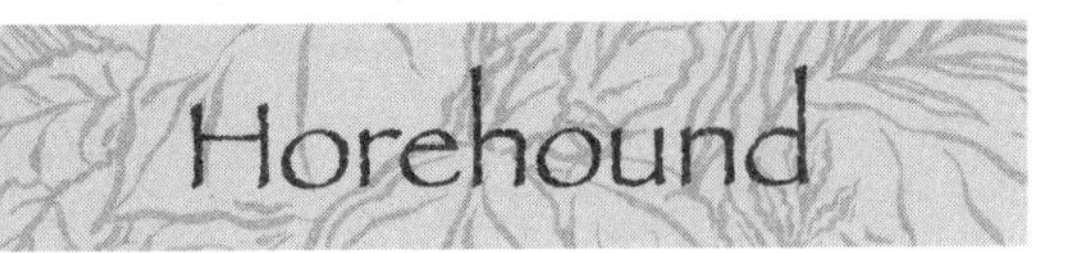

Profile

Common Names: Hoarhound, white horehound
Family: Labiatae/Lamiaceae. Horehound is a member of the mint family.
Genus & Species: *Marrubium vulgare*
Description: Horehound is an aromatic perennial that is covered with soft hairs, giving it a downy or woolly appearance. The stems are square with rounded, wrinkled and deeply veined leaves and white, hairy flowers at the leaf stalk junction. The plant reaches about 18 inches in height.
Historical Use: Horehound was used first by the Egyptians as a cough remedy and expectorant. In colonial America, horehound was used to treat respiratory problems, including tuberculosis. Horehound is one of the five bitter herbs traditionally eaten at the feast of Passover.
Parts to Use: Whole plant.

What It Does

Horehound acts as a cough suppressant, an expectorant in cough syrups and lozenges, and a flavoring in food manufacturing.

What It Might Help Treat

- Loss of appetite.
- Bloating and gas.

Research Insights

Horehound might have weak antioxidant properties, may stimulate bile secretions and may decrease GI spasms. It also may play a role in regulating some types of irregular heartbeat (however, excess may cause an irregular heartbeat).

How It Is Used

As a tea, liquid extract, tincture or pressed juice.

Growing

Horehound is a perennial and, much like its other
family members, grows and spreads quite easily. It needs little water and tolerates poor soil.

Harvesting

Horehound does not bloom until it is 2 years old, but the leaves of the plant may be harvested the first year. Subsequently, the plant is harvested when flowering.

Preserving

Dry leaves and flower tops.

Best Herbal Remedy Forms

Tea, commercially prepared lozenges, juice pressed from leaves, tincture or liquid extract.

Making the Remedy & Dosage

- **Extract,** 1:1. Take 1/4 to 3/4 teaspoon in a small amount of water, 3 times daily.
- **Tinctures,** 1:10. Take 1/2 teaspoon in a small amount of water, 3 times a day.
- **Tea** may be made by steeping 1 to 2 grams dried above-ground parts in 150 mL hot, not boiling, water for 5 to 10 minutes, and strain. Drink 1 cup before

meals as a bile stimulant, or up to 3 cups between meals as an expectorant.
- **Dried herb** may be used for any of the above preparations.
- **Fresh** pressed juice from the leaves and stems, 30 to 60 mL a day. Use a food processor or juicer to pulverize the plant; strain into a clean airtight glass jar. Large quantities of herb are needed for preparing juices.

Safety & Effectiveness

There are no reported, reliable clinical studies that support the suggested medicinal properties of horehound.

Interactions

Drugs. No known interactions or adverse reactions.
Other Herbs. No known interactions or adverse reactions.
Foods. No known interactions or adverse reactions.
Vitamins or Minerals. No known interactions or adverse reactions.

Effects In Laboratory Tests

No known interactions or adverse reactions.

Adverse Reactions

- There appear to be no reports of adverse effects from horehound; however, large doses may cause nausea and vomiting.
- Excessive doses may cause irregular heartbeat.
- Skin contact with the juice may cause allergic reactions in some people.

Who Should Not Use Horehound

- Pregnant women should avoid using in medicinal doses, but may use as a flavoring component in food. It has not been proven safe as a medicinal during pregnancy and lactation.
- Do not give to children under 2 years.

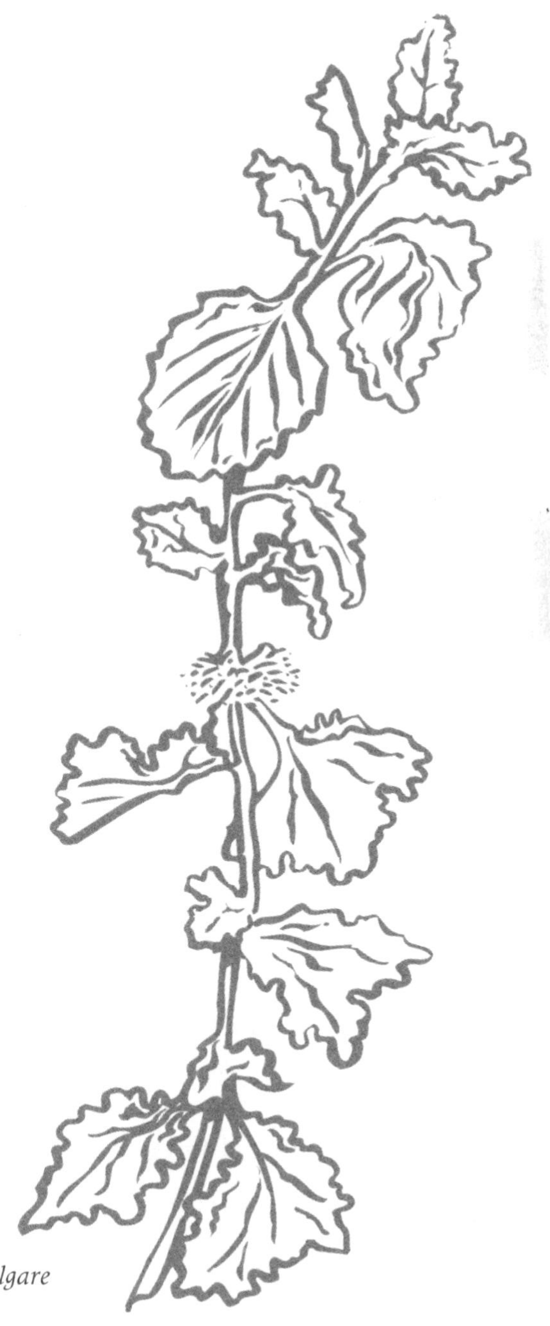

Horehound
Marrubium vulgare

Horse Chestnut Seed

Profile

Common Names: Buckeye, chestnut
Family: Hippocastanaceae
Genus & species: *Aesculus hippocastanum*
Description: Horse chestnut seed comes from a deciduous tree that grows up to 75 feet tall. The ancients who named it believed the large seeds looked like a horse's eyes. The common name buckeye, arose from the seeds' resemblance to the eyes of stags.
Historical Use: All parts of the horse chestnut tree are considered poisonous. Native Americans understood how to detoxify the seeds and used them for food. Native Americans in California used fresh seeds to poison fish in lakes to make them easy to catch. In the late 1890s, its value as an extract for treating hemorrhoids brought it to the forefront for treating vascular ailments.
Parts to Use: Extract of seeds and topical preparations, both made commercially. Because of the toxicity of the plant, home preparations are not recommended.

What It Does

Use horse chestnut seeds for symptomatic treatment of chronic venous insufficiency (CVS), such as varicose veins. It is also used for relieving pain, tiredness, tension, swelling, itching and edema in the legs.

What It Might Help Treat

- Arthritis.
- Hemorrhoids, which are varicosities in the anal area.

Research Insights

Horse chestnut, as an adjunct to compression stockings, reduces lower-leg edema in patients with CVS. It strengthens veins, resulting in decreased leaking from veins—a precursor to varicose veins.

How It Is Used

As a commercially prepared extract.

Growing

Horse chestnut is a lovely shade tree that grows well in many parts of the United States. Because of its size, it is not a candidate for most home gardens. More important, because of its toxic potential if not used appropriately, harvesting, preserving and preparations will not be discussed here.

Best Herbal Remedy Forms

To ensure that you have the correct product and that it contains the recommended active ingredients, it is better to purchase horse extract.

Making the Remedy & Dosage

Horse chestnut seed must be commercially detoxified before being manufactured into a supplement to be taken internally. Do not take any part of the fresh plant internally as ingestion may result in poisoning.

Safety & Effectiveness

Horse chestnut seed is considered safe when used orally as the standardized extract product. European preparations of horse chestnut extracts have removed the primary poison, called esculin, and are generally considered safe. Horse chestnut seed preparations are considered effective in reducing the pain, swelling and tenderness in legs with varicose veins.

Interactions

Drugs. Horse chestnut seeds can have hypoglycemic effects, so persons with diabetes should monitor their blood sugar closely. Horse chestnut seed can have additive and adverse effects with drugs that thin the blood.
Other Herbs. Simultaneous use of horse chestnut seed with herbs that have coumarin ingredients or which affect the ability of blood to clot, may increase the risk of bleeding in some people.
Foods. No known interactions or adverse reactions.
Vitamins or Minerals. No known interactions or adverse reactions.

Effects In Laboratory Tests

No known interactions or adverse reactions.

Adverse Reactions

Horse chestnut seed, when taken orally, can cause stomach upset and possible kidney damage. Symptoms of toxicity include muscle twitching, weakness, loss of coordination, dilated pupils, vomiting, diarrhea, depression, paralysis and unconsciousness.

Who Should Not Use Horse Chestnut

Pregnant or lactating women should not use horse chestnut. Topical applications may be safe for use on varicose veins during pregnancy and lactation. Before using even topical doses, check with your physician.

Comments

People considering using horse chestnut should consult with their healthcare provider. If symptoms are not relieved within the time frame suggested on the label (3 to 6 weeks), horse chestnut may not be the most effective treatment option for you.

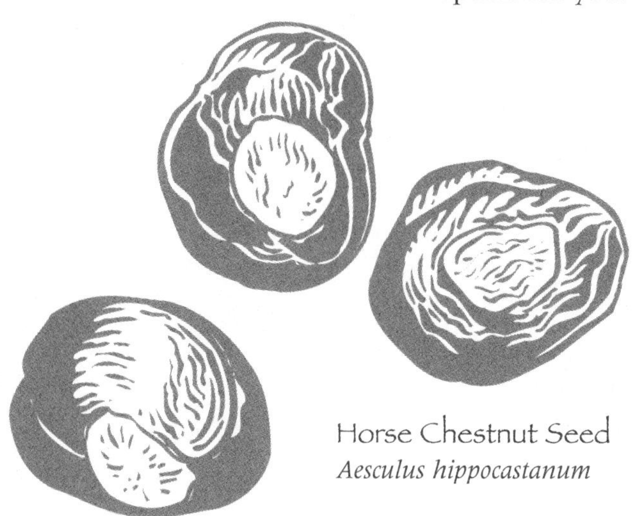

Horse Chestnut Seed
Aesculus hippocastanum

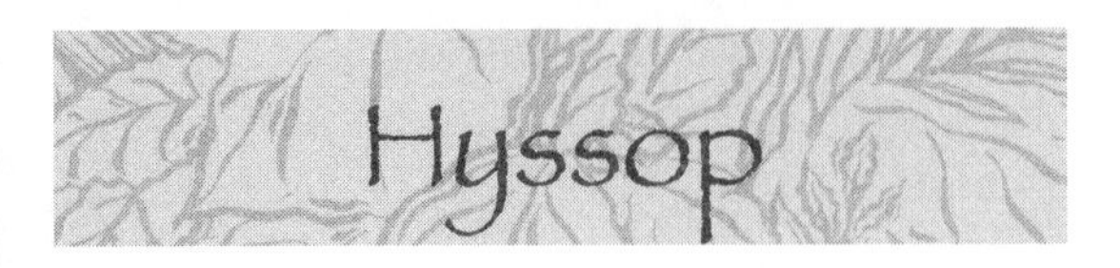

Profile

Common Names: No other name, but many other plants also are called hyssop.
Family: Labiatae/Lamiaceae. Hyssop is also a member of the mint family.
Genus & Species: *Hyssopus officinalis*
Description: Hyssop is a semi-evergreen shrub with small, lance-shaped leaves. It has the characteristic square stems of the mint family, and it produces dense spikes of blue or violet flowers in late summer.
Historical Use: Hyssop has a long history that dates back thousands of years. It is referred to quite often in the Bible, with the most well known reference in the Book of Psalms (51:9) where David proclaimed, "Purge me with hyssop and I shall be clean." Hyssop has been used for respiratory ailments, as an aromatic nasal and chest decongestant and as a poultice for wounds. During the 17th century in Europe, it was used as an air freshener to mask body odor, as people seldom bathed, and to mask the odors of livestock that often shared human living quarters.
Parts to Use: Whole plant, leaves, flowers and oil.

What It Does

Hyssop may be a reasonably effective treatment for respiratory complaints. It is antiviral, especially toward the herpes simplex virus, which causes genital herpes and cold sores. Hyssop is antibacterial. The oil and extract are used as flavorings in foods. The oil is also used as a fragrance in soaps and cosmetics.

What It Might Help Treat

Hyssop has been studied for its use in treating AIDS, but data is inconclusive and cannot be considered a treatment at this time.

Research Insights

Antiviral activity against herpes simplex and HIV in laboratory tests (no human testing).

How It Is Used

As a compress for herpes sores, as an infusion, tincture or commercial preparation.

Growing

Like other members of the mint family, hyssop is relatively easy to grow, is hardy and attractive. If you want bees to visit your garden, make sure to include hyssop.

Harvesting

Leaves may be picked at any time. If the flowers are not going to be used, cut the plant back severely (to about 4 inches) just before it blooms.

Preserving

Drying is the preferred method. The dried herb should be stored in opaque, airtight containers. See standard instructions for leaves.

Caution

Several North American plants are referred to as hyssop, but they should not be taken internally. Purchase hyssop that is clearly labeled *Hyssopus officinalis*.

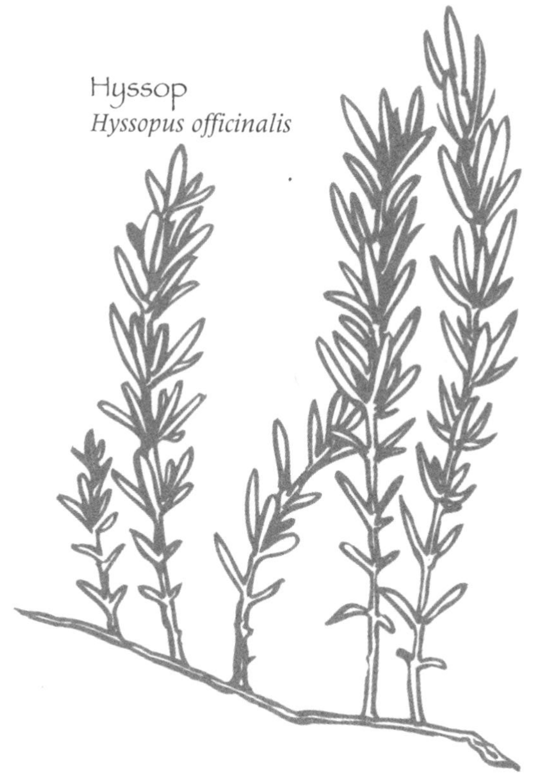

Best Herbal Remedy Forms
Poultices, infusions or tinctures.

Making the Remedy & Dosage
- **Tinctures**, 1:5. Take 1 teaspoon in a small amount of water, up to 3 times a day.
- **Tea** is made by steeping 2 teaspoons of the herb in 1 cup of hot, not boiling, water for 10 minutes. Drink up to 3 cups a day. Because of its bitter camphor-like flavor, it may need to be sweetened with honey.
- **Compresses** can be made by using 1 ounce of dried herb in 1 pint of boiling water. Steep for 15 minutes and cool. Using a clean cloth soaked in the mixture, apply it to cold sores and genital sores as needed.
- **Dried** is the preferred way of using the herb. The whole herb may be dried.

Safety & Effectiveness
If used as directed and in amounts normally consumed or as food, hyssop is considered relatively safe. Hyssop is thought to be reasonably effective as a cough suppressant and expectorant when used as directed. There is not enough reliable, definitive information regarding its use for other conditions at this time.

Interactions
Drugs. There are currently no known reported drug interactions with hyssop.
Other Herbs. There are no known reported interactions or adverse reactions.
Foods. There are no known reported interactions or adverse reactions.
Vitamins or Minerals. There are no known reported interactions or adverse reactions.

Effects In Laboratory Tests
There are no known reported interactions or adverse reactions.

Adverse Reactions
Hyssop's essential oil has been shown to cause seizures in laboratory rats that have been injected with it.

Who Should Not Use Hyssop
- Pregnant women should avoid hyssop in quantities that exceed what might be eaten in food. Historically, hyssop has been used to promote menstruation and abortion, so theoretically, it may be harmful.
- Avoid using during lactation, as sufficient reliable information is not known about its effects on nursing infants.

Lavender

Profile

Common Names: True lavender, spike lavender, lavandin, French lavender, English lavender
Family: Labiatae/Lamiaceae. Lavender is also a member of the mint family.
Genus & Species: *Lavandula angustifolia, Lavandula dentata, Lavandula officinalis and Lavandula spica* are those known for their medicinal value among the 28 or more different species of lavender.
Description: Lavenders are shrubby evergreen plants that may reach up to 3 feet tall. The leaves and flowers span a wide range of shapes and colors. Flowers range from blue to violet and the stem and leaves may be deep bluish gray to green to brown.
Historical Use: Lavender is usually thought of as an aromatic herb used to freshen the air. Its name originated in ancient Rome from the Latin "lavare," which means to wash. Lavender has a long history of use as a digestion and sleep aid, an anti-depressant and for anxiousness and restlessness. It is an important Ayurvedic herb used for treating digestive dysfunctions and depressive states. Lavender infusions and tinctures were used until World War I as a disinfectant for wounds. Lavender oil is considered the premier oil for numerous ailments.
Parts to Use: Flowers, flower spikes and essential oil (commercially prepared).

What It Does

As an aromatic herb, its oil benefits those who suffer from insomnia, anxiety and pain. Internally, lavender has been shown to help with digestion by soothing the smooth muscles of the digestive tract; it is also helpful for bloating and gas.

It is approved for use by the German Commission E for restlessness, nervous stomach, intestines and bloating. Lavender is licensed as a standard medicinal tea for sleep disorders and nervous stomach in Germany. Lavender oil may help to repel insects.

What It Might Help Treat

- Menstrual cramps.
- A compound in lavender, perillyl alcohol, is being studied for its chemo protective and chemotherapeutic value in advanced breast, ovarian and prostate cancers.

Research Insights

Topically, when used in combination with other essential oils, for alopecia areata. Some studies have shown that lavender oil, in combination with essential oils from thyme, rosemary and cedarwood, may improve hair growth. Lavender is effective when used as aromatherapy for insomnia.

How It Is Used

As an infusion, tea, tincture, oil, in baths or in pillows.

Growing

Lavender is native to the Mediterranean, but has been cultivated throughout the world. *Lavandula angustifolia* is considered the best species to grow for medicinal purposes and is among the hardiest of the lavenders.

Harvesting

Pick flowers as they begin to open.

Lavender
Lavandula officinalis

Preserving

If not using fresh, dry lavender.

Best Herbal Remedy Forms

Fresh for teas, but may also be used for jams, jellies, in salads and flavoring of various foods.

Making the Remedy & Dosage

- **Tinctures**, 1:5. Take 1 teaspoon in a small amount of water internally, up to 3 times a day. Tinctures may also be applied to wounds and burns.
- **Tea** may be made using 1 to 3 teaspoons of lavender flowers steeped in 1 cup of hot, not boiling, water for 10 minutes, then strained. Drink up to 3 cups a day.
- **Dried lavender** may be powdered and placed in a cloth bag inside a pillowcase as a sleep aid.
- **Compresses** of lavender may be made with the lavender tea or infusion and applied to a minor wound or burn with a clean cloth.
- **Aromatherapy** uses include:
  - A relaxing bath: Put 1 cup of flowers in a cloth bag and hang it under running water. Add infusions, tinctures or oils to bath water.
  - Apply a few drops of the essential oil to the skin or add to commercial massage oil (10 drops of oil per ounce of lotion).

Safety & Effectiveness

Lavender is considered safe when taken in amounts usually found in foods and beverages, and when used orally and/or topically as recommended.

Lavender is generally effective for treatment of insomnia, anxiety and digestive upsets, including gas and bloating. However, much of the data is anecdotal regarding its benefits when used orally.

Interactions

Drugs

- Lavender may increase the effects of barbiturates.
- Lavender may enhance the therapeutic and adverse effects of CNS depressants.
- Lavender may increase the effects of drugs that affect the enzymes that control cholesterol synthesis. Theoretically, lavender may decrease cholesterol, especially if used in combination with these drugs.

Other Herbs. The use of lavender, in combination with other sedative and/or herbs used for gas, may be beneficial.
Foods. There are no known reported interactions or adverse reactions.
Vitamins or Minerals. There are no known reported interactions or adverse reactions.

Effects in Laboratory Tests

There are no known reported interactions or adverse reactions.

Adverse Reactions

May cause allergic skin reactions when used topically.

Who Should Not Use Lavender

Lavender should not be used internally during pregnancy and lactation, because there is insufficient information regarding its effects on a fetus or nursing child.

Comments

Lavender oil may be toxic, especially for children and the elderly, if taken in amounts greater than one or two drops.

Lemon Balm

Profile

Common Names: Bee balm, balm, Melissa
Family: Labiatae/Lamiaceae. Lemon Balm is also a member of the mint family.
Genus & Species: *Melissa officinalis*
Description: Lemon balm is a low-growing, 1- to 2-foot tall, perennial with a distinct lemon scent. Typical of this family, it grows on a square stem with oval-shaped leaves. In the summer, it bears small, pale yellow flower clusters.
Historical Use: Lemon balm has been cultivated and used medicinally for more than 2,000 years. It was originally cultivated to attract bees, thus the name Melissa, which in Greek means "bee." In ancient Greek and Roman times, lemon balm was steeped in wine and used topically for wounds and bites, and used internally for a number of ailments. It is used in combination with other herbal preparations as a sedative. Lemon balm is recognized by the German Commission E as a treatment for nervous sleep disorders and GI disturbances. It is also on the GRAS (generally recommended as safe) list in the United States.
Parts to Use: Leaves.

What It Does

Lemon balm contains significant antioxidant and immune-enhancing components, as demonstrated in laboratory animals. Used as a sedative, in combination with other herbal sedatives, such as valerian. The extract reduces the duration and severity of genital and oral herpes symptoms.

What It Might Help Treat

- Based on its historical use, lemon balm has sedative, antibacterial and antiviral activities.
- It may be useful in treatment of bloating, gas and spasms of the GI tract.

Research Insights

No significant clinical human studies have been published in English; however, data from German research support its use with other herbal sedatives. Some animal studies have demonstrated its effect on the activity of thyroid-stimulating hormone, which suggests it may be useful in treating Graves' disease and an overactive thyroid (hyperthyroidism).

How It Is Used

Internally or externally, as a tea or infusion and tincture. Standardized topical and tincture preparations are available commercially.

Growing

As with other members of the Labiatae/Lamiaceae family, bee balm is relatively easy to grow and adapts to most climates. It prefers partial shade and a well-drained neutral soil. It may be grown from seeds, nursery stock or root divisions.

Harvesting

Harvest the leaves before the plant flowers, cutting back the plant to a height of 2 to 3 inches above the ground.

Preserving

Leaves must be dried quickly, or they will turn brown. After drying, grind the leaves to a powder and store them in a tightly sealed dark glass container.

Best Herbal Remedy Forms

As tea, dried in capsule form, or commercially prepared creams.

Making the Remedy & Dosage

- **Tinctures,** 1:5. Take ½ to 1½ teaspoons, 3 times a day.
- **Tea** can be made using 2 teaspoons of leaf steeped in 1 cup of hot, not boiling, water for 10 minutes, then strained. Up to 3 cups a day is considered safe.
- **Dried herb** may be taken in capsule form in doses of 1½ to 4½ grams a day.
- **Compresses** can be made using 2 teaspoons of leaves boiled in 1 cup of water for 10 minutes, then cooled and applied with a clean cloth to wounds or herpes sores.
- **Fresh leaves** may be crushed and applied directly to minor cuts.
- Creams and topical **extracts** sold commercially should be applied as directed. Creams should contain 1 percent of a standardized 70:1 extract, as stated on the label.

Safety & Effectiveness

Lemon balm is considered safe when taken in amounts commonly found in foods, or when used as recommended orally and topically as a medicinal herb. Using in combination with other sedative herbs or herbs that treat excess gas and bloating can be beneficial.

Interactions

Caution should be observed when using lemon balm as an herbal medicinal.

Drugs. May interfere with thyroid hormone replacement. May have additive side effects when used with barbiturates or other drugs with sedative properties.

Other Herbs. Use of lemon balm with herbs that have sedative properties might enhance therapeutic and adverse effects of any/all herbs in the preparation.
Foods. There are no known reported interactions or adverse reactions.
Vitamins or Minerals. There are no known reported interactions or adverse reactions.

Effects in Laboratory Tests

There are no known reported interactions or adverse reactions.

Adverse Reactions

Skin hypersensitivity has been reported when lemon balm has been used topically.

Who Should Not Use Lemon Balm

- People who are being treated for hypothyroid conditions, as lemon balm may interfere with drug therapy.
- Women should not use lemon balm as a medicinal herbal during pregnancy and lactation because there is insufficient information regarding its safety.

Lemon Balm
Melissa officinalis

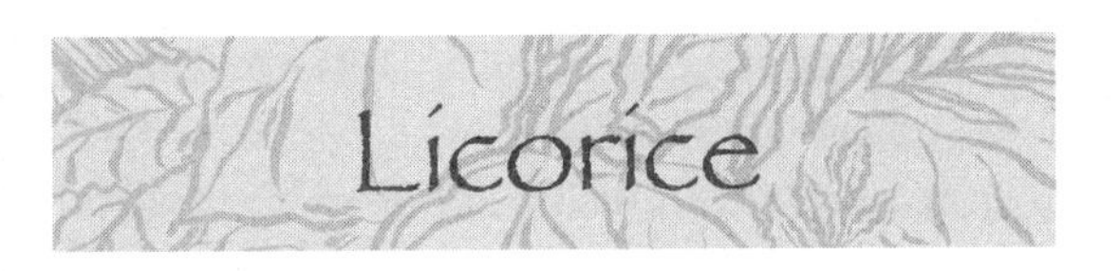

Licorice

Profile

Common Name: Licorice root
Family: Leguminosae. Beans, peas and other legumes belong to this family.
Genus & Species: *Glycyrrhiza glabra*
Description: Licorice is a perennial with very long roots that send out shoots and rhizomes, creating a massive underground network. Its leaves are small; pale blue to violet pea-like flowers in midsummer give rise to oblong pods with kidney-shaped seeds.
Historical Use: Use of licorice as a medicinal has been documented as far back as 3000 B.C.E. It is steeped in history in Chinese and Ayurvedic medicine and extolled for its effectiveness in treating a variety of complaints related to the respiratory and GI tracts. Licorice was a component of Lydia E. Pinkham's Vegetable Compound, which was used in the 1800s for treating "female hysteria" or menstrual and menopausal complaints. Licorice extracts are widely used for flavorings, with about 90 percent of it used for flavoring tobacco products.
Parts to Use: Roots and rhizomes.

What It Does

In Ayurvedic practices, licorice is used as an expectorant, demeculant, anti-inflammatory, adrenal agent and as a mild laxative. In Germany, licorice root is available as a tea to treat bronchitis and upset stomach, and to act as a laxative. It is licensed as a standard medicinal tea for bronchitis and gastritis. It may be efficacious in treating subacute hepatic failure, chronic hepatitis, infectious hepatitis and HIV infection. (If you have any of these conditions, consult with your physician before using.) In Traditional Chinese Medicine, licorice is used for sore throats, abdominal pain, infectious hepatitis, malaria, tuberculosis, sores, abscesses, food poisoning and contact dermatitis.

What It Might Help Treat

- Prostate cancer.
- Arthritis.
- Herpes simplex virus and canker sores.
- Menopausal symptoms.
- Using licorice with aspirin or NSAIDs might protect the stomach lining against aspirin-induced damage.

Research Insights

Licorice, used in combination with seven other herbs (PC-SPES), significantly decreases prostate-specific antigen (PSA) levels in prostate cancer patients. Licorice components are clinically valuable in treatment of gastric ulcers. Although a preliminary report showed that viral replication was inhibited temporarily in patients with HIV, this has not been substantiated since its original report more than 10 years ago.

How It Is Used

Cut or powdered root.

Growing

Licorice is a relatively hardy perennial but is destroyed if it freezes. It will grow in warm climates, Zone 7 or above. It is propagated from root cuttings and requires little care after it is established.

Harvesting

Harvest roots in the fall of the third and fourth years after planting. When harvest is anticipated, pinch back the flowers to allow maximum sap in the roots.

Preserving

Thick roots must be cut into more manageable sections to dry. Roots should be dried in the shade for up to 6 months, depending on drying conditions. Dried root will keep indefinitely if protected from strong sunlight.

Best Herbal Remedy Forms

Powdered root, infusion, tea, decoction or commercially prepared tablets.

Making the Remedy & Dosage

- Make fluid **extracts** by taking equal parts of fresh chopped root and water; let the root dissolve in the water until a strong extract is produced, which may take up to 2 weeks. This extract may be used in decoctions or syrups in a dose of ½ to 1 teaspoon, up to 3 times a day, after meals.
- **Tinctures,** 1:5. May be taken in ½- to 1-teaspoon doses in a small amount of water, up to 2 times a day.
- **Tea** may be made using 2 to 4 grams of root in 150 mL water, after meals, up to 3 times a day.
- Make a **decoction** to use for canker sores by boiling ½ teaspoon of root powder in 1 cup of water for 10 minutes; strain. Take up to 2 cups a day, holding the solution in your mouth so it bathes all sores.
- **Syrup** can be made by adding 500 mL of tea or decoction to 500 grams of honey. Heat it, stirring constantly, until the honey is liquefied and the mixture blended. Allow the syrup to cool and pour into a dark glass bottle. Use a cork for sealing, as syrups have a tendency to ferment, and screw-top bottles may explode.

Safety & Effectiveness

Licorice appears to be safe when used in amounts commonly found in foods. When used in amounts over 20 to 50 grams a day, true licorice can have serious side effects.

One of the most active components of licorice, glycyrrhizin, is responsible for its healing properties as well as its side effects. It is metabolized by the body to substances that interfere with normal functioning of the adrenal gland. The adrenal gland produces hormones, including cortisol and aldosterone. Aldosterone is important to the regulation of mineral balance in the body. Chronic use of whole licorice root interferes with the balance of the minerals sodium and potassium in the body and can lead to high blood pressure, potassium loss, edema and even heart failure in some people.

In the United States most "licorice" candies are not made with true licorice, but with anise oil, which imparts a flavor like licorice. Most true licorice products are manufactured in Europe and only found in specialty shops in the United States. Root and supplements, however, may be purchased in natural foods stores.

Licorice may be effective when used orally in a specific herbal combination for prostate cancer (PC-SPES). Many of the other claims made for licorice's medicinal properties have not been evaluated on humans in a clinical setting; however, history provides us with many possible beneficial uses.

Interactions

Many of the interactions are theoretical based on the historical use of licorice; however, some significant side effects can occur if it is used in excessive amounts.

Drugs

- Licorice may reduce the effect of drugs used to treat high blood pressure. Large amounts of licorice can cause sodium and water retention, and high blood pressure.
- Overuse of licorice, when taking corti costeroids, might increase the duration of the activity of the corticosteroid.
- Using excess licorice while taking cardiac glycosides (digoxin) may result in drug toxicity due to loss of potassium.
- Potassium loss may be exacerbated by licorice overuse when taken with some diuretic and potassium-depleting drugs.
- Licorice is believed to have estrogenic and anti-estrogenic properties; therefore, using it with estrogen and anti-estrogen therapies is not recommended.
- In some people, use of licorice with blood-thinning drugs may increase the risk of bleeding.
- It may interfere with numerous other drugs, including drugs to treat high cholesterol, allergies and antifungal medications. If in doubt, ask your pharmacist or healthcare provider.

Other Herbs. In some people, use of licorice with blood-thinning herbs may increase the risk of bleeding.

Foods. Grapefruit juice might interfere with the proposed anti-inflammatory benefits of licorice.

Vitamins or Minerals. In some people, use of licorice with vitamin E may increase the risk of bleeding.

Effects In Laboratory Tests

Excessive use of licorice can increase blood pressure and blood pressure readings. Excessive licorice can also reduce serum potassium levels. Licorice can decrease blood testosterone levels.

Adverse Reactions

- The use of licorice has been shown to cause amenorrhea (cessation of menstruation).
- More than 20 to 50 grams of licorice candy made with true licorice root a day, or chronic use longer than 6 weeks, can result in high blood pressure, lethargy, headache, sodium and water retention, and edema. Left untreated, severe congestive heart failure with pulmonary edema, lower-extremity weakness, hypertensive encephalopathy and quadriplegia can occur.
- Large amounts of licorice might cause decreased libido and sexual dysfunction in men.
- Chewing tobacco flavored with true licorice has been associated with toxicity.

Who Should Not Use True Licorice or Products Containing True Licorice as a Flavoring

- People with diabetes.
- People with renal insufficiency or liver disease.
- People with congestive heart disease.
- People with low blood potassium levels or persons on diuretic therapy.
- Women with hormone-sensitive cancers, uterine fibroids or endometriosis.
- Children under the age of 2.
- Pregnant women should not use licorice. Insufficient information is known about safety in lactating women.

Comments

Glycyrrhetic acid, which is used outside the United States for treating diseases of the stomach and GI tract, appears to be the active constituent in licorice that results in adverse reactions and interactions. Deglycyrrizinated licorice (DGL), licorice in which the offending compound is removed, is usually free of adverse reactions and interactions.

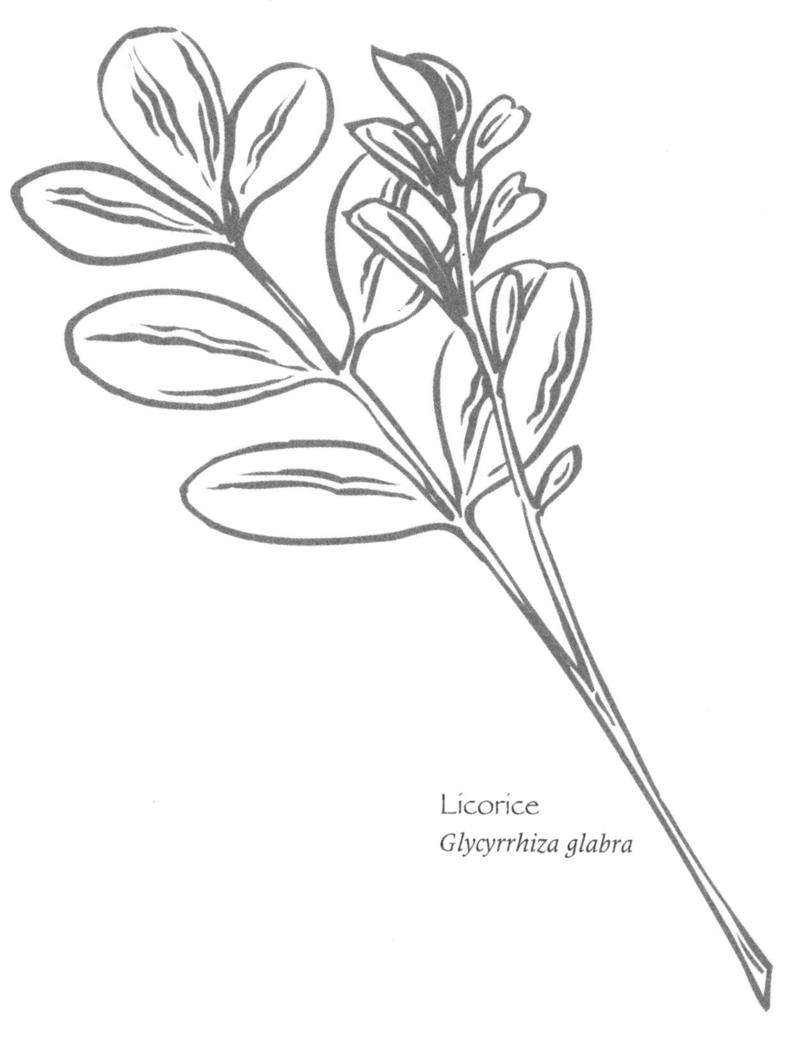

Licorice
Glycyrrhiza glabra

Marsh Mallow

Profile

Common Names: Althea leaf, cheeses
Family: Malvaceae
Genus & Species: *Althaea officinalis*
Description: Marsh mallow is a perennial that grows to a height of 3 to 5 feet with a fleshy taproot, downy stems and velvety oval leaves. It blooms in the summer, giving rise to round fruits referred to as cheeses, hence one of its names.
Historical Use: Marsh mallow's use as an herbal medicine goes back as far as 900 B.C.E. It has been used to treat bruises and blood loss from wounds and as a poultice for inflammation. Marsh mallow is a mucilage herb, meaning that when it comes in contact with water, it absorbs liquid, swells and forms a gel. Marsh mallow has been used as a food in times of famine. Early settlers brought marsh mallow to North America, where the root was used for colds, hoarseness, diarrhea, gonorrhea, GI upset and afflictions of the kidney and bladder. Today's confectionary marshmallow has its "roots" in the marsh mallow root. The French boiled peeled roots to soften it and release it sweetness, then added sugar. This confection evolved over time to become the well-known marshmallow.
Parts to Use: Primarily roots; also leaves and flowers.

What It Does

The German Commission E has approved marsh mallow root and leaf for irritation of the throat and dry coughs, and the root for mild irritation of the stomach. Marsh mallow leaf and root are used topically for abscesses, varicose veins and thrombotic ulcers and as a poultice for skin inflammation, burns and other wounds. Insect bites may be treated with marsh mallow leaf. Marsh mallow leaf is used in foods and beverages as a flavoring.

What It Might Help Treat

High blood sugar.

Research Insights

Research is lacking regarding the use of marsh mallow for conditions other than those mentioned.

How It Is Used

Fresh or dried roots and leaves.

Growing

Marsh mallow grows relatively easily, given the right amount of water. It thrives in marshy areas in full sun and can be grown from seeds, cuttings or root divisions. Now naturalized in North America, it is hardy from Zones 3 to 9.

Harvesting

Roots should not be harvested until they are at least 2 years old. Mature roots should be dug in the fall when the top growth has died and only the lateral roots removed to save the main plant for the next year. Leaves may be picked right before flowering.

Preserving

Wash, peel and dry roots either whole or in slices. Leaves may be dried.

Marsh Mallow
Althaea officinalis

Best Herbal Remedy Forms

Decoction, poultice or dried herb.

Making the Remedy & Dosage

- **Extract,** by cold maceration using 1 to 2 grams of bruised leaves in cold water for 60 minutes, stirring occasionally; strain and warm before drinking. Take 2 to 3 times a day. Extract of root by cold maceration using 2 to 5 grams of ground fresh root in 150 mL of water for 30 minutes, stirring frequently; strain and warm before drinking. Take 150 mL up to 3 times a day.
- **Tincture,** 1:5. Take 1 to 2 teaspoons, 2 to 3 times a day. Tincture made from root, 1:5, 2 to 5 teaspoons, up to 3 times a day.
- **Decoction** made by gently boiling 5 grams of chopped or crushed root for 10 minutes in 1 cup of water. Drink up to 3 cups a day.
- **Dried root** may be taken in amounts of 2 to 5 grams, up to 3 times a day.
- **Gel** can be made from the root by chopping it very fine and adding enough water to make a gel. Apply the gel to minor sunburns or wounds.
- **Syrup** can be made or purchased commercially. Use 500 mL of decoction to 500 grams of honey, heat gently and stir constantly until dissolved. Cool the mixture and pour into a dark glass bottle with a stopper. Because syrup may ferment, using a screw-top bottle may cause the bottle to explode. Use ½ to 2 teaspoons of syrup for mouth and throat irritation and associated cough.

Safety & Effectiveness

Marsh mallow is generally safe when consumed in amounts commonly used in food or when taken as recommended. Marsh mallow preparations are likely effective when used for soothing an irritated mouth and throat, for dry cough and for an irritated stomach.

Interactions

Drugs.

- May interfere with the anti-inflammatory properties of Decadron.
- In people with diabetes, may interfere with the ability to control blood sugar.
- The fiber in marsh mallow may interfere with the absorption of drugs.

Other Herbs. Marsh mallow can retard the absorption of other herbs or supplements if used simultaneously.

Foods. There are no known reported interactions or adverse reactions.

Vitamins or Minerals. There are no known reported interactions or adverse reactions.

Effects in Laboratory Tests

Marsh mallow can theoretically interfere with lab tests for blood sugar.

Adverse Reactions

Marsh mallow can cause low blood sugar.

Who Should Not Use Marsh Mallow

Marsh mallow has no reported adverse reactions in adults, pregnant or lactating women. Marsh mallow syrup contains simple sugars and should not be used by persons with diabetes without consulting their healthcare provider.

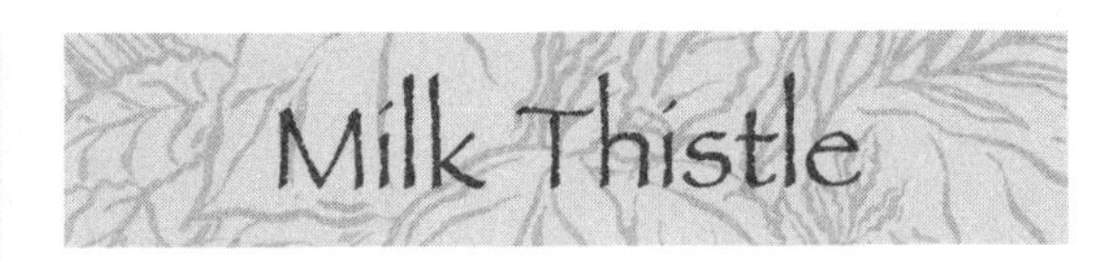

Profile

Common Names: Silybum and holy thistle
Family: Compositae
Genus & Species: *Silybum marianum*
Description: Milk thistle is a tall biennial herb with hard, prickly leaves. It bears one flower head that is reddish purple with bracts ending in sharp spines. It yields small, hard fruits that resemble seeds and are the medicinal part of the plant.
Historical Use: Milk thistle has long been known as a liver protector and detoxifying herb. Records from the first century C.E. claim that milk thistle benefits the flow of bile. Milk thistle is not just an herbal medicinal; Europeans have used its leaves, flowers and roots as a vegetable. Its small fruits have been roasted and ground as a coffee substitute. Milk thistle has long been known as an antidote for death-cap mushrooms.
Parts to Use: The seeds are used for medicinal purposes. Leaves and roots may be used fresh in salads and as a substitute for spinach. The flower heads may be served like an artichoke.

What It Does

Milk thistle appears to protect the liver from harmful chemicals, drugs and pollution; also protects the kidneys. It is useful for treatment of hepatitis. Milk thistle is an antioxidant and a uterine stimulant.

What It Might Help Treat

- High blood cholesterol
- Diabetes

Research Insights

European clinical studies have shown the effectiveness of the standardized active ingredient, silymarin, for toxic and metabolic liver damage and acute and chronic hepatitis. It has been shown to be effective for treating exposure to hazardous chemicals. It has a curative and protective effect on the liver after the exposure to death-cap and possibly other poisonous mushrooms.

How It Is Used

Seeds, extract, decoction or infusion.

Growing

When the English colonists came to America, they brought with them a useful and attractive plant: thistle. Today, milk thistle is considered a noxious weed in many parts of the country. Take care when picking it in the wild to make sure it has not been sprayed with an herbicide. It grows and spreads easily from its parachute-like seeds.

Harvesting

Milk thistle leaves, flower buds and roots can be harvested when tender and used fresh. Seeds should be harvested when ripe.

Preserving

Dry leaves, fruits and seeds.

Best Herbal Remedy Forms

Commercially prepared, standardized milk thistle products are recommended rather than homemade preparations if you want therapeutic levels of silymarin.

Making the Remedy & Dosage

Silymarin is not very water soluble, so water infusions, teas and water-based decoctions do not provide very high doses of it.

- Standardized **extracts** that are commercially available and concentrated provide the most benefits for the liver. For therapeutic use, use standardized milk thistle containing 70 to 80 percent silymarin, in divided doses equal to 420 mg per day, for 8 to 12 weeks, then decrease to 280 mg a day (280 mg is also considered a prophylactic dose).
- **Teas** may be made from ground seeds, 12 to 15 grams in 1 cup of water. These preparations may provide prophylactic, but not therapeutic, benefits.

Safety & Effectiveness

Milk thistle has been used as a food and medicinal herb for centuries without side effects when used as recommended and in clinical trials. Initially, it may have a mild laxative effect.

Milk thistle may be effective in cases of cirrhosis of the liver, hepatitis and possibly for alcoholic cirrhosis when used after cessation of alcohol consumption. It may reduce insulin resistance in people with diabetes and alcoholic cirrhosis.

Interactions

Drugs. People taking drugs that are metabolized by the liver should be cautious when using milk thistle, as it may interfere with its effectiveness.

Other Herbs. Insufficient clinical information about interactions or reactions is available.

Foods. There are no known reported interactions or adverse reactions.

Vitamins or Minerals. There are no known reported interactions or adverse reactions.

Effects in Laboratory Tests

There are no known reported interactions or adverse reactions.

Adverse Reactions

- Can cause an allergic reaction in persons sensitive to the Asteraceae/Compositae family, including ragweed, chrysanthemums, marigolds, daisies and many other herbs.
- A mild laxative effect may occur within the first few weeks.

Who Should Not Use Milk Thistle

- Because milk thistle has a weak estrogenic effect, persons with hormone-sensitive cancers should avoid using it.
- Safety for pregnant and lactating women has not been determined, although it is presumed safe based on its use as a food for thousands of years.

Comments

Because of its history and known benefits, persons with established liver disease or those at risk for liver disease should still have regular liver function tests conducted to determine efficacy.

Motherwort

Profile

Common Names: Lion's tail and heartwort
Family: Labiatae/Lamiaceae. Lemon balm, mints and catnip belong to this family.
Genus & Species: *Leonurus cardiaca*
Description: As a member of the Labiatae/Lamiaceae family, motherwort has the characteristic square stem with a red-violet tint. It grows to a height of 4 feet. Its lower leaves are shaped much like a small maple leaf with mauve to pink or white flowers that bloom from midsummer through mid-fall.
Historical Use: Motherwort began as a treatment for diseases in cattle in the 1500s. As a folk remedy, motherwort was used for female reproductive complaints. Native Americans recognized that motherwort stimulated the uterus and used it to stimulate labor and menstruation and to relax the uterus during pregnancy and after childbirth. It has been used as a tonic or treatment for heart ailments and nervous disorders.
Parts to Use: Whole plant.

What It Does

Motherwort relaxes the cells of heart muscle and is a treatment, according to the German Commission E, for nervous cardiac disorders. It has a mild sedative action. Also stimulates uterine contractions.

What It Might Help Treat

- May be an adjuvant treatment for hypothyroidism.
- May have anti-blood clotting properties.

Research Insights

No current research identified.

How It Is used

Teas usually prepared from dried herb, or dried herb itself.

Growing
As with many of its other family members, motherwort grows very easily and may become a garden pest. It may be grown from seed planted in the spring or from nursery stock.

Harvesting
The entire plant may be harvested after it blooms.

Preserving
Drying.

Best Herbal Remedy Forms
Teas or infusion, commercially prepared fluid extract or tincture.

Making the Remedy & Dosage

- **Tinctures,** 1:5. Take up to 10 mL (2 teaspoons) in a small amount of water, up to 2 times a day.
- **Tea** may be made with 2 to 4½ grams of the dried above-ground part, steeped in 150 mL of hot, not boiling, water for 10 minutes, then strained. Take up to 3 cups a day.
- **Dried herb** may be powdered and taken in capsule form. Suggested dosage is 2 grams of herb, up to 3 times a day.

Safety & Effectiveness

Motherwort is considered safe when taken orally as recommended. Motherwort may be effective for nervous cardiac disorders when taken as recommended.

Interactions

Drugs. Motherwort can increase the effectiveness of the sedative and tranquilizing effects of central nervous system depressants.

Other Herbs. Use of motherwort with herbs and supplements that contain cardiac glycosides can increase the toxicity of cardiac glycosides.

Foods. There are no known reported interactions or adverse reactions.

Vitamins or Minerals. There are no known reported interactions or adverse reactions.

Effects In Laboratory Tests

Motherwort might improve thyroid function test results in persons with underfunctioning thyroids.

Adverse Reactions

- Amounts greater than 3 grams can cause diarrhea, stomach irritation and uterine bleeding.
- Leaves can cause skin rash if they come in contact with the skin.
- May cause allergic reactions in sensitive persons. May cause sensitivity to the sun if used on skin exposed to the sun.

Who Should Not Use Motherwort

- People with heart disease.
- Pregnant women.
- Women with excessive menstrual or uterine bleeding.
- Lactating women; insufficient clinical data is available regarding its effects on the infant.
- Children under 2 years of age.
- For children under 2 and persons over 65, begin with low-strength preparations and increase the strength if needed. Always consult your healthcare professional before using the herb for children or those over 65.

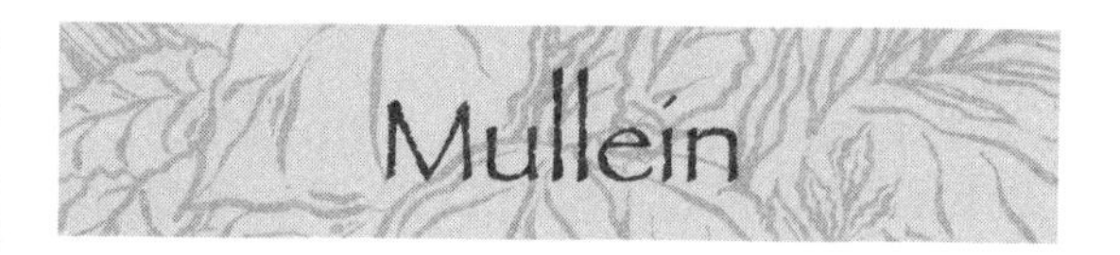

Mullein

Profile

Common Names: Aaron's rod, American Mullein, Beggar's Blanket, Blanket Herb, Blanket Leaf, Candlewick, Feltwort, Flannelflower, Longwort, Orange Mullein, Our Lady's Flannel, Shepherd's Staff, Torch Weed, Velvet Plant and more.
Family: Scrophulariaceae. Other family members include figwort, foxglove and eyebright.
Genus & Species: *Verbascum thapsus*
Description: The first year, the plant does not reach maturity but possesses a rosette of 6- to 15-inch tongue-shaped, hairy, greenish leaves. In its second year, it develops a distinctive 6- to 8-foot flower stem with a cylindrical spike of small, dense, yellow, honey-scented flowers.
Historical Use: The mullein plant has been used as a medicine for hundreds, if not thousands, of years. During the Middle Ages, it was used to treat skin and respiratory problems in humans and cattle. The dried stems and flowers were dipped in suet and burned as torches. It has been used for candlewicking because it burns readily when lit. When introduced to Native Americans by the colonists, the common way to take mullein was by smoking it. It has been used for stomach and respiratory ailments and externally for the treatment of hemorrhoids.
Parts to Use: Leaves and flowers.

Do not confuse mullein with goldenrod (*Solidago virgaurea*), which is one of mullein's common names.

What It Does

When taken orally, it treats respiratory tract mucous membrane inflammations and coughs. Used topically, it is good for wounds, burns, hemorrhoids, frostbite and inflamed mucosa. The leaves soften and protect the skin. It is used as a flavoring ingredient in alcoholic beverages.

What It Might Help Treat

- Diarrhea
- External inflammations
- Herpes and cold sores

Research Insights

There has been little clinical research on the applications of mullein in humans. Much of the support for its use is based on its long history in established traditional and conventional medical systems, research on its phytochemical properties and studies on animals.

How It Is Used

Fresh or dried flowers and/or leaves.

Growing
Mullein is easy to grow and may be directly seeded in the early spring.

Harvesting
Harvest during the second year. Gather leaves before the plant flowers; gather flowers as they appear in mid- to late summer.

Preserving
Mullein leaves and flowers may be used fresh or dry.

Best Herbal Remedy Forms

Infusion or tea, oil infusion, tincture or fluid extract.

Making the Remedy & Dosage

- **Fluid extract,** 1:1. Use 1½ to 2 mL, up to 2 times a day.
- **Tinctures,** 1:5. Use 1½ to 2 teaspoons (7 to 10 mL) diluted in a small amount of water, up to 2 times a day.
- **Teas** are made by steeping 1 to 2 teaspoons of dried leaves or flowers in 1 cup of hot, not boiling, water for 10 minutes, then straining. Drink up to 3 cups a day.
- **Oil infusions** may be made using enough flower heads to pack a canning jar. Cover with cold pressed oil. Let steep in a sunny location for 2 to 3 weeks. Strain, using cheesecloth, squeezing the oil through the cloth. Leave to settle for another week, then strain again.

Safety & Effectiveness

When used as recommended, mullein appears to be safe. Mullein is considered effective when used orally for treating inflammation of the respiratory tract mucous membranes, cough and sore throat.

Interactions

Drugs. There are no known reported interactions or adverse reactions.
Other Herbs. There are no known reported interactions or adverse reactions.
Foods. There are no known reported interactions or adverse reactions.
Vitamins or Minerals. There are no known reported interactions or adverse reactions.

Effects In Laboratory Tests

There are no known reported interactions or adverse reactions.

Adverse Reactions

- Mullein seeds may be poisonous if ingested.
- There have been no reports of adverse reactions to mullein leaf, flower or even root use.
- If taken in large doses, it may cause upset stomach and diarrhea.

Who Should Not Use Mullein

- Pregnant and nursing women may want to avoid mullein as there is insufficient clinical data regarding its safety.
- Use caution in children under age 2. If you would like to try mullein, begin with ½ the adult dose to help sooth coughs. Always inform your physician when trying an herbal remedy in children or yourself.

Mullein
Verbascum thapsus

Pennyroyal

Profile

Common Names: Fleabane, tickweed, mosquito plant and squawmint
Family: Lamiaceae/Labiatae; the mint family.
Genus & Species: *Mentha pulegium* (European), *Hedeoma pulegioides* (American)
Description: Although their botanical qualities differ, both European and American pennyroyals contain similar oils and are used interchangeably. European pennyroyal is a perennial with many of the characteristics of its other family members. It spreads underground by runners, has square stems and oval, hairy leaves. Its flowers are lilac and appear in midsummer. American pennyroyal, on the other hand, is an annual with a square stem, about 3 inches taller than the European's 12 inches, and has bluish flowers. It is one of the most aromatic of the mints.
Historical Use: Pennyroyal has been a popular herb since the first century C.E., so it warrants a brief discussion here. Unfortunately, if used inappropriately, it can be toxic or even fatal. Pennyroyal has been used for coughs and to aid digestion. It is also popular, when used topically, as an insect repellant, hence several of the common names.
Parts to Use: Leaves and flowers.

What It Does

It repels pesky insects—flies, fleas, mosquitoes and ticks. Pennyroyal acts as a decongestant and acts as a digestive aid. It may stimulate menstruation.

What It Might Help Treat

Excessive mucus.

Research Insights

There are no observable clinical trials on pennyroyal. The documentation that exists is based on reported uses and adverse reactions.

How It Is Used

Only the leaves and flowers should be used, and only as directed. The oil should not be used.

Growing

Like other members of the mint family, it grows with ease. The European pennyroyal, being a perennial, will spread and can become a pest. It can be grown from nursery stock and root cuttings. American pennyroyal can be sown from seed in the spring.

Harvesting

Cut leaves during the growing season. Cut whole plants just as flowering begins.

Preserving

Drying.

Best Herbal Remedy Forms

Tea or fresh plant topically.

Making the Remedy & Dosage

Do not attempt to make oils, tinctures or extracts from pennyroyal.

- Make a **tea or infusion** by steeping 1 to 2 teaspoons of dried herb in 1 cup of hot, not boiling, water; steep for 10 minutes and strain. Drink up to 2 cups a day. Use for coughs, congestion or stomach upsets.

- Crush **fresh plant** and rub on your body to repel insects. Crushed fresh plant may be added to petroleum jelly or creams and applied.
- A **fresh** collar of pennyroyal may be used as a flea and tick repellant for animals. (Pennyroyal is often the active ingredient in herbal dog collars.) Do not apply the oil to your pet's skin, because they may get a toxic dose by licking it off their fur.

Safety & Effectiveness

Pennyroyal is likely to be unsafe when the alcoholic extract and oil is used orally; its use has been linked to death. There is insufficient reliable clinical information available about the safety of using pennyroyal leaf as tea. Effectiveness is only known from historical use.

Interactions

Drugs. There are no known reported interactions or adverse reactions.
Other Herbs. There are no known reported interactions or adverse reactions.
Foods. There are no known reported interactions or adverse reactions.
Vitamins or Minerals. There are no known reported interactions or adverse reactions.

Effects In Laboratory Tests

There are no known reported interactions or adverse reactions.

Adverse Reactions

When used internally, the oil can cause:

- Kidney and/or liver failure.
- Abdominal cramping, nausea and vomiting (possibly bloody).
- Dizziness.
- Hallucinations.
- Elevated blood pressure and pulse rate.
- Abortion.
- Respiratory failure.
- Death.
- When used topically, the oil or fresh plant may cause skin rash.

Who Should Not Use Pennyroyal

- Pregnant women should not use the tea or the oil, as it may stimulate menstruation and cause abortion.
- Lactating women; insufficient information about the safety of the tea or oil is available.
- Do not use in children under age 2.
- For older children and elderly individuals, use with caution and begin doses at less than half the typical adult dose. Watch for adverse reactions.
- Consult with your healthcare provider before using pennyroyal.

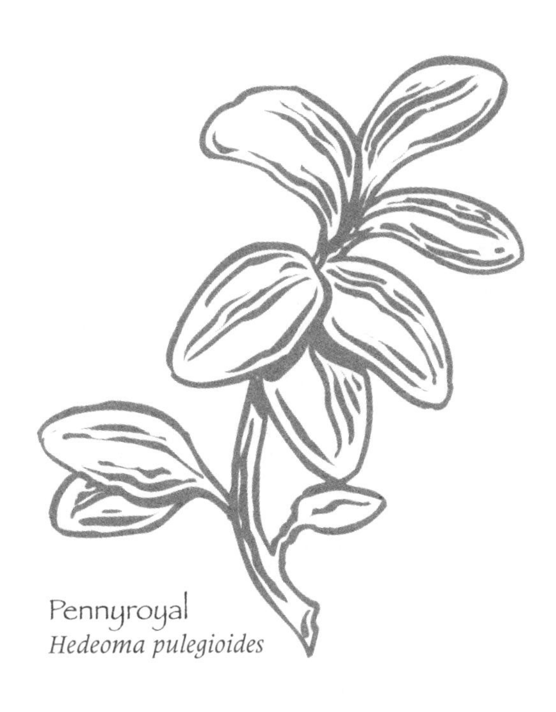

Pennyroyal
Hedeoma pulegioides

Peppermint

Profile

Common Name: Mint
Family: Labiatae/Lamiaceae. (Lemon balm and catnip belong to this family.)
Genus & Species: *Mentha piperita*
Description: Peppermint grows about 3 feet high, spreading underground by root runners. It has square, purplish stems and wrinkled leaves with lilac-pink spiked flowers.
Historical Use: The many aromatic herbs in the Labiatae/Lamiaceae family are commonly referred to as Menthas because of their active ingredients, which include menthol. The most commonly known and used is peppermint. Mints have been used for centuries as flavorings, in aromatherapy and medications. Peppermint leaf and oil is one of the most widely used and recognized herbs in European pharmacopoeias. The FDA generally recognizes it as safe for use in foods and medication, but it may cause side effects in persons with reflux and heartburn.
Parts to Use: Whole plants, leaves and oil.

What It Does

It soothes skin and throat irritation. It relieves respiratory symptoms and is beneficial in some bowel conditions, including gas.

What It Might Help Treat

Irritable bowel syndrome (IBS).

Peppermint
Mentha piperita

Research Insights

People using peppermint report feeling better, but there is no verified decongestant effect. Peppermint improves emptying of the stomach and relieves nausea. Topical oil reduces intensity of headache pain.

How It Is Used

As a tea or oil.

Growing

Peppermint is easy to grow in open garden space or containers. Anyone who has grown mint knows that it can quickly take over the garden if not tamed.

Harvesting

Cut leaves during the growing season. Cut whole plants just as flowering begins.

Preserving

Use fresh or dry.

Best Herbal Remedy Forms

Infusions, teas, powders or ointments.

Making the Remedy & Dosage

- **Fluid extracts** are available commercially and usually measured to precise pharmaceutical specifications. Take 1/4 teaspoon (2 mL) up to 3 times a day.
- **Tinctures** are available commercially or may be made at home (1:5). Take 2 teaspoons, up to 3 times a day.
- **Tea** is one of the most popular ways of taking peppermint. Use 3 to 6 grams of cut leaf, or 1 to 2 teaspoons of dried herb, in 1 cup of hot, not boiling, water. Drink 1 cup up to 3 times a day.
- **Ointments** can be made using 500 grams petroleum jelly or lanolin and 60 grams of dried peppermint. Warm the jelly or lanolin over a pan of boiling water, stir

in the herbs and heat for about 2 hours. Strain the mixture through double layers of cheesecloth, and using rubber gloves, squeeze it through the cloth into a jug. Quickly pour the warm strained mixture into clean, dark glass jars.

- **Essential oil** is made by steam distillation of freshly harvested flowering sprigs. Purchase commercially and use in small doses internally and externally. Average dose of oil for internal use is 6 to 12 drops. For decongested airways, put 3 to 4 drops of essential oil in very hot water; inhale the vapor.
- **Essential oil** may be used in ointments prepared with 5 to 20 percent of the essential oil to jelly or lanolin. A few drops mixed with a small amount of warm water or vegetable oil may be rubbed into areas of skin that are affected.

Safety & Effectiveness

Peppermint leaf is safe when used in amounts commonly found in food and when used as directed for medicinal purposes.
Peppermint oil is safe when used appropriately, but should not be used on the face, particularly the nose of infants and small children, as it may cause them to stop breathing.

Peppermint leaves are considered effective for GI, gallbladder and bile duct spasms. When taken orally, peppermint oil helps relieve spasms of the upper GI tract, respiratory tract inflammation and excess mucus. When used externally according to safety guidelines, peppermint oil is also effective for coughs, colds, myalgia and neuralgia.

Interactions

Drugs. People taking drugs that block stomach acid should use peppermint oil with caution, as it might irritate the stomach. There are no known reported interactions or adverse reactions to peppermint leaf.
Other Herbs. There are no known reported interactions or adverse reactions to peppermint leaf or oil.
Foods. Food may interfere with the absorption of enteric-coated peppermint oil capsules taken for irritable bowel. Take capsules between meals. There are no known reported interactions or adverse reactions to peppermint leaf.
Vitamins or Minerals. There are no known reported interactions or adverse reactions to peppermint leaf or oil.

Effects In Laboratory Tests

There are no known interactions or adverse reactions to peppermint leaf or oil.

Adverse Reactions

- In persons with gallstones, peppermint leaf taken orally may cause spasms in the bile tract.
- Peppermint leaf may cause a choking sensation in infants and young children.
- Oil of peppermint can result in heartburn and allergic reactions.
- Oil of peppermint may worsen symptoms of hiatal hernia.
- Topically, peppermint oil can cause skin irritation.
- Inhaled peppermint oil vapors may cause an allergic reaction in sensitive individuals.

Who Should Not Use Peppermint

- People with gallstones or hiatal hernias should not use peppermint leaf or oil.
- People who produce little or no hydrochloric acid should not take peppermint oil internally.
- People with bile duct obstruction, severe liver disease or a swollen gallbladder should not use peppermint oil.

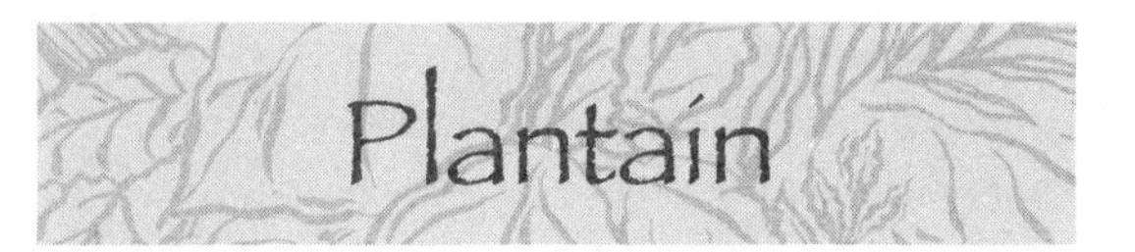

Profile

Common Names: Great plantain, general plantain
Family: Plantaginaceae
Genus & Species: *Plantago major*
Description: Plantain is an annual with linear gray-green leaves mostly arranged in a circular shape around the base of the plant. Its flowers are tiny, yellow-green and are produced on cylindrical stalks.
Historical Use: Plantain belongs to a family of approximately 250 members, many of which are considered weeds. A number of plantains are used for their medicinal properties, some for their seeds and some for their leaves and roots. The main ingredients in the leaf are tannin and a glycoside, which stimulates uric acid secretion of the kidneys. Historically, it has been used for urinary tract infections, bronchitis, colds, irritated or bleeding hemorrhoids and skin conditions. Plantain is an excellent source of vitamin K, beta-carotene and calcium.
Parts to Use: Leaves.

What It Does

Treats bronchitis, as well as symptoms of the common cold.

What It Might Help Treat

Wounds and minor abrasions.

Do not confuse this plantain with its other family members, the blond psyllium and black psyllium.

Research Insights

In animals it has been shown to lower blood pressure and decrease cholesterol and triglycerides.

How It Is Used

The leaves are used both orally and topically.

Growing
This weed is relatively easy to grow and is self-seeding. It is a common plant in the wild and in home gardens in the United States.

Harvesting
Cut leaves before flowering.

Preserving
Use leaves fresh, or dry them for future use.

Best Herbal Remedy Forms
Dried herb, liquid extract or tincture.

Making the Remedy & Dosage
- **Tea** is made by adding 2 to 4 grams of dried leaf to 150 mL of boiling water; steep for 5 to 10 minutes and strain. Take 3 times a day.
- **Fluid extract,** 1:1. Take ½ to 1 teaspoon in a small amount of water, 3 times a day.
- **Tincture,** 1:5. Take ½ to 1 teaspoon in a small amount of water, 3 times a day.

Safety & Effectiveness

Considered safe and effective for bronchitis and the common cold.

Interactions

Drugs. Use with anticoagulants—especially Coumadin—may increase risk of blood clots.
Other Herbs. Use with herbs that have anticoagulant properties may increase risk of blood clots.
Foods. No interactions are known to occur.
Vitamins or Minerals. No interactions are known to occur.

Effects In Laboratory Tests

May reduce clotting time in blood-clotting tests.

Adverse Reactions

- Excess amounts taken orally have a laxative effect and may lower blood pressure.
- Topical use may cause dermatitis.

Who Should Not Use Plantain

- People with plantain hypersensitivity.
- People with melon sensitivities, as plantain may cross-pollinate with melons.
- Avoid using during pregnancy and lactation because of its possible effects on uterine tone.

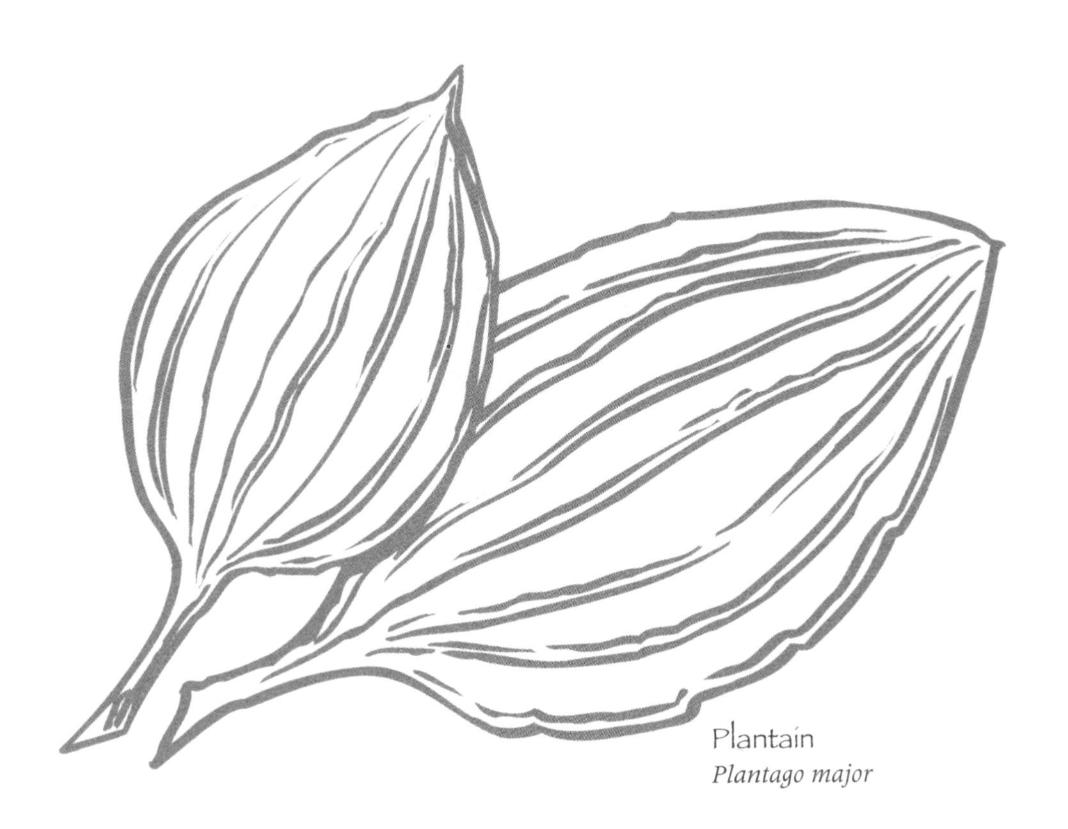

Plantain
Plantago major

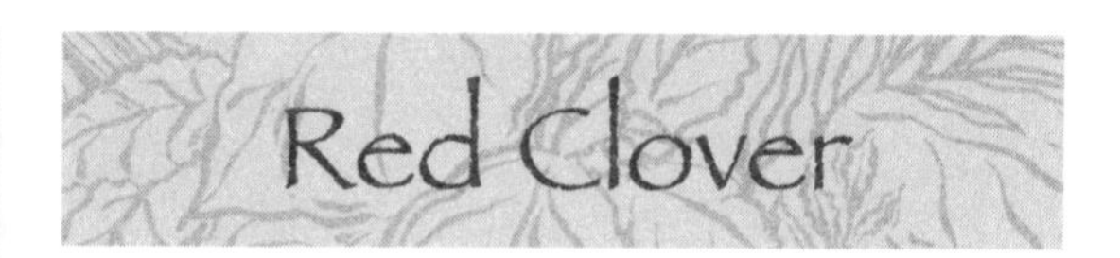

Profile

Common Names: Wild clover, purple clover, Missouri milk vetch, Trefoil, cow clover, beebread
Family: Leguminosae; the bean and pea family.
Genus & Species: *Trifolium pratense*
Description: Red clover is a three-leafed, short-lived perennial that grows to 3 feet. The flowers are ball-shaped, purple-pink and sometimes cream florets.
Historical Use: Red clover's history is long and varied. It has been used since ancient Grecian time. It has had religious connotations and was considered a charm against witchcraft. It has been used in combination with other herbs to treat skin disorders and syphilis, and as part of the controversial alternative cancer treatment, Hoxey Cancer Formula. In more recent history, red clover has been used topically for eczema and psoriasis, and orally for digestion, menopausal complaints and respiratory ailments.
Parts to Use: Flowers.

What It Does

Although no placebo-controlled human trials have been reported, some small trials have been conducted that show some promise for its health benefits. Many of the benefits of red clover have been extrapolated from the research on soy. Red clover contains the same isoflavones, genistein and daidzein, that are thought to convey benefits from soy. Red clover has antioxidant and blood-thinning properties. It is used as a flavoring in food products.

What It Might Help Treat

- Menopausal symptoms
- High blood cholesterol

Research Insights

Red clover may help prevent the development of osteoporosis in pre- and peri-menopausal women. It may reduce symptoms of benign prostatic hyperplasia (BPH), including urinary frequency during the night.

How It Is Used

In preparations made from dried herb.

Growing

Red clover is relatively easy to grow and is often seen growing wild in the country. Plant it in a sunny location with well-drained but moist soil.

Harvesting

Flower heads with upper leaves should be picked as they open during the summer.

Preserving

Drying.

Best Herbal Remedy Forms

Teas, tinctures, capsules and vinegar. May also be purchased already prepared as tablets or capsules.

Making the Remedy & Dosage

- **Fluid extract,** 1:1. Take 1/4 to 1/2 teaspoon, up to 3 times per day.
- **Tinctures,** 1:10. Take 15 to 30 drops, up to 4 times a day.
- **Teas** can be made using 1 to 3 teaspoons of dried flowers per cup of hot, not boiling, water, steeped for 10 minutes and strained. Drink up to 3 cups a day.

- **Dried flowers** may be taken in 4-gram doses, up to 3 times a day.
- **Vinegar** may be made by submerging fresh red clover leaves and flowers in enough apple cider vinegar to cover the herb in a glass jar. Cover the jar; place in a cool, dark place for 1 week. Strain, refrigerate and use for salads, pasta or by the spoonful.

Safety & Effectiveness

Red clover is safe when used in amounts commonly found in foods or as recommended as an herbal remedy.

Red clover may be effective against osteoporosis in peri- and menopausal women when used up to 1 year. It might also help reduce hot flashes associated with menopause. It may be effective for men suffering from BPH.

Interactions

Drugs. Using red clover with anticoagulant or antiplatelet drugs may increase the risk of bleeding. Because of its theoretical estrogenic activity, red clover may interfere with estrogen or oral contraceptive therapy. Theoretically, red clover might also increase levels of drugs used to treat high cholesterol, fungal infections and allergies, to name a few. Use red clover cautiously or avoid if you are taking these drugs.
Other Herbs. Use of red clover with other herbs that affect coagulation or platelets may increase the risk of bleeding. Theoretically, red clover could have a cumulative or compounding effect or work against other herbs that have weak estrogen properties.
Foods. There are no known reported interactions or adverse reactions.
Vitamins or Minerals. Do not use if you are taking more than 400 IU of vitamin E, as it may increase the risk of bleeding.

Effects In Laboratory Tests

There are no known reported interactions or adverse reactions.

Adverse Reactions

- Rash
- Estrogenic activity

Who Should Not Use Red Clover

- During pregnancy and lactation, red clover should not be used in medicinal amounts; red clover has estrogenic activity. There is not enough reliable information available about the safety of topical use of red clover during pregnancy and lactation.
- People treated for coagulation disorders.
- People with hormone-sensitive cancers.

Comments

- In excess amounts red clover has caused sterility in livestock animals and reproductive and liver failure in cheetahs in a zoo population.
- If you pick wild red clover, make sure your source is free of pesticides or herbicides.

Red Clover
Trifolium pratense

St. John's Wort

Profile

Common Names: Hypericum, SJW
Family: Hypericaceae
Genus & Species: *Hypericum perforatum*
Description: St. John's wort is a woody perennial that spreads wildly. It has blunt, oblong leaves with glands that produce red oil. The flowers are yellow, five-petaled and also gland-dotted.
Historical Use: St. John's wort was used in traditional Greek medicine to treat neuralgias, anxiety, neurosis and depression. Europeans of the time believed that it possessed magical and protective powers against evil and disease. Early colonists from Europe introduced the plant to North America, where it became popular for wound-healing and as an antidepressant.
Parts to Use: Whole plant.

What It Does

It acts as a mild antidepressant. SJW may relieve anxiety and insomnia and may help persons with seasonal affective disorder (SAD). Externally, it helps treat wounds, bruises and first-degree burns.

What It Might Help Treat

Viral infections.

Research Insights

May treat obsessive-compulsive disorders. It may be beneficial in treating premenstrual syndrome (PMS).

St John's Wort
Hypericum perforatum

How It Is Used

As a standardized extract, tincture, powdered extract or fresh.

Growing

SJW is relatively easy to grow from nursery stock or root divisions in the spring or fall. It will spread unless contained. It should be replanted every few years to maintain healthy and effectual plants.

Harvesting

Cut plants as flowering begins.

Preserving

May be used fresh or dried. If taken in amounts greater than recommended for medicinal purposes, it may be harmful.

Best Herbal Remedy Forms

A standardized extract from a reliable manufacturer will provide the most consistent results. However, in recent evaluations of commercially available products, more than 90 percent were found to contain less than what was listed on the label, and some contained virtually none.

Making the Remedy & Dosage

- **Fluid extracts,** 1:1. Take 2 mL, up to 2 times a day.
- **Tinctures,** 1:5. Take 20 to 30 drops, up to 3 times a day.
- **Infusions** have been used traditionally, but they have been withdrawn from the market in Germany because efficacy data were lacking.
- **Dried herb**, in doses of 2 to 4 grams, chopped or powdered, a day.
- **Chopped fresh flowering tops** may be added to oils, petroleum jelly and creams for topical preparations. Or they may be crushed and applied directly to the cleaned affected area.

Safety & Effectiveness

St. John's wort is considered safe and well tolerated by most people. There are no reports of major side effects with doses taken as recommended. There have been limited reports of sun sensitivity in some persons using SJW. SJW is believed to be effective for mild to moderate depression and possibly for some viral infections, including herpes virus.

Interactions

Drugs. St. John's wort may interact with certain drugs metabolized by the same liver enzyme system as the herb. The list of drugs that SJW may interact with is lengthy. Most interactions result in an increased or decreased effect of the prescription drug. Since some interactions can be severe, be sure to check with your healthcare provider before using St. John's wort. These drugs include but are not limited to:

- Selective Serotonin Agonists
- Amitriptyline
- Antidepressants
- Barbiturates
- Transplant anti-rejection medications
- Blood-thinning medications
- Monoamine oxidase inhibitors (MAOIs) (Theoretically, SJW may have additive adverse effects, including hypertension, sensitivity to cold, agitation, confusion and coma.)
- Digoxin (digitalis)
- Oral contraceptives
- Many drugs used for treating AIDS/HIV

Other Herbs. Therapeutic effects of herbs with sedative properties may be enhanced and adverse reactions increased.

Foods. Theoretically, use of large amounts of SJW and tyramine-containing foods might exacerbate high blood pressure.

Vitamins or Minerals. May reduce absorption of medicinal levels of iron.

Effects in Laboratory Tests

St. John's wort can decrease PT/INR lab results in patients treated with the blood-thinning drug Coumadin.

Adverse Reactions

- Healthy individuals who are not taking any prescription drugs or herbs usually tolerate St. John's wort.
- Mild stomach upset appears to be the most common side effect, followed by allergic reactions, tiredness, insomnia and restlessness.
- Although sun sensitivity does not appear to be a problem in humans, it would be wise to avoid excess exposure to sun, especially for those who are sun-sensitive.

Who Should Not Use St. John's Wort

People who:

- have Alzheimer's disease.
- have bipolar disease or schizophrenia.
- have major clinical depression.
- are having difficulty conceiving.
- are pregnant or lactating.

Comments

If you are currently taking antidepressants, do not change or discontinue your dosage without the advice of your healthcare provider. SJW or other herbs are not substitutes for medical treatment in cases of serious illness. Many conditions should not be self-diagnosed or self-medicated.

It may take 2 to 4 weeks of regular use before antidepressant effects are seen. To avoid risk of withdrawal effects, do not abruptly discontinue using SJW.

Saw Palmetto

Profile

Common Names: American dwarf palm, cabbage palm, sabal
Family: Palmae (other family members include various palms).
Genus & Species: *Serenoa repens*
Description: Saw palmetto is a small clump-forming palm tree with fan-shaped blue-green to yellow-green leaves. Small fragrant cream-colored flowers in summer give rise to 1-inch ovoid, oily blue-black fruits.
Historical Use: Native Americans depended on saw palmetto as a food and as a diuretic, and also used its leaves for mattress stuffing, roof thatching and for weaving hats and baskets. Its primary use was as an aphrodisiac, for breast enhancement in women, and for benign prostate enlargement. In the 1800s and 1900s, saw palmetto was known for its use for prostatic conditions and was used by mainstream American doctors until the 1940s.
Parts to Use: Fruits.

What It Does

Saw palmetto helps maintain prostate health. It may relieve mild to moderate benign prostatic hyperplasia (BPH). It also may relieve chronic inflammation of the prostate (prostatitis).

What It Might Help Treat

- Inflammation
- Poor sperm production
- Edema

Research Insights

The potential for saw palmetto to inhibit prostate cancer is being explored.

How It Is Used

The most reliable way to use it is in its standardized extract form that may be purchased commercially.

Growing

Saw palmetto grows easily in the south-eastern United States in areas with sandy soil. It has been found as far west as Alabama and Missouri.

Harvesting

Collect the fruits when ripe.

Preserving

Drying.

Best Herbal Remedy Forms

Infusions, teas, liquid extracts, tinctures and dried.

Making the Remedy & Dosage

- **Fluid extract,** 1:1. Take 1 to 2 mL 2 times a day.
- **Tincture,** 1:2. Take 2 to 4 mL 2 times a day.
- Make a **tea** by simmering ½ to 1 gram of dried berry in 150 mL hot, not boiling, water for 5 to 10 minutes. strain; take 3 times a day.
  Brewed teas or other hydrophilic (water) preparations might not contain adequate active constituents, as it is not soluble in water.
- **Dried standardized extract,** 160 mg, 2 times a day. One dose of 320 mg has also been shown to be effective. It is typically standardized to contain 85 to 95 percent fatty acids and sterols.

- **Fresh cut fruit** from the saw palmetto tree has been suggested in an amount of 1 to 2 grams a day.

Safety & Effectiveness

The German Commission E has approved the oral use of saw palmetto. When used as recommended, saw palmetto is considered safe. Saw palmetto has been researched in European countries quite extensively and been found to be safe and effective. Men over age 40 should schedule a yearly prostate exam to check for prostate enlargement, even if they are using saw palmetto on a regular basis.

Interactions

Drugs. Use of saw palmetto may interfere with hormone therapy or oral contraceptives.
Other herbs. There are no known reported interactions or adverse reactions.
Foods. There are no known reported interactions or adverse reactions.
Vitamins or Minerals. Potential for decreased absorption of iron supplements due to formation of tannin-iron complex.

Effects In Laboratory Tests

Contrary to earlier reports, saw palmetto does not affect the standard blood test for or concentrations of prostate-specific antigen (PSA).

Adverse Reactions

Adverse reactions are generally mild and may include dizziness, nausea, vomiting, constipation and diarrhea.

Who Should Not Use Saw Palmetto

Pregnant and lactating women should not use it because of its potential estrogenic and anti-androgenic activity.

Comments

Length of therapy varies. Some men see improvement in 1 month, while others require 45 to 90 days to see the benefits. The course of therapy is generally recommended for 4 to 6 months with a reevaluation by a healthcare professional at that time.

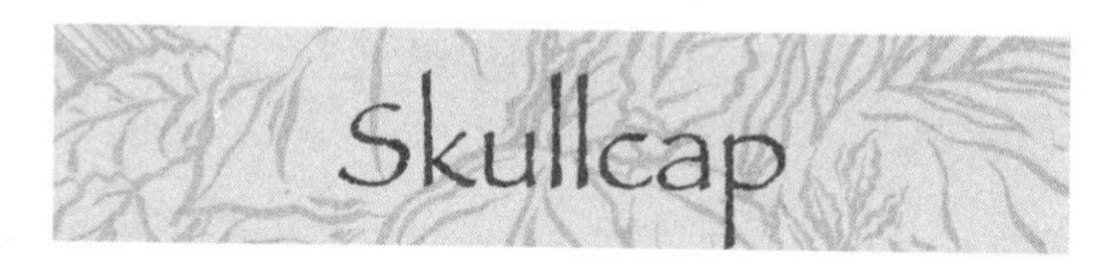

Skullcap

Profile

Common Names: Skullcap, Virginia scullcap
Family: Labiatae/Lamiaceae; other family members include mints.
Genus & Species: *Scutellaria lateriflora*
Description: It is a bushy perennial with arrow-shaped leaves and blue-purple tubular flowers produced on one side of the flower stalk.
Historical Use: Skullcap has been used as a sedative in Chinese medicine for centuries. In the 1800s, it was used for insomnia, nervousness, malaria, convulsions and delirium tremens of alcoholism. It has been used for female complaints, including PMS.
Parts to Use: Plant and flowers.

What It Does

It decreases PSA in men with BPH when used in combination with seven other herbs (PC-SPES). It decreases testosterone. Scullcap acts as a tranquilizer.

What It Might Help Treat

- Inflammation
- Increases HDL ("good") cholesterol

Research Insights

Scullcap may decrease PSA levels, cause tumor cell death and decrease testosterone levels.

How It Is Used

Dried or commercially prepared.

Growing

Skullcap may be grown from seeds planted in fall or root divisions planted in early spring. It requires little care and grows in most conditions under full sun. This perennial lasts only about 3 years.

Harvesting

Cut plants when flowering.

Preserving

Dry plant parts and flowers.

Best Herbal Remedy Forms

Infusions, teas, liquid extracts and tinctures.

Making the Remedy & Dosage

- **Teas** are made with 1 to 2 grams of dried herb in 150 mL of boiling water, steeped for 5 to 10 minutes and strained. Drink 3 times a day.
- **Extract** 1:1. Take 2- to 4-mL doses, 3 times a day.
- **Tincture,** 1:5. Take in 1- to 2-mL doses, 3 times a day.

Safety & Effectiveness

Considered safe when used in the PC-SPES formula to treat BPH; however, at this writing, PC-SPES is not commonly available. Believed to be effective when used orally as directed.

Interactions

Drugs. There are no known reported interactions or adverse reactions.
Other Herbs. Use with herbs that have sedative properties may enhance therapeutic and adverse reactions.
Foods. There are no known reported interactions or adverse reactions.
Vitamins or Minerals. There are no known reported interactions or adverse reactions.

Effects In Laboratory Tests

There are no known medical reports of interactions or adverse reactions.

Adverse Reactions

Large amounts may cause giddiness, stupor, confusion, limb twitching or seizures.

Who Should Not Use Skullcap

- People with liver disorders.
- Women who are pregnant or lactating.

Comments

Skullcap has been adulterated with other herbs and drugs. There was a recall of a PC-SPES product containing skullcap in early 2002 because of contamination with prescription drugs, resulting in potential adverse effects.

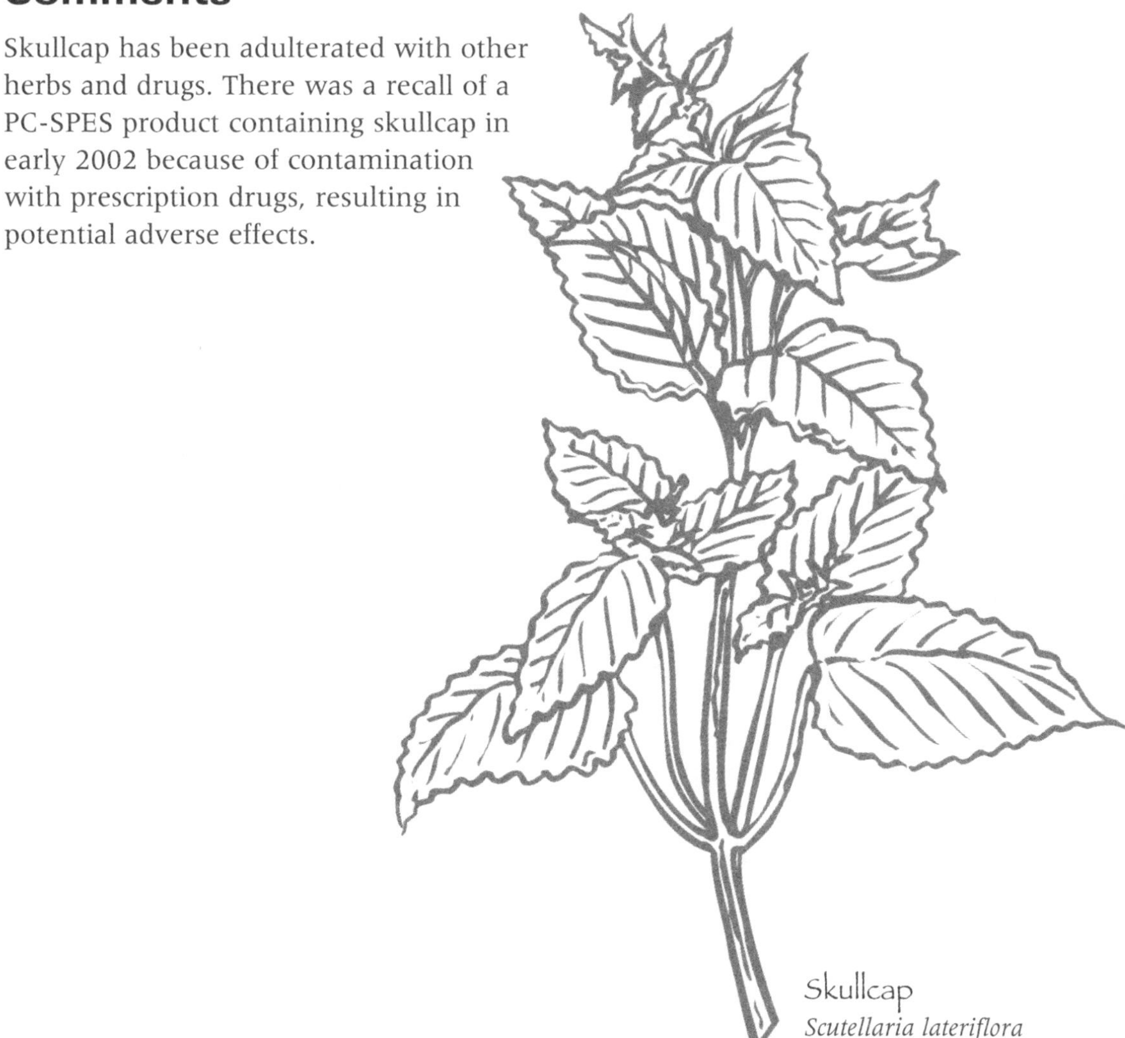

Skullcap
Scutellaria lateriflora

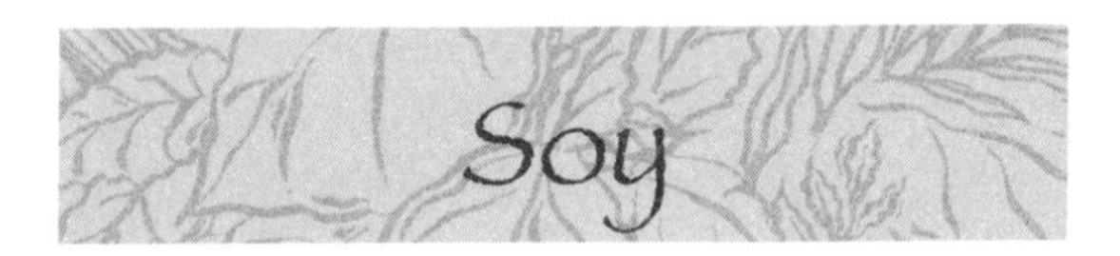

Profile

Common Names: Soybean, soya, tofu, soybean curd, soy protein, soy isoflavones
Family: Leguminosae (other members include beans and peas).
Genus & Species: *Glycine max*
Description: The soybean is an annual plant that looks and grows much like the familiar garden green bean. It can get up to 5 feet tall with stems, leaves and beans that are covered in small, fine hairs. The seeds generally come four to a pod.
Historical Use: Soy and its products have been a food staple in Asia for thousands of years. Chinese immigrants brought soybeans to America in the 1800s. Soybeans became a major agricultural crop, raised almost exclusively for livestock feed and export, until the 1970s, when its potential benefits for humans began to surface. Many of today's claims and research are based on what has been observed in the Asian population: relief of menopausal complaints and high blood cholesterol, prevention of osteoporosis, heart disease and more.
Parts Used: Seeds.

What It Does

May help reduce blood cholesterol when used in combination with a low-fat diet.

What It Might Help Treat

- Menopausal symptoms, including hot flashes
- Heart disease and osteoporosis in post-menopausal women

Research Insights

- Data associating breast cancer risk reduction with soy intake are promising, but are conflicting and controversial in both human and animal trials.
- The protective effect of soy against breast cancer appears to be strongest in individuals raised in Asia and who have immigrated to the United States. The same protective effect has not been observed in United States–born Asians.
- Animal studies and human intervention trials provide promising evidence regarding soy's potential for reducing the risk of prostate cancer; however, epidemiological studies do not support its use.

How It Is Used

Use the seeds, either fresh or dried, for food. Numerous commercial preparations that contain soy and its products are available in today's marketplace.

Growing

It is relatively easy to grow from seed, but requires considerable space to produce usable amounts in the home garden.

Harvesting

Pick pods when fully developed. Allow pods to dry on the vine and pick before frost when the plant has died and dried.

Preserving

Separate beans from pods. Dry in a well-ventilated area and store in a tightly sealed container when thoroughly dry.

Best Herbal Remedy Forms

Soy is best used as a food rather than a supplement. Some powdered soy products may be beneficial when used as directed for additives to foods and beverages.

Using Soy

- For lowering cholesterol, the typical recommended dose is 20 to 50 grams of soy protein a day.
- For reducing the severity of menopausal symptoms, including hot flashes, the typical dose is 20 to 60 grams of soy protein a day.
- For diarrhea in infants, soy-fortified formula that contains 18 to 20 grams of soy protein may be beneficial.

Safety & Effectiveness

Soy is believed to be safe when consumed in recommended amounts in food. Soy is considered effective for reducing cholesterol and possibly easing menopausal symptoms.

Interactions

Drugs. Soy's weak estrogenic properties may interfere with estrogen replacement therapy.
Other Herbs. No interactions are known to occur.
Foods. Soy protein isolate reduces the absorption of iron from non-animal products.
Vitamins or Minerals. No interactions are known to occur.

Effects In Laboratory Tests

None known.

Adverse Reactions

When taken internally, soy can cause GI upset including constipation if adequate fluids are not taken. Allergic reactions, including skin rash, have been seen in some people.

Who Should Not Use Soy

- People with asthma or allergic rhinitis, as they may be at risk for soy hull allergy.
- Soy may be contraindicated in breast cancer because of its estrogenic properties. Therapeutic use of soy should be approached cautiously in women with a personal or family history of breast cancer.
- Children with cystic fibrosis.
- People with hypothyroid disorders.
- Infants with elevated bilirubin levels.

Valerian

Profile

Common Names: Garden valerian, garden heliotrope, phu, all-heal, Mexican valerian, Pacific valerian
Family: Valerianaceae
Genus & Species: *Valeriana officinalis*
Description: Valerian is a clump-forming perennial with roots consisting of long cylindrical fibers growing out of its rhizomes. It grows to 5 feet in height with an erect, grooved and hollow stem. Its leaves are fernlike. Its blooms in the summer consist of small tubular pink or white flower clusters followed by tiny seeds with a tuft of white hairs.
Historical Use: Valerian's use can be traced back to Hippocrates, who prescribed it for insomnia. It was referred to in 1 C.E. as "phu" because of its offensive odor. Use in the 1500s and 1600s included treatment of epilepsy and the plague, and to stimulate menstruation, to treat women's hysteria (menstrual complaints), and for sores and wounds. Colonists found Native Americans using the American form of valerian to treat wounds. In Germany, valerian is an active ingredient in more than 100 over-the-counter medications and sleep aids.
Parts to Use: Rhizomes, roots and oil.

What It Does

The current use of valerian appears to be supported based on its long history in traditional and conventional medicine, phytochemical research, in vitro and in vivo experiments in animals and in some human clinical investigations. Most of the information is based on the use of pharmaceutical-grade products.

Valerian is a sedative and useful in treating anxiety. It calms a nervous stomach. Used as a bath additive, it relieves restlessness and sleep disorders. Extracts and essential oil of valerian are used as flavoring in foods and beverages.

What It Might Help Treat

- Epilepsy
- Tumors
- High blood pressure

Research Insights

Valerian may improve poor appetite. Taking valerian may reduce muscular pain and spasms. Valerian used by itself or in combination with other sedative herbs decreases the time it takes to fall asleep, improves sleep and decreases restlessness.

How It Is Used

Fresh or dried root or commercially prepared, standardized extracts.

Growing

Valerian is a hardy perennial and may be grown from seeds, root divisions or nursery stock. Once established, the plants propagate by self-seeding or through their root runners. As plants age, they lose their medicinal properties, so they should be thinned as they are harvested.

Harvesting

Dig rhizomes and roots in the fall of the second year, after the leaves have died.

Preserving

Dried.

Best Herbal Remedy Forms

Liquid extracts, infusions or teas, tinctures or dried root capsules.

Valerian
Valeriana officinalis

Making the Remedy & Dosage

- **Extract** or simple maceration is made by soaking 25 grams of chopped, preferably fresh root in 500 mL of cold water for 10 hours; strain. Drink 1 cup for anxiety or insomnia. These preparations have a foul taste that may need to be masked by the addition of 2 to 3 drops of peppermint water.
- **Tinctures,** 1:5. Begin with 15 to 20 drops in water and gradually increase, if necessary, to several times a day.
- **Tea** is prepared by steeping 2 to 3 grams of the root in 150 mL of hot, not boiling, water for 5 to 10 minutes and then straining. Take several times a day.
- **Dried root** maximum dose is 15 grams a day.
- **As a bath,** mix 100 grams of the root with 2 L of hot water; add to a full bath.
- For children and elderly adults, start with low-strength doses and increase the strength if necessary. Always consult with your physician prior to using herbal remedies.

Safety & Effectiveness

Valerian is considered safe when used in amounts commonly found in foods, when used orally and as recommended on a short-term basis for medicinal purposes. Excessive amounts of valerian may cause headache, blurred vision, restlessness, nausea and morning wooziness. Valerian is considered effective for insomnia. There is insufficient clinical data to support the other proposed uses.

Interactions

Drugs. Use with alcohol, barbiturates, benzodiazepines and other sedative drugs may compound the effects of these drugs resulting in adverse reactions. Studies have reported that valerian may interact with certain drugs metabolized by the same liver enzyme system as the herb. These include some calcium channel-blockers, chemotherapeutic agents, antifungals, glucocorticoids, proton pump inhibitors and allergy medications, to name a few.

Other Herbs. Use of valerian with herbs and supplements that have sedative properties may cause compounding or cumulative effects and adverse reactions to valerian or other drugs.

Foods. There are no known reported interactions or adverse reactions.

Vitamins or Minerals. Potential for decreased absorption of iron supplements due to formation of tannin-iron complex.

Effects In Laboratory Tests

There are no known medical or scientific reports of interactions or adverse reactions.

Adverse Reactions

- When taken orally, valerian has been observed to cause headache, excitability, uneasiness, cardiac disturbances and insomnia.
- Impaired alertness and information-processing has been reported, with impairment being dose-dependent and peaking within the first few hours after taking valerian. Persons should not drive or operate dangerous machinery after taking valerian.
- Signs of valerian toxicity include difficulty walking, hypothermia and increased muscle relaxation. Extended use can cause withdrawal symptoms when treatment is discontinued, so doses should be tapered slowly after extended use.
- There have been reports of liver toxicity in persons taking combination products containing valerian, and single valerian supplements.

Who Should Not Use Valerian

- Women who are pregnant and lactating because of insufficient safety and reliability information.
- Children under 2 years of age.

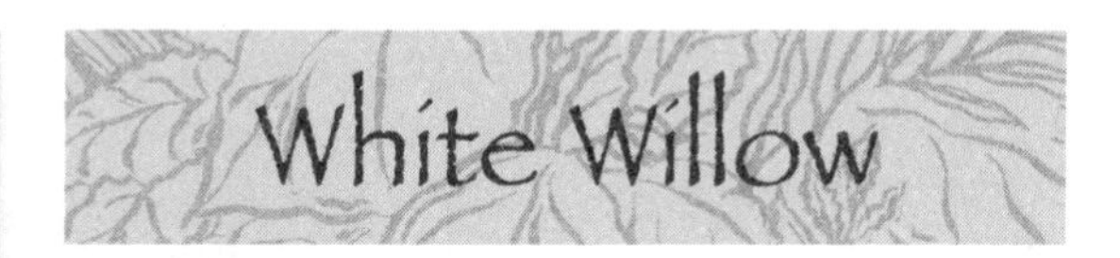

Profile

Common Names: Willow, white willow bark, salicin willow
Family: Salicaceae (other family members include poplars).
Genus & Species: *Salix alba*
Description: Willow is a deciduous tree or shrub that is common in wetlands and near watercourses. White willow is a large tree with deeply fissured bark, with a gray-brown color and long, thin leaves on flexible branches. Male flowers are yellow in color, while female flowers tend to have a more yellow-green color.
Historical Use: There are more than 300 species of willow trees found in North America and Europe. Several of the species possess medicinal value. However, the one referred to most often is white willow (*Salix alba*). Willow bark has been used since 500 B.C.E. for pain relief. Through the centuries, willow bark has been used for numerous ailments, including gout, warts, vomiting and fever. In the mid-1800s, salicin, the precursor of aspirin, was isolated from white willow. Despite the knowledge of white willow's properties, the first aspirin was actually made from meadowsweet, which contains the same chemical.
Parts to Use: Leaves and bark.

What It Does

It reduces fever and pain. It also reduces inflammation in joint disease.

What It Might Help Treat

- May be a substitute for aspirin in heart attack and stroke prevention.
- May help prevent certain kinds of cancers, although studies are preliminary at this time.
- Headaches.
- Menstrual cramps.

Research Insights

There have been no clinical trials evaluating its effectiveness in treating disorders other than fever and inflammation in the last 100 years. It is an analgesic pain killer, especially effective for back pain. White willow treats fevers. Used topically, willow bark may reduce symptoms of migraine headache.

How It Is Used

Fresh or dried.

Growing

White willow is a hardy tree that may grow up to 30 feet in height. It grows best where it can get plenty of water in deep soil and sun.

Harvesting

Harvest the leaves during the growing season. Bark may be removed throughout the summer; make sure the tree is not damaged by the bark's removal.

Preserving

Leaves may be used fresh or dried. Bark is dried.

Best Herbal Remedy Forms

Decoction, fluid extract, tincture, powder and infusion or tea.

Making the Remedy & Dosage

- **Fluid extracts** are generally purchased, as they are made to pharmaceutical specifications. A fluid extract can be made 1:1. Take 1 to 3 mL, 3 times a day.
- **Decoction** of 1 teaspoon powdered bark in 8 ounces cold water soaked for 8 hours, then strained. Drink up to 3 cups per day.

- **Tinctures,** 1:5. Take up to 15 mL, up to 3 times a day.
- **For a tea or infusion,** steep 1 to 3 grams of bark in 150 mL of hot, not boiling, water for 5 minutes, and strain. Take up to 3 or 4 times a day.
- **Leaf tea** may be made with 30 grams of dried, or 75 grams fresh, leaf steeped in 1 cup hot, not boiling, water for 10 minutes and strained. Drink after meals as needed.
- **Dried powdered bark** can be taken in doses up to 15 grams a day, in split doses of 3 grams each.

Safety & Effectiveness

White willow appears to be safe for adults when used up to 4 weeks in recommended amounts. White willow appears to be effective when used internally for conditions accompanied by fever, rheumatic ailments and headaches, although the effectiveness depends on the actual salicin content in the product.

Interactions

Drugs. It is unlikely that use of white willow will interact with antiplatelet or anticoagulant drugs. There is not enough information available to determine if there is enough salicylate in willow bark to cause drug interactions common to aspirin.

Other Herbs.

- Using white willow with other herbs that contain salicylates may increase their effects and potential for adverse reactions.
- Although evidence is only theoretical, using white willow with herbs that have anticoagulant or antiplatelet activity may increase risk of bleeding.
- Herbs such as willow bark contain high percentages of tannins, which might bind with other herbs and/or drugs and prevent their absorption.

Foods. There are no known reported interactions or adverse reactions.

Vitamins or Minerals. Theoretically, using white willow might interfere with absorption of some nutrients, particularly iron, due to the high tannin content of willow bark.

Effects In Laboratory Tests

There are no known medical or scientific reports of interactions or adverse reactions.

Adverse Reactions

- Plants with high tannin content are reported to have the potential to cause kidney damage.
- If you have aspirin hypersensitivity, asthma, active peptic ulcer disease, diabetes, gout, hemophilia, hypoprothrombinemia, kidney or liver disease, avoid white willow or use it cautiously.

Who Should Not Use White Willow

- Pregnant women, as there is insufficient information regarding its safety.
- Women who are nursing should not use willow bark, as it contains salicylates, which are excreted in breast milk and have been linked to rashes in breastfed infants.
- Children and youth under age 16 who have the flu or chicken pox should avoid willow bark because of the risk of Reye's syndrome.

Comments

The salicylate content of the species varies significantly. It is estimated that 1.5 gallons of willow bark tea a day is needed to obtain the pain relief of 4.5 grams of aspirin, which is the average daily dose used to treat arthritic-rheumatic disorders.

Witch Hazel

Profile

Common Names: Winterbloom, snapping hazelnut, hazel
Family: Hamamelidaceae
Genus & Species: *Hamamelis virginiana*
Description: Witch hazel is a bushy perennial herb with broad, oval leaves that turn yellow and drop in the fall. Flowers appear in clusters of two to four, followed by woody seedpods that survive the winter. The pods do not open until the plant begins to flower the next year, and then do so with a discernable pop that may propel their seeds up to 25 feet.
Historical Use: Witch hazel was a valuable treatment in Native American healing. It was used for various irritations and to stop internal bleeding, prevent miscarriages, treat colds, fevers, sore throats and menstrual pain. The branches of the plant were used for making bows.
Parts to Use: Leaves, branches and bark.

What It Does

When used topically, it provides temporary relief for itching, irritations and burning due to disorders around the anus, including hemorrhoids.

What It Might Help Treat

- May help treat minor skin injuries, local skin and mucous membrane inflammation.
- May help relieve inflammation of varicose veins.
- Minor sunburn.

Research Insights

May be effective for the treatment of sunburns.

How It Is Used

Orally or topically. Topically for minor skin irritations. Internally as a gargle for inflammation of the throat and to treat diarrhea.

Witch Hazel
Hamamelis virginiana

Growing

Witch hazel grows from seeds or cut twigs. Seeds do best if refrigerated prior to their planting; they may take up to 2 years to germinate. It likes moist, rich, sandy soil best but will tolerate other conditions.

Harvesting

Cut branches and twigs in the spring. Pick leaves in summer.

Preserving

Dry leaves and plant parts in a well-ventilated area and store in a tightly sealed container when thoroughly dry.

Best Herbal Remedy Forms

Tea, dried leaves, compresses and commercially prepared products.

Making the Remedy & Dosage

- **Teas** can be made with 2 grams of dried leaves steeped for 5 to 10 minutes in 150 mL boiling water then strained. Take 3 times a day.
- **Dried leaves** can be taken orally in 2-gram doses, 3 times a day. These dried leaves may be put in capsule form to make them easier and more convenient to take.
- A **compress** for topical applications is made using 5 to 10 grams of leaf and bark in 250 mL of water. Soak a clean cloth in the solution and apply to the affected area.

Safety & Effectiveness

Witch hazel is considered safe when used externally and as directed. Oral preparations may be safe if used as directed. Witch hazel is effective when the solution is applied topically for relief of itching, burning and irritations, especially around the anal area.

Interactions

Drugs. No interactions are known to occur.
Other Herbs. No interactions are known to occur.
Foods. No interactions are known to occur.
Vitamins or Minerals. No interactions are known to occur.

Effects In Laboratory Tests

None known.

Adverse Reactions

- When taken internally, can cause GI upset especially if taken in amounts greater than 1 gram. Large amounts may cause nausea, vomiting and possibly fecal impaction.
- In rare cases, liver damage has been known to occur.
- May cause contact dermatitis

Who Should Not Use Witch Hazel

Avoid using internally during pregnancy and lactation because of insufficient reliable information about its safety.

Culinary Herbs & Spices

Not only do herbs have a long history as medicinals, but they are also important in the kitchen. Different from herbs, spices are difficult to define and the two are often confused. Spices tend to come from tropical plants (but not always) and are the dried parts of plants including buds, bark, roots, stems and seeds. Garlic and ginger are thought of as an herb, but they could be a spice as well because they represent the root and rhizome rather than the herbaceous or leafy parts of the plant. As you will discover in the pages that follow, spices, along with herbs, offer some interesting possibilities for health enhancement.

Preserving Your Bounty

Most herbs and some spices used for cooking can be preserved in the same manner: drying or freezing. Rather than discussing the method under each herb, the methods of preserving are described here.

Rosemary
Rosmarinus officinalis

Harvesting

- Pick herbs at their peak of flavor, which is usually just before they bloom.
- Remember that the flowers of some herbs are very flavorful.
- Before using or preserving the herbs, wash them and pat them dry with a paper towel.
- If the stems of the herbs are woody, strip the leaves from them.
- If stems are soft and pliable, use them, too; they are very flavorful.

Freezing Herbs

Option 1

Herbs that freeze well are basil, chives, dill, fennel, oregano, parsley, peppermint, rosemary, sage, tarragon and thyme. Wash and dry them thoroughly. Chop with a knife or cut into small pieces with scissors. Place them in a sealable plastic bag, squeezing out as much air as possible, label and freeze. They can be stored in screw-top jars as well.

Option 2

Chop herbs very fine. Place about 1 tablespoon of herb in each section of an ice cube tray, cover with water and freeze. Whole leaves and flowers can also be frozen. When solid, transfer cubes to a sealable plastic bag, label and return to the freezer.

Drying Herbs

Microwave

Wash the leaves, pat dry and place between paper towels. Dry the herbs on your microwave's lowest power setting for 2 to 3 minutes. Allow to cool. Store the herb in tightly covered containers, preferably glass jars.

Oven

Wash the herbs and blot them dry. Remove leaves from the stems. Place herbs in a single layer on baking sheets. Place in an oven heated to 100°F, propping the door open to let moisture escape. After 2 hours, check to see if they are dry. If not, continue drying, checking periodically, and remove the leaves before they turn brown. Cool herbs and store in tightly covered containers, preferably glass jars.

Tips

- Avoid storing herbs and spices near a window or above the stove. Air, heat and light shorten their flavor.
- When substituting dried herbs for fresh, 1 teaspoon of dried equals 1 tablespoon of fresh.

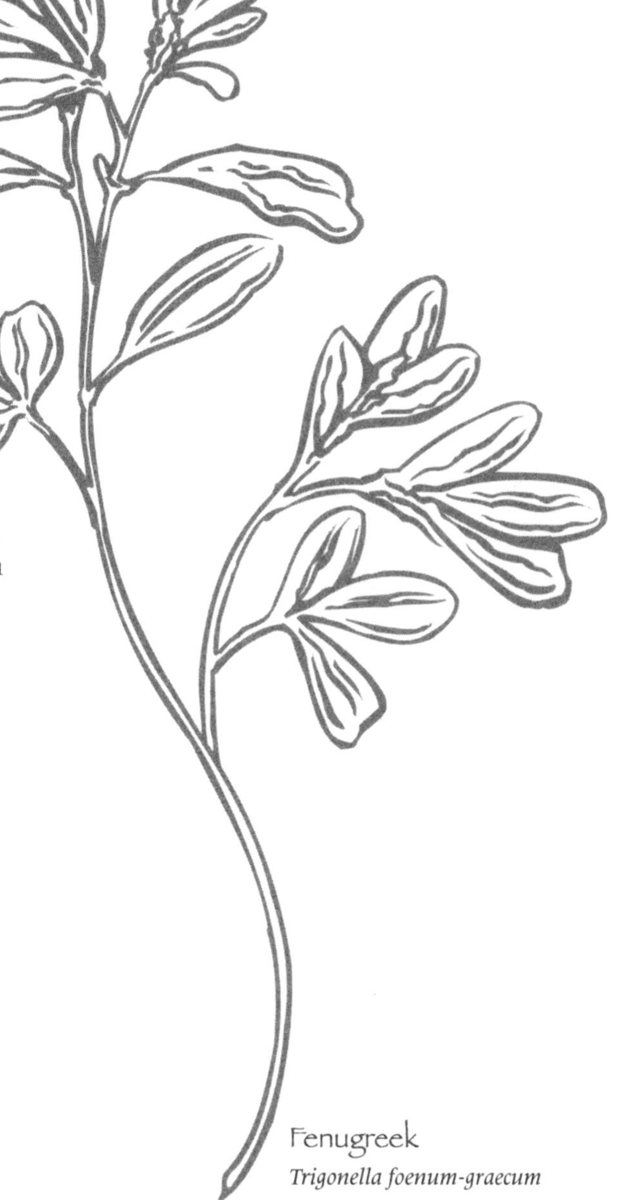

Fenugreek
Trigonella foenum-graecum

Artichoke

Profile

Common Name: Globe artichoke
Family: Asteraceae/Compositae; other family members are chamomile, feverfew, echinacea and milk thistle.
Genus & Species: *Cynara scolymus*
Description: Artichokes are giant clump-forming perennials with gray-green, leather leaves. When allowed to flower, they look like their cousin the milk thistle, with blue-violet flowers.
Historical Use: Artichokes are thought of as a vegetable rather than an herb. Their history goes back at least 2,000 years. Artichoke leaf has been used to stimulate bile and as a diuretic in traditional European medicine since Roman times. During the 1700s and 1800s in Europe, it was used to treat jaundice, liver disease, arthritis and urinary tract infections.
Parts to Use: Leaves, roots and flower heads.

What It Does

Artichoke stimulates bile secretion. It reduces symptoms of diseases of the liver or bile duct (bloating, gas, abdominal pain and nausea). It contains antioxidants that protect the liver from free-radical damage. It is used as a food.

What It Might Help Treat

High cholesterol.

Research Insights

Research supports the use of artichoke as a bile stimulant, liver protectant and for digestive upsets.

How It Is Used

Fresh, dried or as a purchased extract.

Growing

Artichoke is available in supermarkets and grocery stores. It is grown primarily in California, Texas and Florida, where the nighttime temperatures do not get below 20°F. It can be cultivated elsewhere with care, but it is not a hardy plant.

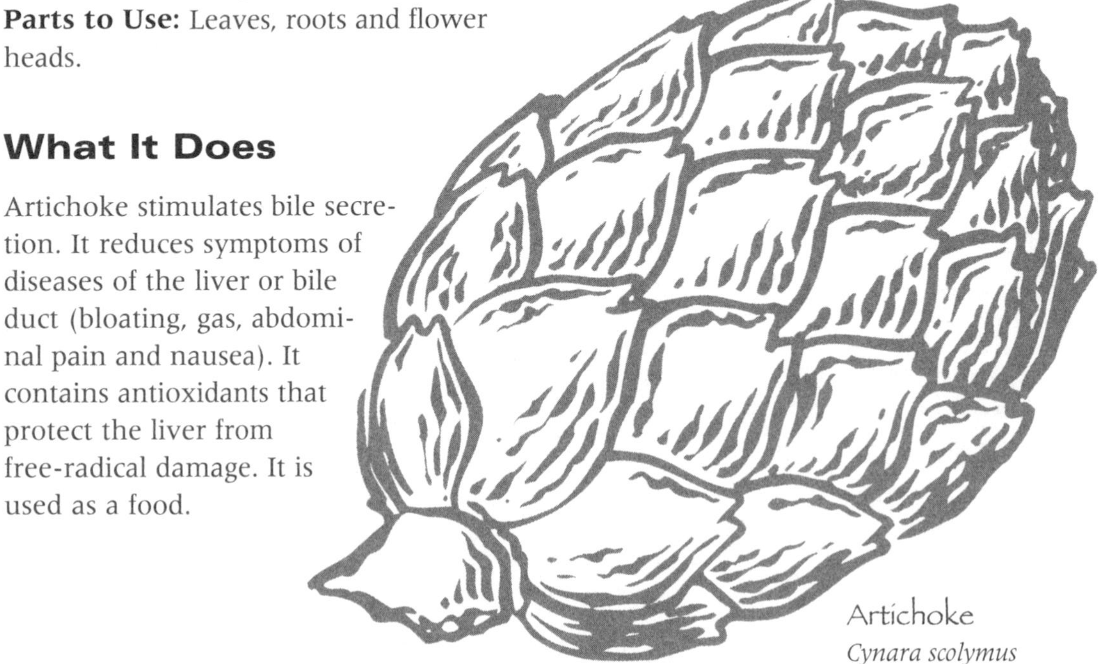

Artichoke
Cynara scolymus

Best Herbal Remedy Forms

Fresh or dried.

Making the Remedy & Dosage

- **Artichoke root** may be dug and dried as any other root. Use 1 to 4 grams, 3 times a day.
- Dry leaf **extract** that is purchased in a ratio of 12:1 is dosed at 500 mg a day. Standardized extracts contain 2.5 to 15 percent 3-caffeoylquinic acid (including cynarin).

Safety & Effectiveness

Artichoke is safe when used in the amounts found in foods. Both artichoke leaf and extract have been effective in treating the feeling of fullness after meals and with bile duct disease. It has also been effective in relieving nausea, vomiting, gas and abdominal pain.

Interactions

No interactions with drugs, other herbs, foods, vitamins or minerals, or adverse effects in laboratory tests have been known to occur. There is no reason to believe that such reactions will occur when used as a food or in appropriate medicinal amounts.

Adverse reactions

People with allergies to other members of the Asteraceae/Compositae family may be allergic to artichokes.

Who Should Not Use Artichoke

- People with bile duct obstruction and/or gallstones.
- There are no suggested limits when consumed as a food; however, persons with bile duct obstruction or gallbladder disease would do well to limit or avoid eating artichokes.
- Women who are pregnant or lactating should avoid using artichoke as an herbal medicinal.

Basil

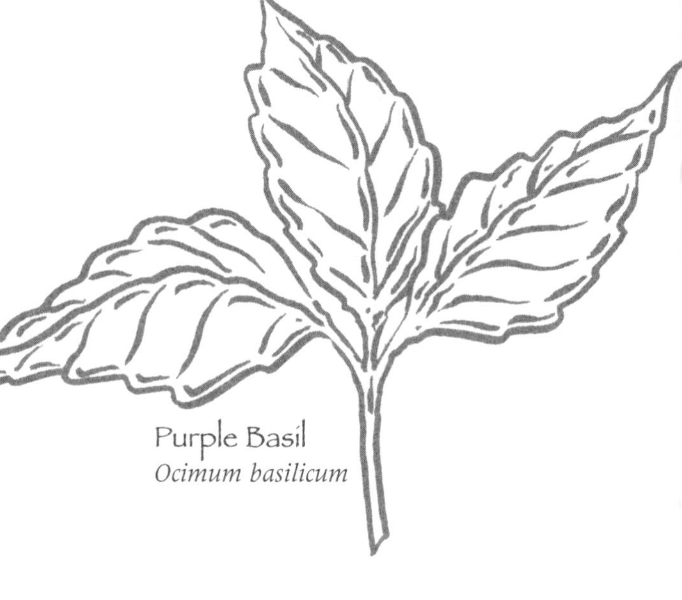

Profile

Common Names: Common basil, holy basil, sweet basil
Family: Labiatae/Lamiaceae
Genus & Species: *Ocimum basilicum*
Description: *Ocimum basilicum,* the most common basil, is a short-lived perennial that stands erect, has many branches with oval bright green, purple or variegated purple and green leaves. Its flowers are white.
Historical Use: There are about 25 species that belong to the same genus. Some basils are important in folklore and religion. In Hindu homes, it is grown for its protective influence. One tropical American member known as the mosquito bush is used to repel its namesake.
Parts to Use: Leaves.

What It Does

It is a rich source of vitamin C, calcium, magnesium, potassium and iron. It repels insects. It relieves gas or bloating.

What It Might Help Treat

There is insufficient information about the effectiveness of basil in treating conditions other than those mentioned.

Research Insights

No clinical trials on the medicinal properties of basil are known.

How It Is Used

Fresh or dried. Fresh in sauces or teas. Dried as a seasoning or a tea.

Growing

Basil is relatively easy to grow, if you have the right conditions. It prefers a rich, light, well-drained to dry soil. Growing tips should be pinched out to encourage bushiness and delay flowering.

Best Herbal Remedy Forms

Teas. Fresh in sauces as pesto and in salads.

Making the Remedy & Dosage

Tea may be made by steeping 2 to 4 grams of leaf in 150 mL of water for 10 to 15 minutes and straining. Drink 1 cup, up to 3 times a day, for up to 8 days, then stop for 14 days and resume.

Safety & Effectiveness

When the leaves are used as a spice in cooking it is considered safe. Basil has GRAS status as a food ingredient in the United States. There is insufficient information regarding effectiveness of basil for medicinal purposes.

Interactions

No interactions with drugs, other herbs, foods, vitamins or minerals, or adverse effects in laboratory tests have been known to occur. There is no reason to believe that such reactions will occur when used as a food or in appropriate medicinal amounts.

Adverse Reactions

- Basil has been known to cause low blood sugar.
- Basil essential oil should not be used, as it is believed to be carcinogenic.

Who Should Not Use Basil

- There are no contraindications when basil is used as a culinary herb.
- Neither very young children nor pregnant or lactating women should take the essential oil.

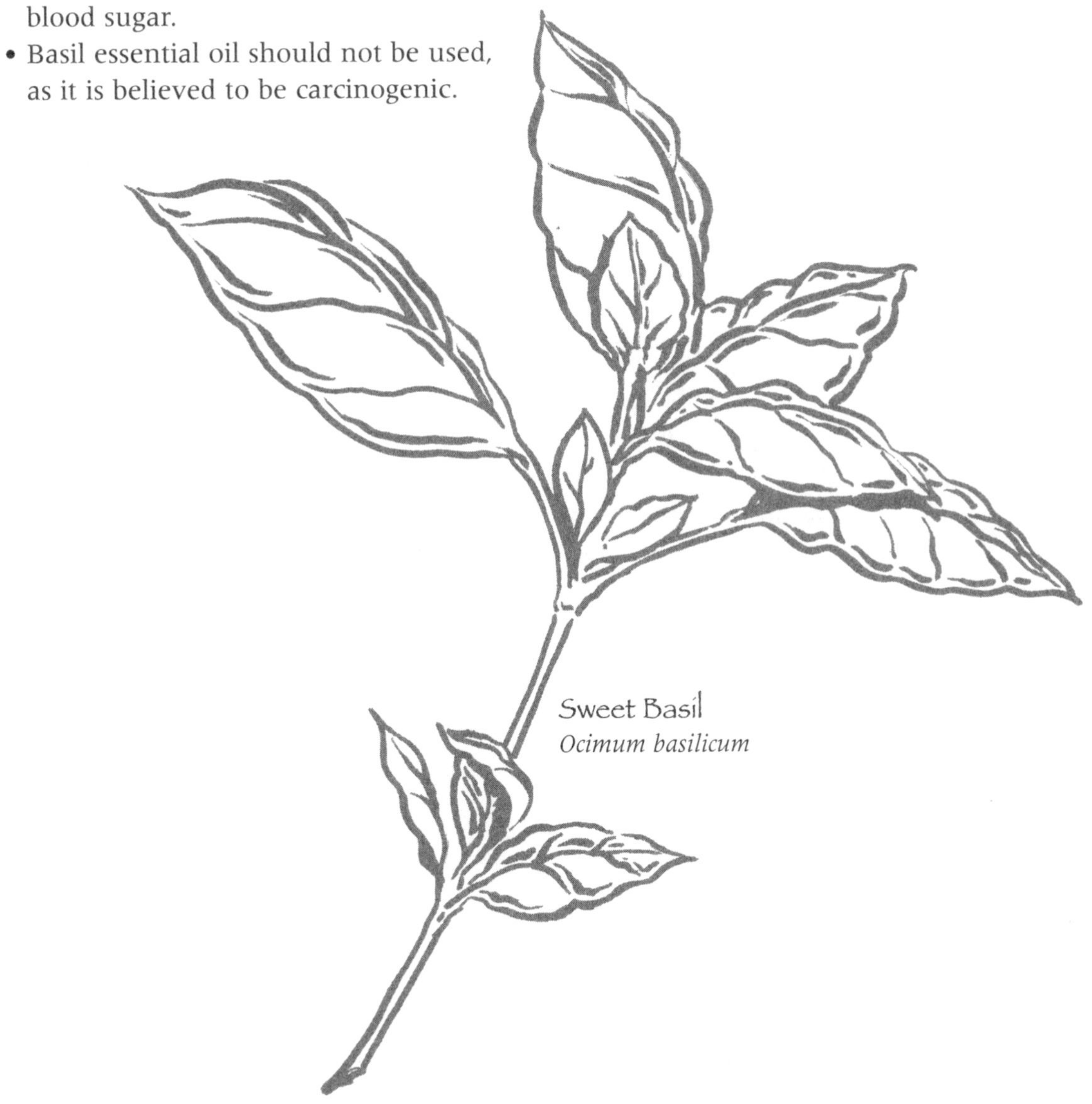

Sweet Basil
Ocimum basilicum

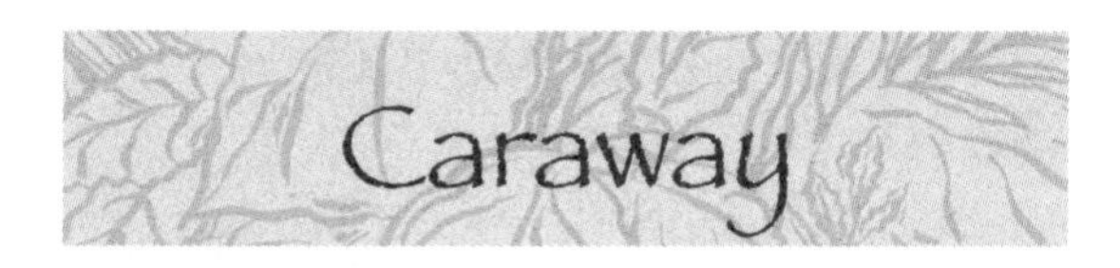

Profile

Common Names: Carvi fructus, cumin des Pres, Kummel, semen cumini
Family: Apiaceae/Umbelliferae
Genus & Species: *Carum carvi*
Description: Caraway is an erect biennial with hollow stems and fern-like leaves. Tiny, white-to-pink rayed flowers give rise to aromatic five-ribbed seeds (fruits).
Historical Use: Traditionally, caraway has been used as an expectorant, to relieve menstrual complaints, to stimulate milk flow in nursing mothers, for incontinence and as a mouthwash. The seeds are used as a spice; the oil is used for flavoring in pharmaceuticals. In folklore, caraway was thought to prevent the theft of any item that contained the seed and to keep lovers from losing interest in each other.
Parts to Use: Leaves, roots, seeds and oil.

What It Does

Caraway relieves gas. It eases spastic conditions of the GI tract including bloating and fullness. It stimulates the appetite. Its oil may relieve mild GI spasms, flatulence and fullness.

What It Might Help Treat

There is insufficient information about the effectiveness of caraway in treating conditions other than those mentioned.

Research Insights

No clinical trials on the medicinal properties of caraway are known.

How It Is Used

Dried seeds or commercially purchased oil.

Growing

Caraway is relatively easy to grow. It is hardy and will self-seed if the fruits are not picked after they ripen.

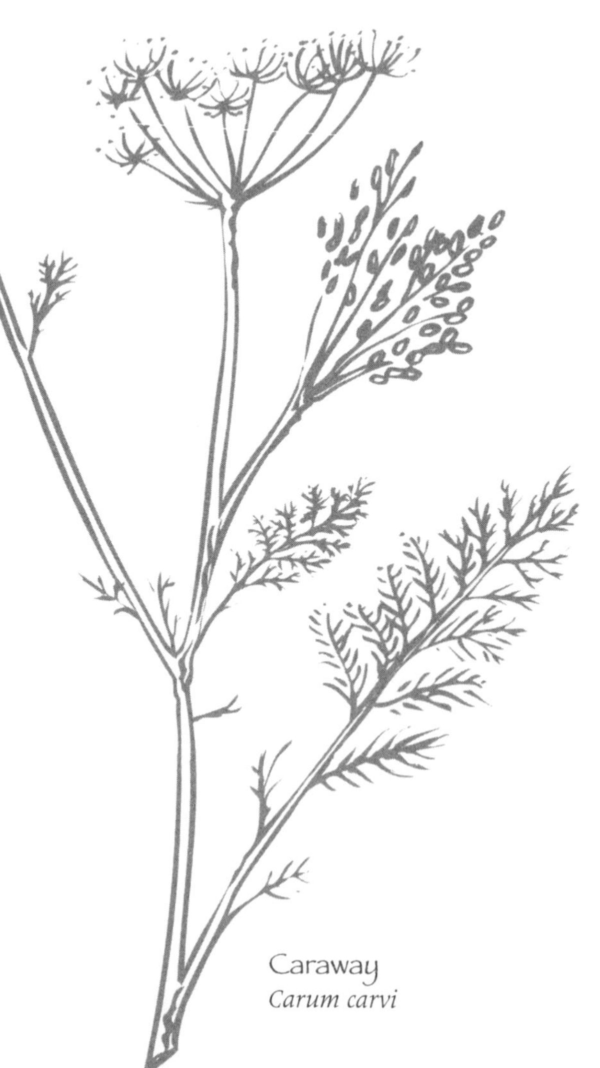

Caraway
Carum carvi

Best Herbal Remedy Forms

Crushed fruits (seeds), tea or commercially prepared oil.

Making the Remedy & Dosage

- **Chew** 1½ to 6 grams of seed for indigestion, 2 to 4 times a day.
- **Tea** is made by steeping 1 to 2 teaspoons of freshly crushed seed in 150 mL hot, not boiling, water for 10 minutes. Strain. Drink 2 to 4 cups a day. The dose for infants and small children is 1 teaspoonful of the tea 2 to 4 times per day.
- The dose for **caraway oil** is 3 to 6 drops per day.

Safety & Effectiveness

Caraway seed and oil are considered safe when used in amounts commonly found in foods and when taken for medicinal purposes as recommended. Caraway is GRAS and approved for food and flavoring in the United States. The seeds and oil are thought to be effective when taken orally for digestive upset, including spasms, gas and fullness, and to stimulate the appetite. Before giving any amount of caraway to children, consult with your healthcare provider.

Interactions

No interactions with drugs, other herbs, foods, vitamins or minerals, or adverse effects in laboratory tests have been known to occur. There is no reason to believe that such reactions will occur when used as a food or in appropriate medicinal amounts.

Adverse Reactions

Caraway plant and oil can cause skin irritation.

Who Should Not Use Caraway

Women who are pregnant or lactating should not use caraway in amounts that exceed what is commonly eaten in food. Caraway oil should be avoided because there is insufficient data regarding its safety.

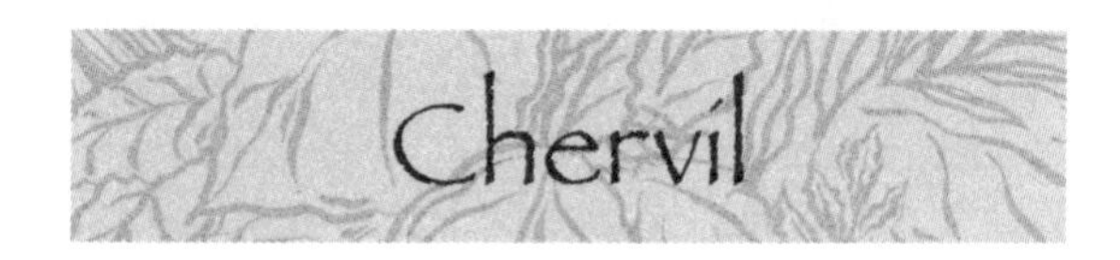

Profile

Common Names: Golden chervil, salad chervil
Family: Apiaceae/Umbelliferae
Genus & Species: *Anthriscus cerefolium*
Description: Chervil grows up to 2 feet tall with hollow, furrowed stems and delicate, bright green leaves. In the summer, it bears tiny white flowers followed by linear fruits.
Historical Use: Chervil has been used since Roman times and has been considered indispensable for culinary and medicinal purposes. In ancient times, it was considered a spring tonic and good for poor memory and mental depression.
Parts to Use: Leaves.

What It Does

Its medicinal uses are based on folklore and historical use. It has been used as a diuretic, expectorant and digestive aid, and to treat rheumatism, jaundice and high blood pressure. The juice pressed from the leaves has been used for eczema, gout and abscesses. It is used as a flavoring agent in foods and beverages.

What It Might Help Treat

There are no known studies or reliable information on the effectiveness of chervil for any specific condition.

Research Insights

The edible parts of chervil are rich in calcium and potassium.

How It Is Used

Fresh or dried.

Growing

Relatively easy to grow. Prefers cooler climates. May be sown from seed in early spring.

Best Herbal Remedy Forms

Fresh in foods or as tea. The delicate flavor of anise that is characteristic to chervil does not withstand drying or long cooking.

Making the Remedy & Dosage

Tea is made using 1 teaspoon fresh or dried herb to 1 cup hot, not boiling, water. Drink 1 cup per day, consumed a mouthful at a time.

Safety & Effectiveness

There is insufficient information on chervil's safety as a medicinal herb. A major constituent of the oil, estragole, is reported to produce tumors in mice. Chervil has GRAS status in the United States and is considered safe when used in amounts found in foods.

Interactions

No interactions with drugs, other herbs, foods, vitamins or minerals, or adverse effects in laboratory tests have been known to occur. There is no reason to believe that such reactions will occur when used as a food or in appropriate medicinal amounts.

Adverse Reactions

None reported.

Who Should Not Use Chervil

Women who are pregnant or lactating should avoid amounts exceeding what is used in foods and the volatile oil due to its potential to be mutagenic.

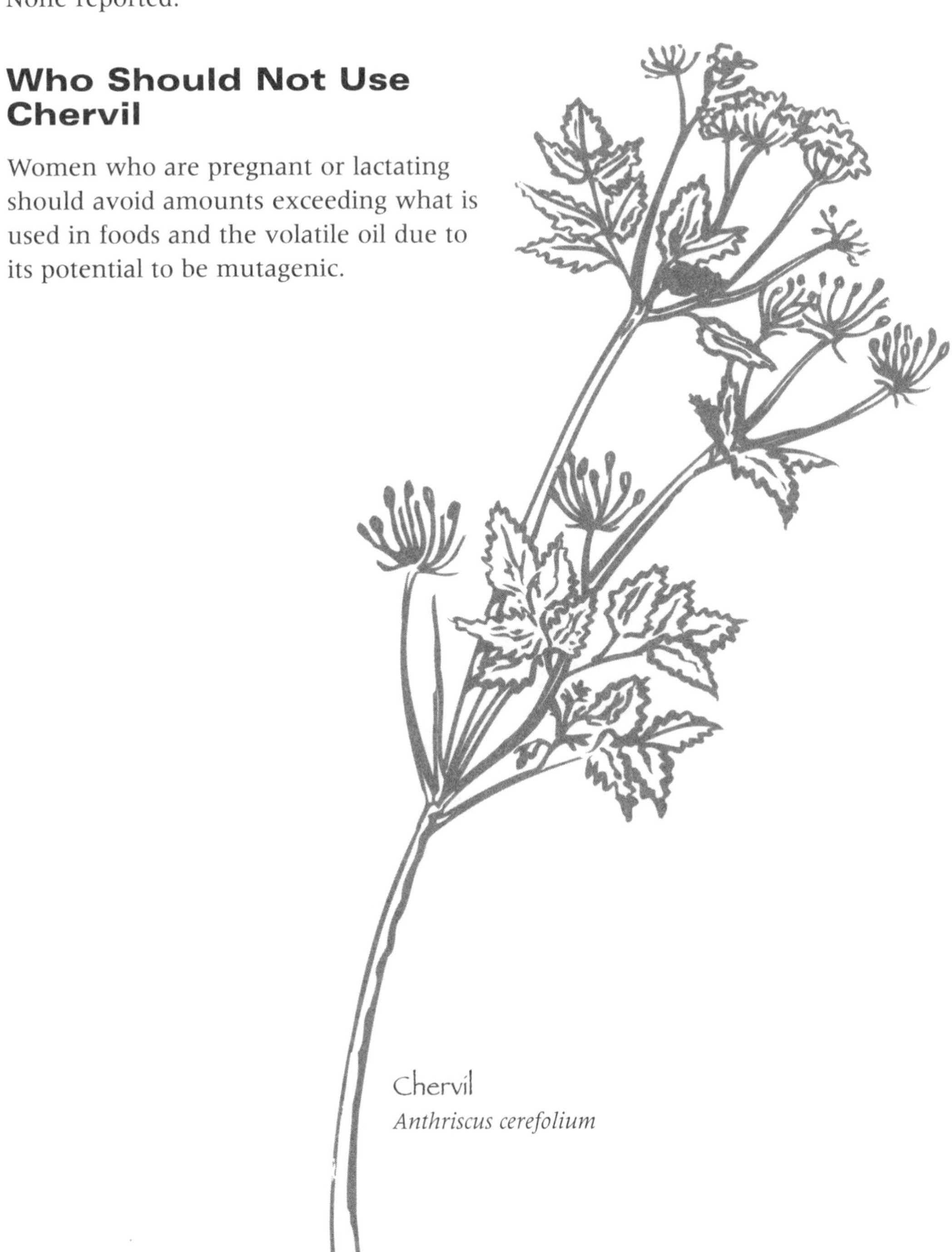

Chervil
Anthriscus cerefolium

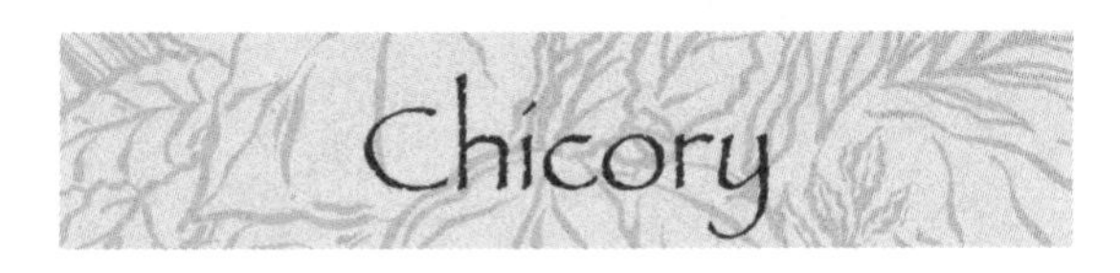

Chicory

Profile

Common Names: Wild chicory, blue sailors, Cichorii Radix
Family: Asteraceae/Compositae; members of this family include daisies, chamomile, marigolds and other herbs.
Genus & Species: *Chichorium intybus*
Historical Use: Chicory was grown as a vegetable in Roman times. The leaves and roots have completely different qualities and purposes. As a folk medicine, it has been used as a laxative for children and irregular heartbeats in adults. It is used as a flavoring component in foods and beverages. The roasted root is ground and used to enhance the richness in coffee and is particularly popular in the southern United States. Within the species are several radicchio-type plants that are used in salads or cooked as a vegetable.
Description: Chicory is a tall clump-forming perennial with a thick taproot. Its flowers are sky-blue to violet and occasionally pink or white. It is often seen growing along roadsides in the summer.
Parts to Use: Leaves, roots, flowers.

What It Does

It has a mild laxative effect. It slows the heart rate. It stimulates bile production. It has a sedative effect.

What It Might Help Treat

There are no known studies or reliable information on the effectiveness of chicory for any specific condition other than those listed.

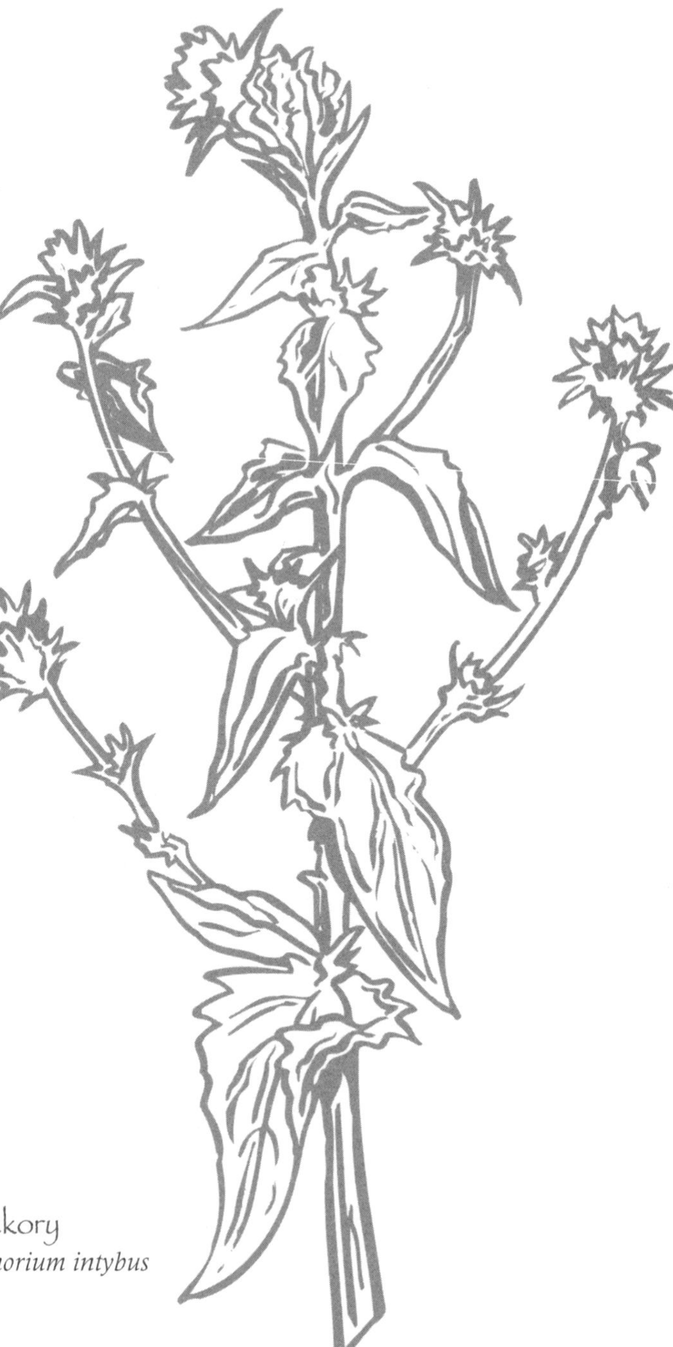

Chickory
Chichorium intybus

Research Insights

The edible parts of chicory are rich in beta-carotene.

How It Is Used

Fresh or dried.

Growing

Chicory is hardy and has been naturalized in North America. It may self-seed and become a weed in dry, alkaline soil.

Best Herbal Remedy Forms

Fresh leaves and flowers for culinary use, dried root for beverages.

Making the Remedy & Dosage

- **Tea** is made by steeping 4 to 6 grams of the root in 1 cup of boiling water for 10 minutes, then straining. Enjoy up to 2 cups per day.
- **Ground chicory root** may also be added to ground coffee before brewing. Allow about 5 grams per cup of water in addition to the ground coffee.

Safety & Effectiveness

Chicory is considered safe when taken in amounts commonly found in foods. It has GRAS status for food use in the United States. It is believed to be effective as an appetite stimulant and for GI distress.

Interactions

No interactions with drugs, other herbs, foods, vitamins or minerals, or adverse effects in laboratory tests have been known to occur. There is no reason to believe that reactions will occur when used as a food or in appropriate medicinal amounts.

Adverse Reactions

- Handling the plant may cause skin rash or eruptions.
- People allergic to other members of the Asteraceae/Compositae family may be allergic to chicory.

Who Should Not Use Chicory

- Women who are pregnant should not use chicory, as there is some concern that it can promote menstruation or miscarriage.
- Women who are lactating should avoid chicory, as there is insufficient reliable information about its effects on infants.
- People with gallstones should avoid chicory because of its bile-stimulating effects.
- People who are allergic to members of the Asteraceae/Compositae family, including daisies and chamomile.

Comments

Chicory can be contaminated, particularly if picked at a roadside, with bacteria, fungicides or herbicides.

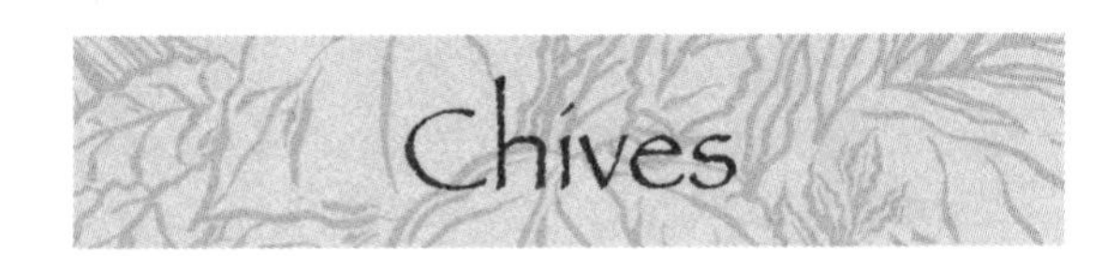

Culinary Herbs

Profile

Common Name: Chives
Family: Liliaceae; other members of this family include onions, garlic
Genus & Species: *Allium schoenoprasum*
Description: Chives are clump-forming perennials with slender leaves and bulbs. They produce pale pink to purple globe-like clusters of flowers in the summer. Chives thrive best when their tops are clipped back for regular culinary use.
Historical Use: Chives have been used for approximately 5,000 years. Their use has been primarily culinary. Chives have many of the same components as other family members, but are much milder. It would take large amounts of chives to produce measurable, if any, medicinal benefits.
Parts to Use: Leaves, flowers and bulbs.

What It Does

There is insufficient information regarding medicinal uses of chives. It is used as a food ingredient and flavoring. It has been used to treat parasitic worms, but information on this use is limited.

What It Might Help Treat

There are no known studies or reliable information on the effectiveness of chives for any specific condition. Theoretically, chives may have some of the same benefits as other family members, garlic and onions.

How It Is Used

For home use, chives are best used fresh, but may be frozen to use in cooked dishes. Commercially dried chives retain their flavor much better than home-dried chives.

Growing

Chives are relatively easy to grow and are a hardy perennial. They may be sown from seed in early spring. They will self-seed if allowed to.

Best Herbal Remedy Forms

Chives are not typically used as an herbal medicine.

Safety & Effectiveness

Chives are safe for consumption in almost any amount. There are no known safety considerations with chives. Chives are not typically used as an herbal medicine, so effectiveness has not been an issue.

Interactions

No interactions with drugs, other herbs, foods, vitamins or minerals, or adverse effects on laboratory tests have been known to occur. There is no reason to believe that such reactions will occur when used as a food or in appropriate medicinal amounts.

Adverse Reactions

Consuming large amounts of chives may cause stomach upset.

Who Should Not Use Chives

It is safe to consume chives during pregnancy and lactation in moderate amounts. There are no known adverse reactions, but there is insufficient data available.

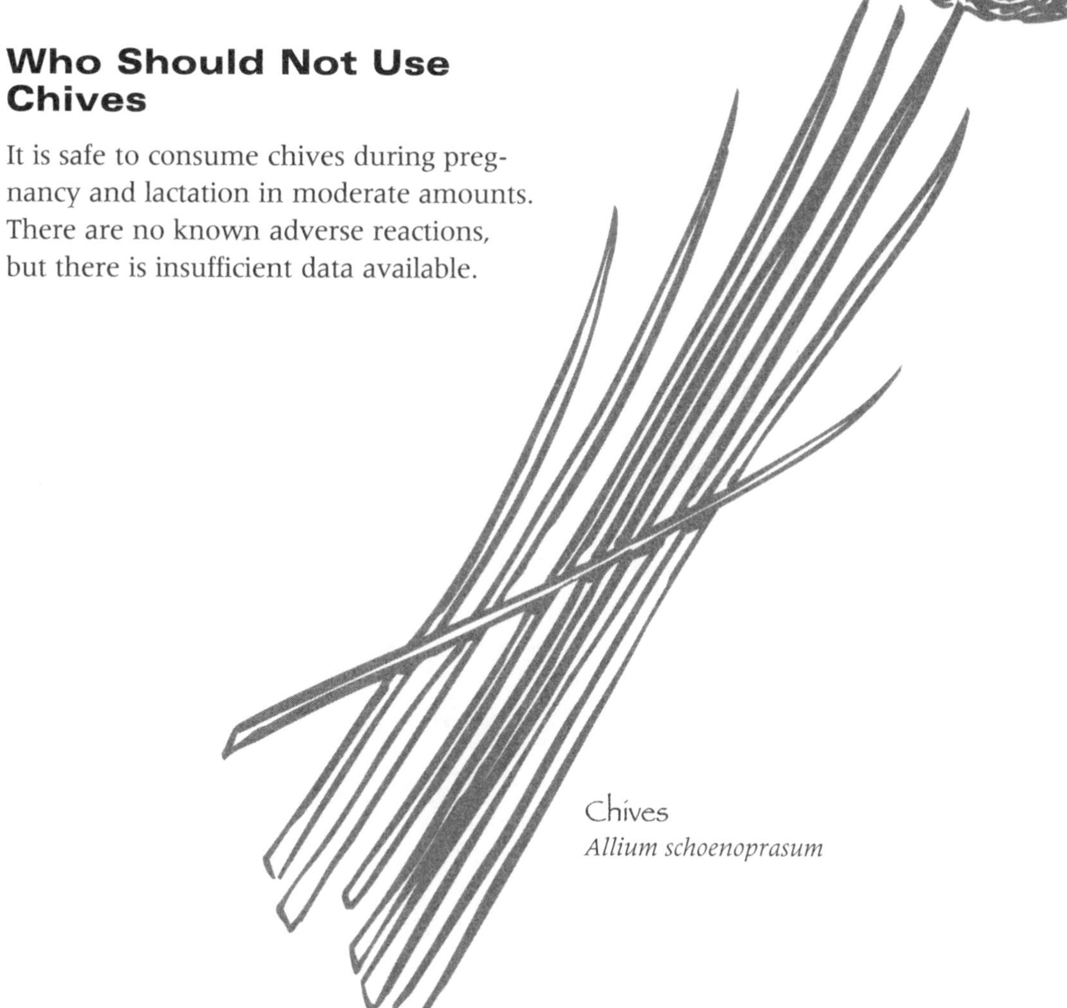

Chives
Allium schoenoprasum

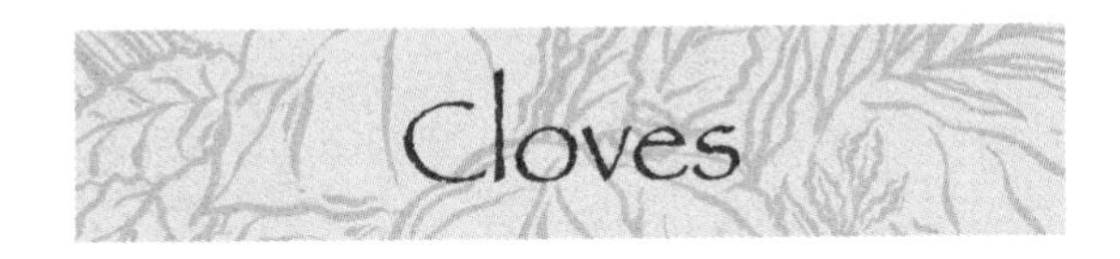

Profile

Common Names: Clavos, caryophyluss
Family: Myrtaceae; other family members include tea tree and eucalyptus.
Genus & Species: *Eugenia caryophillata; syzygium aromaticum*
Description: It is a small, busy evergreen with upward branches and shiny, oval, aromatic leaves. Its flowers are fragrant and give rise to aromatic purple berries.
Historical Use: Clove is the bud of a very aromatic Asian tropical evergreen tree that has been used since before 2200 B.C.E. Cloves have been traditionally used for indigestion, bad breath, diarrhea and fungal infections. It is used as a flavoring in foods and beverages worldwide.
Parts to Use: Berries and oil.

What It Does

As part of a topical multi-herb compound used for treating premature ejaculation. Oil is used in dental applications as a topical analgesic and also used for mouth and throat inflammation. It is used for treating dry socket after tooth extraction.

What It Might Help Treat

- Digestive tract upset
- Parasites
- Infections
- As a complement to medications used for hay fever

Research Insights

There appears to be insufficient reliable information regarding the use of clove for other ailments.

How It Is Used

Cloves, flowerbud, stem, leaf, clove oil.

Growing

Clove does not grow in the United States.

Best Herbal Remedy Forms

- Fluid extract
- Dried
- Food flavoring

Making the Remedy & Dosage

- Dried, ground **clove buds** in doses of 120 to 300 mg a day.
- **Clove oil** is an essential oil and should not be used internally if undiluted. Commercially prepared products with known amounts of clove oil appear safest to use. Read label directions carefully. A typical dose is 5 to 30 drops of oil containing fluid extract or ½ to 1 ounce of mouth rinse containing clove oil.

Safety & Effectiveness

Cloves have GRAS status in the United States. Cloves and clove oil are believed to be safe when used topically and as recommended. Cloves and clove oil are considered safe when taken orally in amounts commonly found in food. Undiluted clove oil should not be used orally or topically. Clove oil is considered effective when used topically as an analgesic for inflammation of the mouth and throat. May also be helpful for dry socket resulting from tooth extraction. Clove cigarettes are sometimes used as an alternative to tobacco for persons wishing to quit smoking.

Interactions

Drugs. Anticoagulant or antiplatelet drug effects may be enhanced when used with cloves.
Other Herbs. Anticoagulant or antiplatelet herb effects may be enhanced when used with clove.
Foods. No known interactions.
Vitamins or Minerals. No known interactions.

Effects in Laboratory Tests

No known adverse effects.

Adverse Reactions

- Cloves can cause respiratory distress when inhaled. Deaths and injuries have been reported when clove cigarettes have been used improperly.
- Multi-ingredient products containing cloves have resulted in adverse effects when applied to the penis for ejaculation problems.
- Clove oil, used internally, can cause CNS depression, seizures and liver problems, and can irritate mucous membranes.
- Topical use of clove oil may irritate the skin.

Who Should Not Use Cloves and Oil

- People with blood platelet problems.
- During pregnancy and lactation, women should avoid using amounts greater than found in foods.

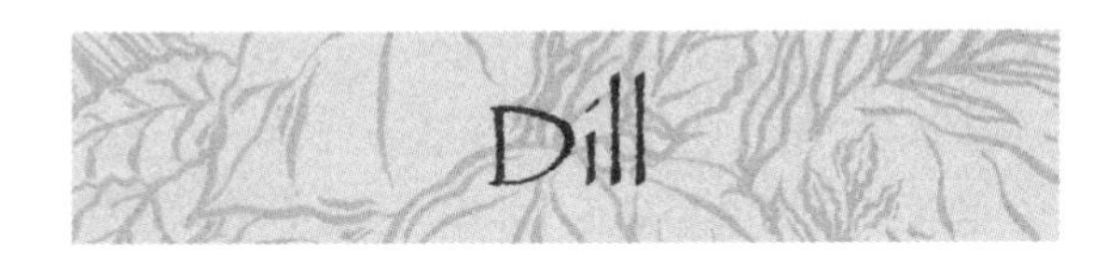

Profile

Common Names: Dill weed, dill seed
Family: Apiaceae/Umbelliferae
Genus & Species: *Anetheum graveolens*
Description: Dill is an annual or biennial that has one upright hollow stem with thin leaves divided into thread-like segments. Its flowers appear at the top of the stem. They are yellow and followed by oval aromatic seeds.
Historical Use: Dill has played an important role as a medicinal herbal since Biblical times. Ancient Jewish law, the Talmud, records that dill was subject to a tithe. In the Middle Ages, it was used as a charm against witchcraft. It has been used for GI upset, gas and stomach distention, to induce sleep in babies with colic, and stimulate milk flow. Dill is used as a culinary spice. The oil is used as a fragrance ingredient in cosmetics.
Parts to Use: Leaves and seeds.

How It Is Used

Fresh or dried.

Growing

Dill is easy to grow. Sow seeds in late fall or early spring. If it's left to bloom and the seeds go unpicked, dill may turn up where you least expect—or want—it.

Best Herbal Remedy Forms

Fresh or dried, above-ground parts and seed. Essential oil may be available for purchase commercially.

Making the Remedy & Dosage

- Chew 1 teaspoon of **dill seed** for a fresher breath up to 3 times daily.
- **Teas** may be made by adding 2 teaspoons of bruised seeds to 1 cup of boiling water. Drink up to 3 cups a day.
- **Tincture** may be made in small batches using dill seed in proportion of 1:1.
- Common dose of the **seeds** is 1 to 4 grams, 3 times a day.
- Typical dose for **dill oil** is 2 to 6 drops a day.

What It Does

Dill relieves stomach upset.

What It Might Help Treat

There are no known studies or reliable information on the effectiveness of dill for any specific condition other than those listed.

Research Insights

Dill leaf is a rich source of beta-carotene, iron and potassium.

Dill
Anetheum graveolens

Safety & Effectiveness

Dill has GRAS status in the United States and is considered safe when consumed in amounts commonly found in foods and when used as recommended for medicinal purposes. Dill seed or oil is believed to be effective when used for GI upset, but its effectiveness for other conditions is not supported.

Interactions

No interactions with drugs, other herbs, foods, vitamins or minerals, or adverse effects in laboratory tests have been known to occur. There is no reason to believe that such reactions will occur with dill if it is used as a food or in appropriate medicinal amounts.

Adverse Reactions

- Sensitivity to the sun may occur after skin contact with juice from freshly harvested plants.
- May cause contact skin rashes.

Who Should Not Use Dill

Pregnant women may use dill in amounts commonly found in foods; excess dill is believed to stimulate menstruation.

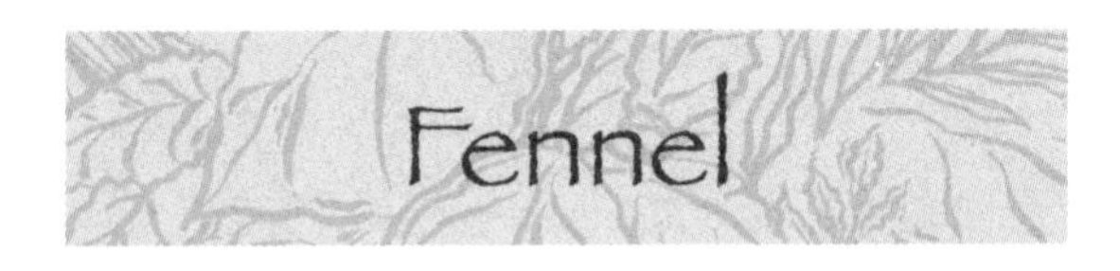

Profile

Common Names: Common fennel, bitter fennel
Family: Apiaceae/Umbelliferae; other family members include carrot, parsley, dill and angelica.
Genus & Species: *Foeniculum vulgare*
Description: Fennel looks much like its relative, dill. It grows up to 6 feet tall with feathery leaves and tall stalks. Its umbrella-like flower heads with tiny clusters of yellow flowers give rise to tiny oval-shaped seeds.
Historical Use: Fennel has been used throughout the centuries both therapeutically and medicinally. It has been—and still is—used in Arabian, Ayurvedic, Chinese and Japanese medicine. Its use is primarily for stomach upset and coughs, and as an expectorant. Early herbalists often mixed fennel with strong laxatives to help soothe the strong intestinal cramps that these laxatives caused. It has also been used to promote lactation. It is used in foods and beverages as a flavoring and has GRAS status in the United States.
Parts to Use: Leaves and seeds.

What It Does

Relieves minor stomach discomfort and gas. It also relieves inflammation of the respiratory tract. It promotes menstruation. It enhances milk production in nursing mothers.

What It Might Help Treat

Fennel has been shown to be a diuretic in laboratory animals, but its use in humans for this purpose has not been documented.

Research Insights

It may have a mild estrogenic effect.

How It Is Used

Fresh or dried.

Growing

Fennel is relatively easy to grow, especially if purchased as nursery plants.

Best Herbal Remedy Forms

Infusion or tea, and commercially purchased oil or syrup.

Making the Remedy & Dosage

When using commercially prepared preparations, including oil, follow package directions.

- **Tea** is made by steeping 1 to 2 grams of crushed seed in 150 mL of boiling water for 5 to 10 minutes; strain. Drink up to 1 cup of tea, 3 times a day.
- A commercially prepared fennel **tincture** may be taken in amounts up to ½ to 1 teaspoon, 3 times a day.
- **Syrup or honey**, taken in amounts up to 20 grams a day.

Safety & Effectiveness

Fennel seed and oil are considered safe when taken in amounts commonly found in food and when used as directed for up to 2 weeks. The major constituent is estragole, a potential carcinogen.

Fennel is believed to be effective when taken internally for mild GI distress, gas and upper respiratory inflammation. There is insufficient information regarding its use for treating other conditions.

Interactions

Drugs. Fennel seed may reduce the effectiveness of the powerful antibiotic ciprofloxacin (Cipro). No interaction of the oil with drugs is known to occur.

Other. No interactions with other herbs, foods, vitamins or minerals, or adverse effects in laboratory tests have been known to occur. There is no reason to believe that such reactions will occur when used as a food or in appropriate medicinal amounts.

Adverse Reactions

- Fennel seed can cause allergic reactions affecting the skin and the respiratory system.
- Exposure to sun light or ultraviolet light when using fennel seed may cause skin reactions.
- Persons allergic to other members of the Apiaceae family may be allergic to fennel seed or fennel oil.

Who Should Not Use Fennel

- During pregnancy and lactation, women should avoid amounts greater than found in foods.
- People with estrogen-dependent cancer.
- Persons with diabetes should exercise caution when using fennel syrup.
- Children under age 2 should not be given fennel preparations without consulting a healthcare provider.

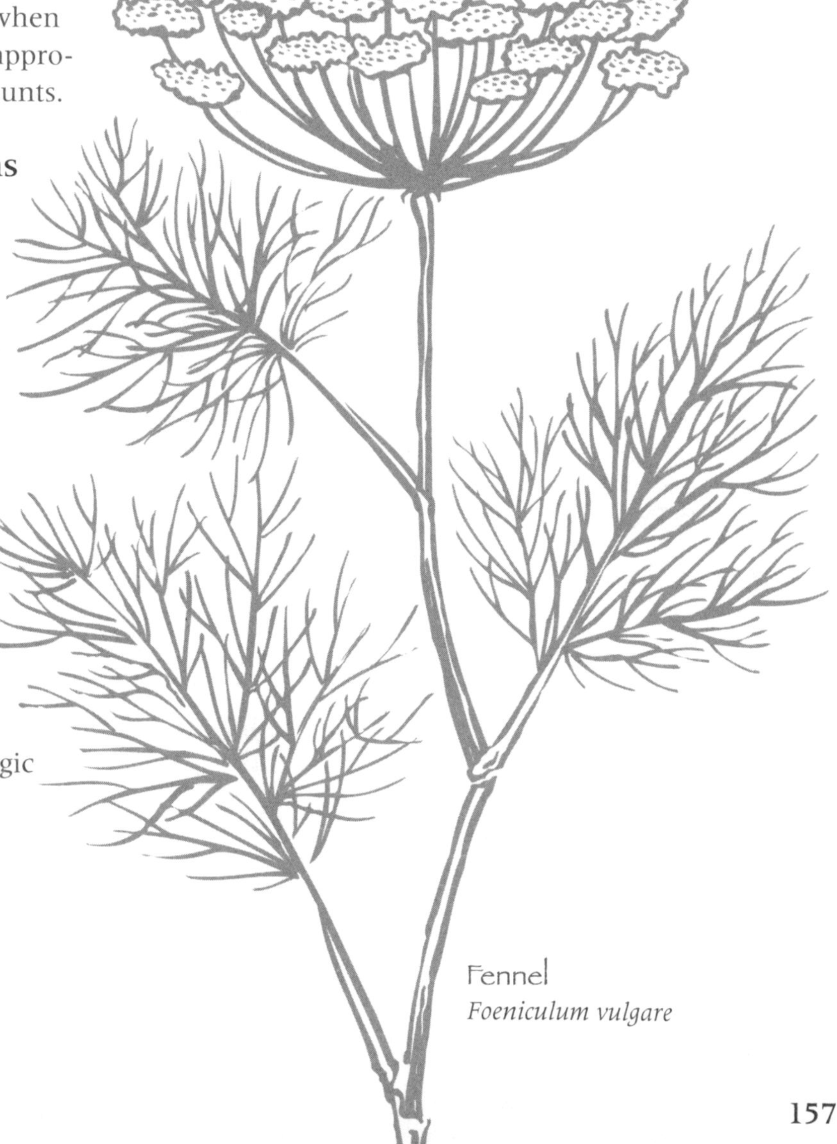

Fennel
Foeniculum vulgare

Culinary Herbs

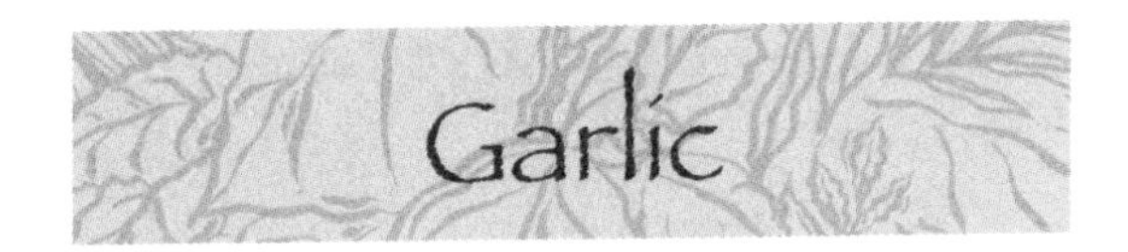

Profile

Common Names: Stinking rose, ajo, allium, heal-all
Family: Amaryllidaceae/Liliaceae
Genus & Species: *Allium sativum*
Description: Garlic is a perennial with a globe-shaped bulb made up of 5 to 15 cloves encased in a papery skin. Its leaves are flat and about 24 inches long. Globes of green-white to pink flowers are produced in summer.
Historical Use: Garlic is one of the oldest herbal remedies and culinary herbs. The history of garlic is rich in myth and reality. The Egyptians, who loved their garlic so much they were referred to as "the stinking ones," believed garlic prevented illness and increased strength and endurance. Garlic has been and is still used in many ancient medicinal practices, including Ayurveda and Traditional Chinese Medicine. Garlic has stood the test of time, and new uses for it seem to be found every day.
Parts to Use: Bulbs.

What It Does

Despite garlic's rich history, the evidence for its medicinal benefits is often conflicting, possibly due in part to poorly controlled studies. The German Commission E and the World Health Organization have recognized the potential supportive benefits of garlic for controlling high blood cholesterol and atherosclerotic vascular changes. Among its many suggested benefits, garlic:

- May reduce cholesterol.
- May inhibit the substances that promote blood clotting, thus reducing the risk of some types of heart disease.
- Improves blood flow in arteries.
- Has antibacterial properties.
- Lowers blood sugar levels.

What It Might Help Treat

- Coughs, colds, respiratory inflammations.
- May help prevent cell damage that ultimately results in cancerous growths.
- Fungus and yeast infections.
- Ulcers.

Research Insights

Garlic may improve the immune system and decrease the severity of herpes sores and diarrhea in persons with AIDS.

How It Is Used

Fresh garlic is most effective, but garlic breath is an unwelcome side effect. Those of you who don't share a love of garlic with friends and family may choose to use commercially prepared concentrated supplements.

Growing

Garlic cloves are the easiest and most reliable to grow bulbs from. Like other members of the Allium family, it is tolerant of colder climates and often does best if planted in the fall, 6 weeks before the final frost.

Best Herbal Remedy Forms

Fresh or commercially prepared powders, tablets, "perles," aged garlic extract, infusion/tea or tincture.

Making the Remedy & Dosage

- Add **fresh garlic** to salads or salad dressings. The recommended dose is up to 10 cloves per day. Using fresh garlic

is the most effective, but the herb does maintain some of its medicinal properties when cooked lightly.
- Make an **infusion or tea** using 6 chopped cloves steeped in 1 cup cold water overnight.
- Make a **tincture** using 1 cup crushed garlic cloves and 1 quart brandy. Place in a clean glass jar in a cool dark place. Shake the mixture once a day for 2 weeks. It will be ready to use then. Take up to 3 tablespoons a day. May take with a small amount of water.

Safety & Effectiveness

Garlic is considered safe when used in amounts commonly found in foods. Garlic, garlic oil and extract have GRAS status in the United States as a food ingredient. Garlic may be effective when used for elevated blood cholesterol, for elevated blood pressure, and for preventing age-related vascular changes and heart disease. There is some evidence from some epidemiological studies that garlic may reduce the risk of some cancers.

Interactions

Drugs

- Garlic can enhance the effect of blood-thinning drugs.
- Garlic may increase effects and adverse effects of insulin or oral hypoglycemic agents in people with diabetes.

Other Herbs and Dietary Supplements

- Garlic can enhance the anti-clot forming effects of fish oils, which help prevent the formation of blood clots.
- Use with herbs that have anticoagulant or antiplatelet potential may increase the risk of bleeding.

Foods. There are no known reported interactions or adverse reactions.

Vitamins or Minerals. There are no known reported interactions or adverse reactions.

Effects in Laboratory Tests

Garlic can lower blood sugar levels and test results. It can increase blood insulin levels and test results. It can alter the PT/INR of people taking anticoagulant or antiplatelet medications.

Adverse Reactions

- Bad breath and body odor.
- Mouth or stomach irritation.
- Gas, heartburn, nausea and vomiting.
- When used topically, fresh garlic may cause skin rash.
- May change intestinal flora.

Who Should Not Use Garlic

- People with bleeding disorders.
- People with diabetes.
- People with GI infections or inflammatory GI conditions.
- People who are having surgery should discontinue using garlic at least 2 weeks prior to surgery, as it can prolong bleeding time.
- Pregnant women should avoid using large (medicinal) amounts of garlic due to its blood-thinning properties; amounts commonly found in foods appear to be safe during pregnancy and lactation.

Comments

Studies have shown that some commercially produced garlic products do not contain as much active constituent as 1 clove of garlic. Some odorless products have been shown to contain no active components at all. When in doubt, fresh garlic is best!

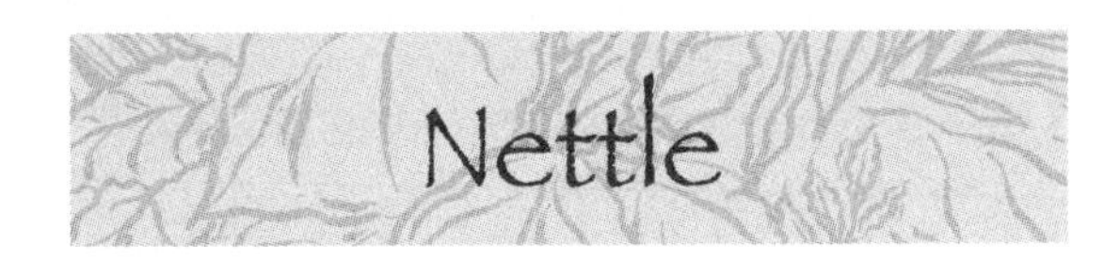

Nettle

Profile

Common Names: Common nettle, stinging nettle, nettle
Family: Urticaceae (other family members are nettles).
Genus & Species: *Urtica dioica*
Historical Use: Urtica, the botanical name meaning "to sting," aptly describes the qualities of the nettle. Coming in contact with nettle results in a painful, itchy skin eruption that can last for several hours. Nettle has been used for a variety of ailments since the 3rd century B.C.E. It has been considered a nutritive tonic that can treat arthritis, allergies, edema and urinary tract conditions, including BPH.
Description: Nettle produces an erect stem from creeping underground yellow rhizomes. It is a coarse perennial with pointed, deeply serrated oval leaves that are covered with the bristly stinging hairs that it is named for. Pendulous clusters of tiny green flowers are born on separate plants: male on one, female on the other.
Parts to Use: Whole plant, leaves and roots.

What It Does

It relieves symptoms of urinary tract inflammation. Nettle promotes diuresis. The root may help relieve painful and frequent urination in men with BPH. It may be used in early stages of inflamed prostate to relieve symptoms including urinary retention. It stimulates uterine contractions.

Nettle
Urtica dioica

What It Might Help Treat

- High blood pressure (by promoting diuresis).
- As additional therapy for congestive heart failure by promoting diuresis.
- May relieve bloating associated with premenstrual syndrome.

Research Insights

Many of the clinical trials have been conducted in Germany and some results may not have been translated. Preliminary information supports its benefits for reducing inflammation in arthritis, for soothing allergic nasal conditions and for BPH.

How It Is Used

Fresh (wear protective clothing and gloves while picking and preparing), commercially prepared freeze-dried capsules and commercially prepared root preparation.

Growing

Nettle is considered a noxious weed in many parts of the country and it grows very easily from seeds or root divisions.

Best Herbal Remedy Forms

Infusion or tea, fresh juice, purchased dried and liquid extracts and alcoholic extracts.

Making the Remedy & Dosage

Nettle root remedies to treat conditions of BPH are best purchased commercially to ensure potency. Follow package directions.

- Make **fresh juice** from macerating the leaves in a blender or food processor and straining. Take 10 to 15 mL, 3 times a day.

- **Fresh nettles** may be steamed (steaming destroys the chemical that causes the sting) and eaten as a vegetable. Pick approximately 1 cup raw nettles per person. Steam in a steaming basket or microwave approximately 1 minute per cup. Season as desired.
- Make **teas** from the leaves or the root. For leaf tea, steep 1⅕ to 5 grams of leaves in 150 mL of hot, not boiling, water for 10 minutes and strain; drink up to 3 times a day. Drink additional fluids throughout the day. For root tea, steep 1½ grams dried, powdered root in 150 mL boiling water for 10 minutes and strain; take up to 6 grams or 2½ (8-ounce) cups or 4 (15-mL) cups a day. Drink additional fluid throughout the day.

Safety & Effectiveness

Nettle leaves, above-ground parts and roots are considered safe when taken as recommended; however, some interactions to be aware of are listed below. Nettle leaf and above-ground parts may be effective for urinary tract conditions, for kidney stones, for supportive therapy in rheumatic ailments and used topically, as supportive therapy for rheumatic ailments. Nettle root may be effective for symptoms associated with BPH (Benign Prostatic Hyperplasia).

Interactions

Drugs

The leaves and above-ground parts used in excessive amounts may interact with:

- Anticoagulant or antiplatelet drugs—in any amount—due to nettle's high vitamin K content.
- Insulin or oral hypoglycemic agents.
- Drugs used to treat high blood pressure.
- Central nervous system depressants (sedatives).
- Some anti-arthritic medications.

Other Herbs. Herbs with sedative properties. Herbs that contain vitamin K, due to the vitamin's role in blood clotting. When taken with other herbs that contain vitamin K, blood clotting may be affected, by decreasing the time it takes blood to clot. These include alfalfa, parsley and plantain.

Vitamins or Minerals. Potential for decreased absorption of iron because of formation of tannin-iron complex.

Other. No interactions with foods, or adverse effects in laboratory tests have been known to occur. There is no reason to believe that such reactions will occur when used as a food or in appropriate medicinal amounts.

Adverse Reactions

- Fresh juice may cause diarrhea.
- Nettle root may cause GI upset, sweating and allergic skin reactions.

Who Should Not Use Nettle

- People with heart or kidney insufficiency.
- People with diabetes.
- People with high or low blood pressure.
- During pregnancy and lactation, women should avoid nettle because of its possible uterine stimulating effects and the lack of reliable information about nettle's safety.

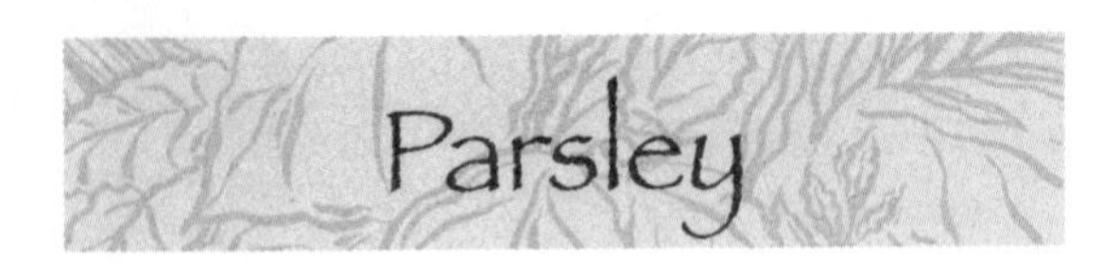

Profile

Common Names: Common parsley, garden parsley
Family: Apiaceae/Umbelliferae
Genus & Species: *Petroselinum crispum*
Description: You probably know what parsley looks like; it's been the throw-away garnish on many a dinner plate. Parsley is dense green and its leaves form a rosette base with tiny greenish yellow flowers in early summer. Two varieties are used medicinally: Italian (or flat-leaved), which has a strong flavor, and the milder curly variety.
Historical Use: Parsley has been used as a medicinal and culinary herb since at least the first century C.E. It has been part of traditional Ayurvedic medicine as a diuretic and expectorant. It is used in foods, beverages and as a garnish.
Parts to Use: Leaf and root.

What It Does

Parsley freshens breath, prevents kidney stones, promotes diuresis, and relieves gas and mild stomach upset.

What It Might Help Treat

When used topically, it may relieve dry, chapped lips and skin, insect bites and bruises.

Research Insights

The current therapeutic applications are based on its history of clinical use, phytochemical research and pharmacologic studies in animals. There are no known investigations on the efficacy of parsley as a medicinal herbal.

How It Is Used

Fresh or dried. Fresh as an ingredient in many foods and tea. Dried as a flavoring or for tea.

Growing

Parsley is easy to grow and even grows wild in some parts of the temperate world. Soak seeds to encourage germination, then sow immediately in warm spring soil. Parsley likes full sun or partial shade and moist soil.

Best Herbal Remedy Forms

Tea, dried (for tea or culinary purposes), or fresh (in foods or as a breath freshener).

Making the Remedy & Dosage

- Make **teas** with 2 grams of chopped dried root in 150 mL of boiling water, steeped for 10 minutes, then strained. Take 2 or 3 cups a day as a mild diuretic. Drink additional water when taking parsley to flush the kidneys.
- Dried parsley may be used for **tea**; 1 to 2 teaspoons per 1 cup of hot, not boiling, water. Take up to 3 cups per day.
- **Dried parsley** is also used as a flavoring for soups, stews and other foods, in varying amounts.
- Chew a few sprigs of **fresh parsley** as a breath freshener—eat the garnish on your plate!

Safety & Effectiveness

Parsley has GRAS status in the United States and is considered safe when taken in amounts commonly used in foods. Large amounts and the oil of parsley are unsafe, as they contain toxic constituents. Parsley is considered effective when used for kidney stone prevention and treatment.

Interactions

Drugs.

- Large amounts of parsley may interfere with anticoagulant therapy because of its vitamin K content.
- Aspirin may increase parsley allergy.
- The effects of prescription diuretics may be compounded by medicinal doses of parsley.
- MAOIs may be inhibited by large amounts of parsley or parsley oil.

Vitamins or Minerals. Avoid more than 400 IU of vitamin E a day when using parsley because parsley and vitamin E both have blood-thinning properties.

Other. No interactions with other herbs or foods, or adverse effects in laboratory tests, have been known to occur. There is no reason to believe that such reactions will occur when used as a food or in appropriate medicinal amounts.

Adverse Reactions

- Occasional allergic skin or mucous membrane reactions.
- Parsley oil can cause skin rash in people exposed to excess sunshine.
- Excessive amounts may cause liver and kidney problems.

Who Should Not Use Parsley

- People with edema, as it might increase sodium retention.
- People with high blood pressure.
- People with kidney disease or inflammation.
- Use of amounts commonly used in food is safe for pregnant women, but larger amounts may stimulate uterine contractions.
- Insufficient information is available on medicinal use during lactation, so parsley should be avoided except in amounts commonly used in food.

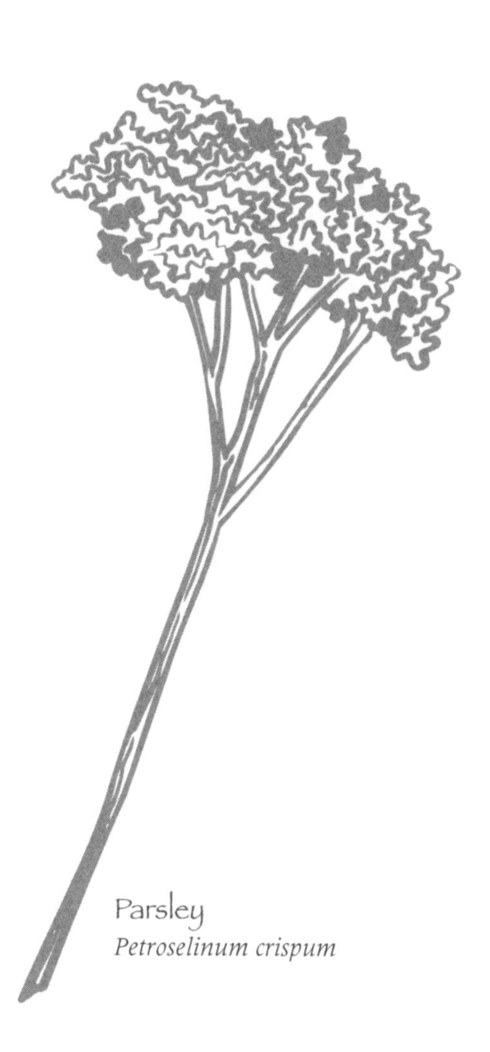

Parsley
Petroselinum crispum

Rosemary

Profile

Common Names: Garden rosemary, compass plant, compass-weed
Family: Labiatae/Lamiaceae; other family members include mints.
Genus & Species: *Rosmarinus officinalis*
Description: Rosemary is an evergreen shrub with needle-like leaves and a pine scent. It can reach 3 feet in height and produces small, pale blue flowers in the summer. It is used in the western United States as a groundcover and tumbles over garden walls. Rosemary leaves are used as a spice and its oil is used as a flavoring in foods and beverages.
Historical Use: Rosemary was one of the first preservatives used, thousands of years ago. People wrapped meats in rosemary to preserve them and give them a pleasant odor. Its meat-preserving ability led to the belief that it preserved memory. Rosemary has been used medicinally in Europe, Traditional Chinese Medicine and Ayurvedic medicine for its memory- and concentration-preserving properties and for headaches. It has also been known for its ability to relieve gas, GI discomfort and joint inflammation.
Parts to Use: Leaves.

What It Does

Rosemary improves liver and gallbladder function. It soothes GI upset. Topically, it is used to relieve muscle aches and joint inflammation.

What It Might Help Treat

- Skin infections and abrasions.
- Congestion.
- Promotes regular menstruation.

Research Insights

Rosemary reduces spasms in the gallbladder and small intestines. It may increase blood flow through the coronary arteries. Its antioxidants may help prevent cancer.

How It Is Used

Leaves fresh or dried.

Growing

Rosemary grows well in temperate climates. It does not like winters where the temperature dips below zero, but it can be grown in containers in colder climates.

Best Herbal Remedy Forms

Infusion or tea, purchased liquid extract or as a bath.

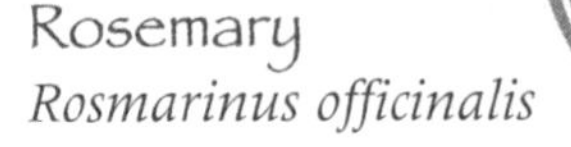

Rosemary
Rosmarinus officinalis

Making the Remedy & Dosage

- Make an **infusion or tea** using 1 teaspoon of crushed herb in 8 ounces of boiling water. Steep for 10 minutes and strain. Drink up to 3 cups a day.
- Use **commercial preparations** according to package directions.
- **Liquid extract**, 1:1, using equal amounts of herb and 45 percent alcohol/water solution, may be taken in doses of 2 to 4 mL, 3 times a day.
- For a rosemary **bath**, use 50 grams of leaf to 1 liter of hot, not boiling, water and add to bath water.

Safety & Effectiveness

Rosemary leaf and oil are considered safe in amounts commonly used in foods. Rosemary has GRAS status for use as a food or ingredient in the United States. Rosemary is considered effective when used internally for GI upset and as supportive therapy for joint or muscle pain and circulatory problems.

Interactions

No interactions with drugs, other herbs, foods, vitamins or minerals, or adverse effects on laboratory tests, have been known to occur when rosemary is used in recommended amounts. There is no reason to believe such reactions will occur when used as a food or in appropriate medicinal amounts.

Adverse Reactions

- Excessive amounts of rosemary leaves containing rosemary oil, taken internally may cause numerous adverse reactions including coma, vomiting, gastroenteritis, kidney irritation, kidney damage, pulmonary edema and even death (amounts greater than what would be recommended in recipes or for typical dose).
- Rosemary, when used topically, may lead to skin irritation, especially when exposed to the sun.
- Occupational asthma has been known to occur in those who are exposed to rosemary in the work environment.

Who Should Not Use Rosemary

- People with seizure disorders.
- During pregnancy or lactation, women should not use rosemary in amounts greater than commonly used in foods. Excessive amounts of leaf or oil are thought to promote menstrual flow.

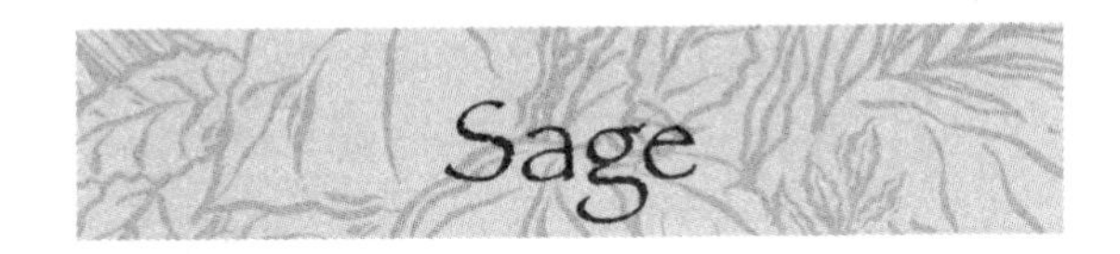

Culinary Herbs

Profile

Common Names: Garden sage, common sage, true sage
Family: Labiatae/Lamiaceae; other family members include mints.
Genus & Species: *Salvia officinalis*
Description: Sage is a perennial evergreen shrub that can grow up to 3 feet tall. Its stems are square, woolly and woody near the bottom, progressing into 2-inch oval, velvety gray leaves with long stalks. Sage's small flowers are pink, blue, white or purple, depending on the species.
Historical Use: Sage has been cultivated since medieval times and was introduced by the colonists to North America in the 1600s. It has been used to treat numerous maladies and was even thought to extend life to the point of immortality. It was used by 16th century Chinese physicians to treat insomnia, depression, GI distress, mental illness and menstrual complaints, just to name a few. Traditional Ayurvedic physicians used sage similarly and also prescribed it for sexually transmitted diseases. Folk healers in America used sage for insomnia, epilepsy, measles, seasickness and intestinal worms.
Parts to Use: Leaves.

What It Does

Sage relieves GI complaints including bloating and gas. It relieves excessive perspiration. When used topically, it relieves inflammation of mucous membranes of the nose and throat. It soothes canker sores, bleeding gums and sore throat. Sage is a rich source of beta-carotene.

What It Might Help Treat

- Wounds
- May help promote regular menstruation

Research Insights

Sage may reduce blood sugar in people with diabetes.

How It Is Used

Fresh, dried or commercially purchased essential oil.

Growing

Sage is easy to grow from seeds or cuttings. It grows in almost any type of soil. It should be replaced every 3 to 4 years because plants become less productive and woodier.

Best Herbal Remedy Forms

Fresh, infusion or tea, commercially prepared essential oil and tincture.

Making the Remedy & Dosage

- Make **tea** by adding 2 to 3 teaspoons of dried leaves to 8 ounces of boiling water. Steep for 10 minutes, strain and drink up to 3 cups a day. If symptoms for which you are drinking sage tea do not subside within 7 to 10 days, consult your physician. The infusion may also be used for a gargle to soothe a sore throat.
- Take dried leaf in **capsule** form in doses of 1 to 3 grams, 3 times a day.
- For **purchased preparations**, follow label directions.

Safety & Effectiveness

Sage is safe in amounts used in food and is approved as a food ingredient in the United States. It may be unsafe if used in amounts that exceed what is commonly used in food. When used internally for GI upset, including gas and bloating, sage is believed to be effective. When used topically, it is considered effective for sore gums and mucous membranes of the mouth.

Interactions

Drugs.

- Might interfere with anticonvulsant therapy; some species of sage can cause convulsions.
- Sage may have an additive (or com pounding) effect with drugs used to treat high blood sugar.
- Sage may have an additive effect when used with sedative drugs.

Other Herbs. Sage may enhance the therapeutic and adverse effects of herbs with sedative properties.

Other. No interactions with foods, vitamins or minerals, or adverse effects in laboratory tests, have been known to occur. There is no reason to believe that such reactions will occur when used as a food or in appropriate medicinal amounts.

Adverse Reactions

- Sage, taken orally by itself, may cause irritation of the mouth.
- Large amounts or prolonged use of sage leaf or oil may cause restlessness, dizziness, vomiting, heart rhythm irregularities and kidney damage.

Who Should Not Use Sage

- People with diabetes should not use sage in medicinal amounts. Amounts in common food intake are considered safe.
- People with seizure disorders should not use sage in medicinal amounts. Amounts in common food intake are considered safe.
- Women who are pregnant should not use sage in amounts that exceed common food intake; it may stimulate menstruation.
- During lactation, women should not use sage in amounts that exceed common food intake; it may reduce milk supply.

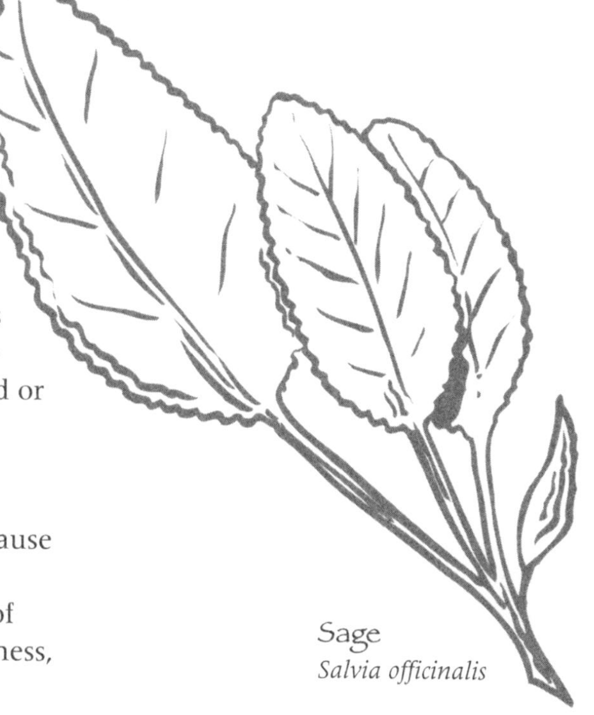

Sage
Salvia officinalis

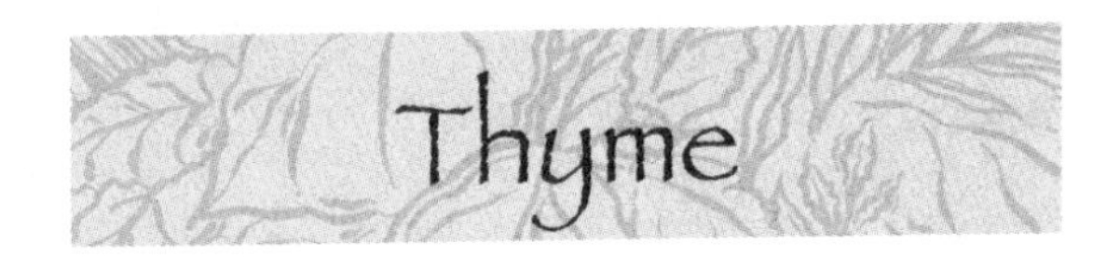

Profile

Common Names: Garden thyme, common thyme, wild thyme, mother thyme
Family: Labiatae/Lamiaceae
Genus & Species: *Thymus vulgaris* and *thymus serpyllum*
Description: Thyme is a perennial shrub that acts as a groundcover. It has many branches with small, almost stalkless leaves and pink-to-violet flowers in mid-summer. It is a very aromatic herb.
Historical Use: Thyme can be found in places you least expect—mouthwashes, decongestants, toothpastes and perfumes, to name a few. Thyme became a culinary herb as an offshoot of its meat-preserving properties. It has been cultivated throughout the world since Roman times. It has been used as an antiseptic during plagues, as a symbol of courage in the Middle Ages, for nervous disorders, headaches, GI disturbances and menstrual complaints. As a folk medicine, it has been used as an appetite stimulant, diuretic and urinary disinfectant, and for parasites. Thyme is used in food as a culinary herb.
Parts to Use: Leaves and flowers.

What It Does

The German Commission E has approved thyme for symptoms of bronchitis, whooping cough and inflamed upper respiratory system. It is also used to improve digestion. Thyme is a rich source of iron.

What It Might Help Treat

- Menstrual cramps.
- Infections.

Research Insights

Thyme may inhibit the growth of the bacteria *(H. pylori)* known to cause stomach ulcers.

How It Is Used

Fresh, dried.

Growing

Thyme is a hardy herb that can be grown from seeds, root cuttings or nursery stock. Once established, thyme does not need a lot of care. To prevent it from becoming woody, divide the roots every few years.

Best Herbal Remedy Forms

Infusions or teas or purchased fluid extract.

Making the Remedy & Dosage

Make **tea** from 1 to 2 grams of dried herb in 150 mL of boiling water, steeped for 10 minutes and strained. Take the tea several times a day, as needed. Do not exceed 10 grams of dried leaf per day.

Safety & Effectiveness

Thyme has GRAS status as a food ingredient and is considered safe when consumed in amounts commonly used in foods and when used as recommended for internal and topical use. Thyme is considered effective when used internally for symptoms of bronchitis and whooping cough. When used topically, it may be effective for upper respiratory tract inflammations and bad breath.

Interactions

No interactions with other herbs, foods, vitamins or minerals, or adverse effects in laboratory tests, have been known to occur. There is no reason to believe that such reactions will occur when used as a food or in appropriate medicinal amounts.

Adverse Reactions

Topically, thyme oil may cause skin irritation. There appear to be no adverse interactions to other herbs, dietary supplements, drugs, foods or in lab tests.

Who Should Not Use Thyme

- People with active urinary tract disease or inflammation.
- People with stomach ulcers or other GI irritations, as it can exacerbate inflammation.
- People who are allergic to other members of the Labiatae/Lamiaceae family, including oregano and mints.
- During pregnancy, women should avoid using amounts greater than amounts used in foods; it may stimulate menstruation. It is considered safe during lactation when taken in amounts commonly used in foods.

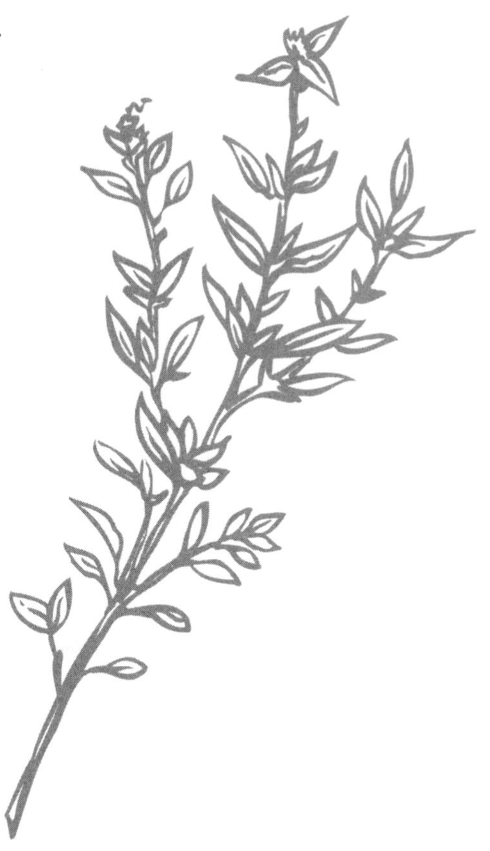

Thyme
Thymus vulgaris

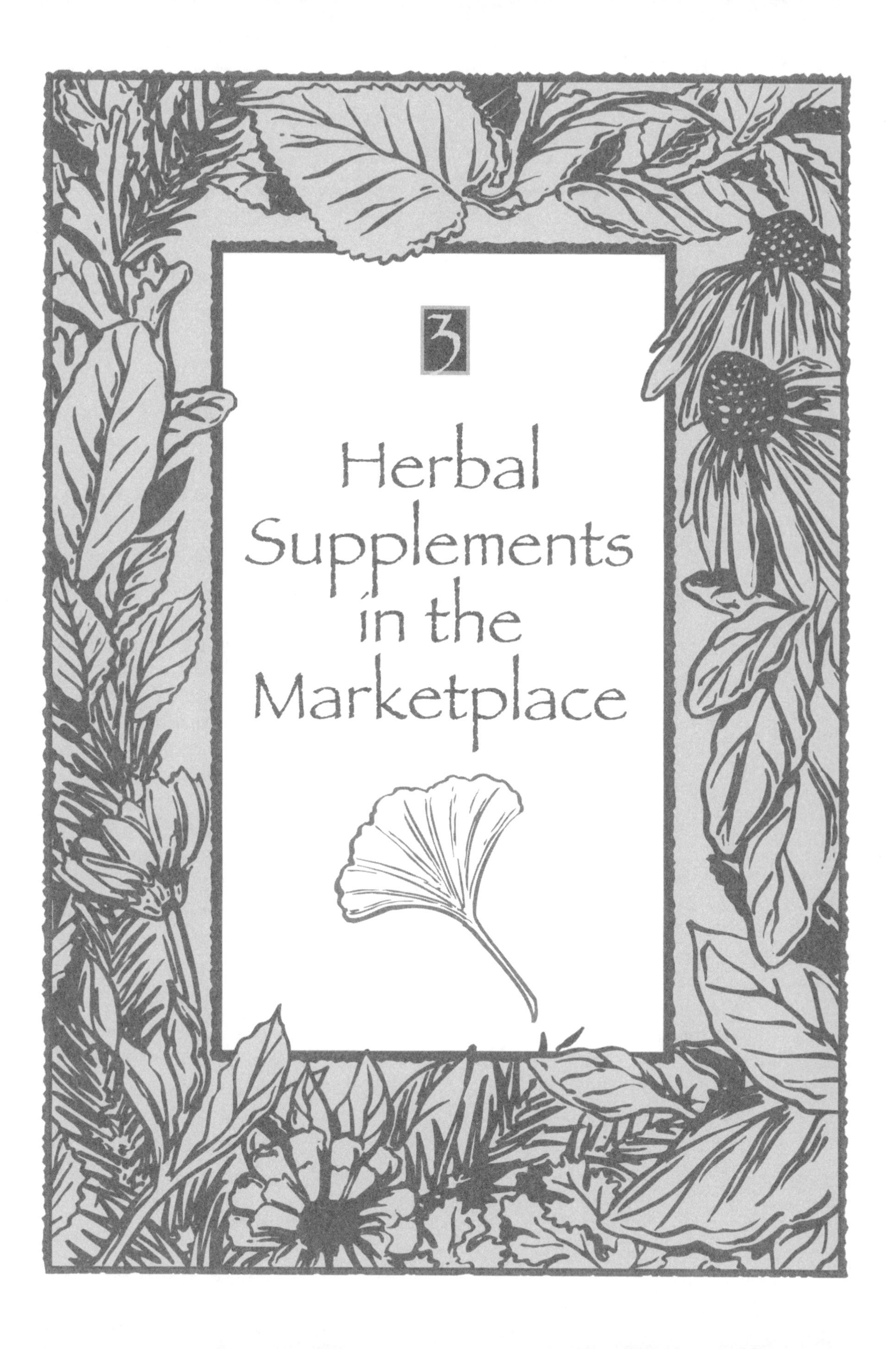

3 Herbal Supplements in the Marketplace

3

Herbal Supplements in the Marketplace

Herbs and herbal supplements are not regulated like drugs. There are no strict requirements for the quality, packaging or dosing of supplements. Because of legislation passed in 1994 (see below), the Food and Drug Administration (FDA) does not require proof from clinical trials regarding the safety and effectiveness of herbal products before they are put on the market. The FDA does limit, however, the claims that can be made regarding the use and efficacy of supplements. Unlike pharmaceutical companies, supplement manufacturers are not required by law to report product or health problems associated with herbal products. The reports of adverse events caused by dietary supplements usually come from people who are not expert in the area, rather than healthcare practitioners. A reporting mechanism is available on the web at the FDA's medical products reporting program site (www.fda.gov/medwatch).

It is important to understand a bit about the regulations governing the manufacture and sales of dietary supplements in order to be able to make wise selections from the numerous options available. A number of third-party, independent companies are beginning to test dietary supplements for accuracy of ingredient labeling, quality and purity. Much of this information is available to consumers to help in the evaluation process.

Current Regulations

Congress enacted the Dietary Supplement Health and Education Act (DSHEA) in 1994. The idea behind the law was to give powers to the federal government to ensure the safety of supplements and the accuracy of health claims. Before DSHEA, the FDA regulated dietary supplements as foods to make sure they were wholesome and that their labeling was not misleading and was truthful. At the same time DSHEA was enacted, the Office of Dietary Supplements (ODS) was established. The ODS is responsible for coordinating funding for scientific studies on the relationship between dietary supplements and disease prevention.

Safety

All herbal medicines are drugs, but not all drugs are herbal medicines. Approximately 25 to 30 percent of modern-day prescription medicines have some relationship with botanicals, either as a constituent or as a laboratory copy, synthesized to have the same properties. The active component of aspirin, for example, was first identified in white willow and later made in the laboratory.

Many botanicals are on the FDA's Generally Recognized as Safe (GRAS) list; most are herbs and spices that have some culinary or flavoring role. Some GRAS botanicals are safer than others, and some should be used with extreme care, preferably under the guidance of a healthcare provider.

Just as over-the-counter (OTC) drugs are restricted to treating conditions that will go away in time, such as a headache, herbal medicines are also intended for conditions that will subside in time. Herbs and dietary supplements are most beneficial when used as support for a healthy diet and lifestyle. Dietary supplements differ from other OTC products because they do not have to be proven safe and effective. There are a few herbs that are the exception, including psyllium, senna and cascara, which are used as laxatives.

According to DSHEA, dietary supplement manufacturers are responsible for making sure that the information about their product is truthful and not misleading, and that all of the ingredients in the supplement are safe. This is a tall order for many of the manufacturers that have products on the market today. Dietary supplements are considered safe unless proven unsafe by the FDA. This is in contrast to how prescription and nonprescription drugs must be proven safe and effective by the manufacturer prior to sale. The FDA does not evaluate scientific evidence concerning the supplement or its possible side effects or interactions because it was not given this charge under DSHEA. The only time the FDA will evaluate a product is when it has been notified that the product is unsafe. Then, before the product is restricted or

What Are Dietary Supplements?

Dietary supplements are products that are intended to supplement, not supplant, a healthy diet. They must meet at least one of the following four criteria:

- It contains one or more of the following dietary ingredients: a vitamin, mineral, herb or other botanical; or an amino acid or dietary substance that supplements the diet by increasing the total dietary intake; or a concentrate, metabolite or constituent, extract or combination of these ingredients.
- It is intended for ingestion in pill, capsule, tablet, softgel, gelcap or liquid form.
- It is labeled as a dietary supplement.
- It cannot be represented for use as a conventional food, as a meal or as a diet replacement.

What is GRAS?

GRAS is the acronym for the term "generally recognized as safe." Substances with the GRAS designation are considered safe for consumption and can be added to foods by manufacturers without establishing their safety through rigorous testing and evaluation. Congress first defined GRAS in 1958 when it passed the Food Additives Amendment to the Food, Drug and Cosmetic Act. The safety of GRAS substances is based on a long history of use in food before 1958 or based on published scientific data. Hundreds of food additives, including numerous culinary herbs, monosodium glutamate (MSG), sugar, spices, salt, vitamins and minerals, are on the list.

banned, the FDA must demonstrate that it is mislabeled or unsafe.

The Science Behind the Claims ... Is There Any?

Health promotion and disease prevention claims for foods and dietary supplements are regulated under the Nutrition Labeling and Education Act of 1990 (NLEA). The NLEA requires that there be pre-market approval of all health claims by the FDA. Claims fall under two categories: structure/function claims and disease claims. The final rule enacting labeling standards for dietary supplements was published in 2000.

Structure/function claims are statements regarding the effect of a nutrient or botanical on a specific function in the human body and describe the conditions under which supplements can make such claims. No reference to disease or medical diagnosis can be specifically stated. For example, a structure/function claim may state that "calcium builds strong bones," but cannot state that "calcium will prevent osteoporosis."

All structure/function claims must bear the disclaimer "This statement has not been evaluated by the Food and Drug Administration. This product is not intended to diagnose, treat, cure or prevent any disease."

Disease claims have different regulations. When disease claims are made, the product will be regulated as a drug unless it has an authorized health claim for which the product qualifies. A disease claim either explicitly or implicitly claims that the product:

- has an effect on a specific disease or class of diseases.
- has an effect on usual signs or symptoms of disease.
- has an effect on an abnormal condition associated with a natural state or process, if that condition is uncommon or can cause significant or permanent harm.
- has an effect on disease through one or more of the following:
  - implies an effect on disease in the name of the product.
  - makes a statement about the formulation of the product, including a claim that the product contains an ingredient regulated by the FDA as a drug and is well known to consumers for its use or claimed use in preventing or treating a disease.
  - cites a publication or reference that refers to a disease if the context of the labeling as a whole implies treatment or prevention of a disease.
  - uses the term *disease* or *diseased*

Currently Allowed Claims for Dietary Supplements

The FDA allows manufacturers to make the following claims about dietary supplements and their possible healthful results:

- Folic acid and a decreased risk of neural tube birth defects.
- Calcium and a lowered risk of osteoporosis.
- Potassium and the reduced risk of high blood pressure and stroke.
- Psyllium seed husk (as part of a diet low in cholesterol and saturated fat) and reduced risk of coronary heart disease.
- Plant sterol/stanol esters and the reduced risk of coronary heart diseases.

except in general statements about disease prevention that do not refer to a specific disease or class of diseases.

- uses pictures or vignettes, symbols or other means to refer to disease, such as a heart symbol.
- is marketed as a substitute for a product that is a therapy for a disease.
- treats, prevents or lessens adverse effects associated with therapy for disease or otherwise suggests an effect on disease.

Critics of herbal therapies maintain that herbs are hazardous because typical preparations do not always yield consistent amounts of active constituents. This is true; there are many things that influence an herb's effectiveness—growing conditions, harvesting and storage, to name a few. Critics fail to recognize, however, that herbal medicines, although not as regulated as pharmaceutical drugs, have much longer histories of use, and usually without the adverse effects

Using Herbs Safely

Herbal medicines can be safely used with the right information. Here are some tips to help you evaluate the safety of the herb you want to use.

- Before you take an herb, or any drug for that matter, learn as much as possible about it.
- Know what the herb looks like if you are growing it or purchasing it in bulk. Use the Latin binomial name—the genus and species—to identify the herb.
- Know what part of the herb is the most effective and safe.
- Don't exceed the recommended dosage; follow typical dosing information on the labels. As with prescription drugs, too little may be ineffective, while too much may be deadly.
- If you prepare your own herbal products, store any leftovers in an opaque glass container that can be sealed well. Air and light are an herbal preparation's worst enemies. Store preparations in a cool, dark place.
- Know your body and be aware of adverse reactions, allergic reactions and other sensitivities. Even if you have not suffered from an allergy before, you may still develop an allergy or be sensitive to one or more herbal medicines.
- If you are over 65 years old, start with small doses of herbs. If you are also taking prescription drugs, make sure you know the potential for interactions.
- Pregnant and lactating women should avoid using herbs that are not intended to be used as a food or food ingredient. Avoid any culinary herb in large amounts.
- Inform your healthcare provider about the herbs and dietary supplements you are taking.
- If you are preparing for any surgery, discontinue using herbal medicines at least two weeks prior. If that is not possible, make sure to tell your physician and surgeon what you have been taking.

observed in those who take prescription medications. Yes, a variation in potency of herbal products may cause adverse effects. Likewise, inappropriate use of prescription products will result in severe adverse effects. Both herbs and drugs rely on the person taking them to make the decision about how little or how much, if any, of either to take. Criticism of herbal medicine may stem from the unknown rather than from knowledge about the herb itself. For example, conventionally trained physicians may not have learned about some of the popular herbs, may be concerned about the lack of rigorously conducted research, may be wary of purity and quality, or may not be certain whether effects are due to the herb or simply a placebo effect.

Statistics bear out the fact that there are more adverse reactions, morbidity and mortality reported with pharmaceutical use than are reported for herbal medicines. Much of this may be due to strict guidelines requiring pharmaceutical manufacturers to report and track all adverse effects. However, when we learn of a problem regarding an herbal medicine, it seems as though it is a bigger deal because it is not mainstream medicine.

Truth in Advertising?

The law does not allow medical claims on dietary supplement labels, but what about the advertising for these products? The Federal Trade Commission (FTC) regulates the advertising of dietary supplements. Realistically, however, with the number of products and the numerous ways they are advertised, it is difficult, if not impossible, for the FTC to be on top of everything that is out there.

Publications are required to meet the following five criteria:

1. The advertising must not be false or misleading;
2. It must not promote a particular brand or manufacturer;
3. It must present a balanced view of available scientific information;
4. It must be physically separate from the product if displayed where the product is sold; and
5. It must not have any information that is changed or removed by a sticker or any other method.

Think back to the last time you surfed the Internet, browsed through a catalog or shopped in a natural foods store. What advertising did you see, and did it meet these criteria?

Choosing the Right Herb or Herbal Medicine

To help consumers understand what they are taking, manufacturers are required to label products with certain information. Just as food that comes to us partially prepared or ready to eat must have a nutrition facts panel, supplements that are ready to use must contain a supplement facts panel. The facts panel is required to carry the name of each ingredient, total quantity of all dietary ingredients and the words *dietary supplement.* (A descriptive statement, like "vitamin and mineral supplement," may replace the words "dietary supplement," as appropriate.) In botanical products, the part of the plant that is used in the supplement must be identified on the label.

Supplement facts panels must contain the following information:

- Statement of identity—what is it you are buying.
- Net quantity of contents, listed by common names in descending order by weight; active ingredients; other ingredients, including binding agents, fillers, artificial flavors and colors; if a product contains a proprietary blend, the total amount of the blend must be listed, although a list of individual ingredients and amounts do not have to be named.
- Appropriate serving size.
- Directions for use.
- Quantity and daily values (DV) for 14 nutrients and any added vitamins or minerals when present in significant amounts; a product with no DV must list the amount per serving (for example, 10 grams).
- Name and place of business of the manufacturer, packager or distributor.
- High potency products must have 100 percent or more of the established Recommended Daily Intake (RDI) for that vitamin or mineral.

If a structure/function claim is made, the following disclaimer must be added: "This statement has not been evaluated by the Food and Drug Administration. This product is not intended to diagnose, treat, cure or prevent any disease."

READING AN HERBAL SUPPLEMENT LABEL

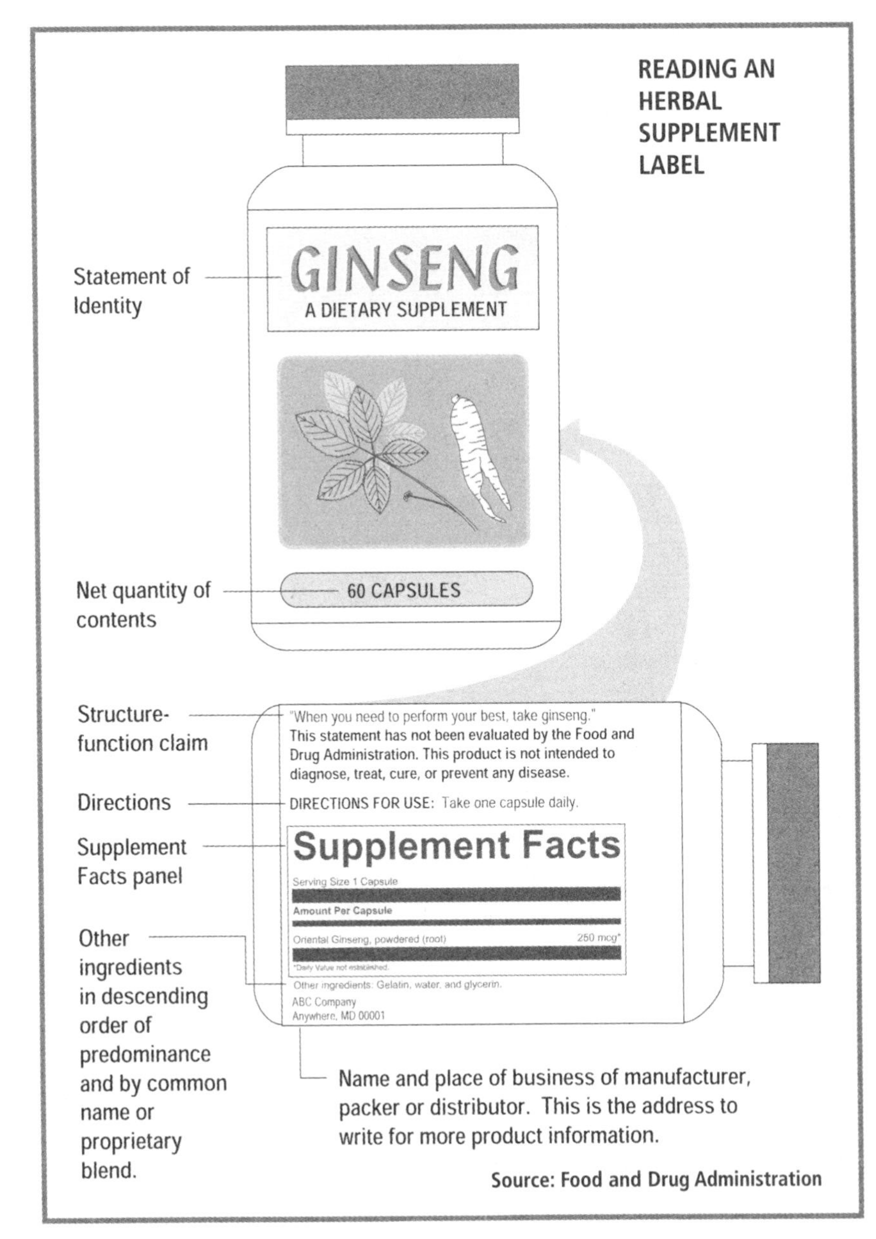

Source: Food and Drug Administration

Ensuring Product Quality & Safety

Let's face it, there are those out there who want to take advantage of the market and the consumer and offer products that are not pure, safe and high quality, or make claims that cannot be substantiated. Under the DSHEA regulations, the FDA cannot mandate testing of supplements prior to marketing. The only time they can require testing is when a product has been determined unsafe. There are numerous companies in the herbal and dietary supplement industry that are ethical and committed to quality, safety and high standards. With that in mind, these companies follow what are called Good Manufacturing Practices (GMPs) that address the uniqueness of the supplement industry. These are steps that the companies take to ensure product quality: good record keeping, laboratory testing, maintaining sanitary and clean conditions and using the appropriate equipment, processing methods and raw materials.

Some manufacturers participate in independent auditing systems that set standards to ensure integrity and uniform quality of drugs and healthcare technology. Standards include product strength, quality, purity, disintegration and dissolution (whether the product dissolves and can be absorbed by the body), packaging, weight variation and labeling. Organizations including United States Pharmacopoeia (USP) and the National Sanitation Foundation (NSF) offer auditing services. The National Nutritional Foods Association (NNFA) requires evaluation by a third party, TruLabel, in order for suppliers to belong to its self-regulatory testing programs. TruLabel's evaluation is based on NNFA's GMPs.

Standards are voluntary, so supplement suppliers can choose whether to participate. If they do participate, the symbols NSF, USP or NNFA may be carried on the label. This tells you that the products have met the requirements to have that designation. Additionally, there are a number of third parties, independent testing laboratories, that test dietary supplements. Several of these have Web sites and are listed in the references section on pages 312-313.

Recently, independent lab testing has found that the contents of preparations containing certain herbs (ginseng and St. John's wort, for example) can vary greatly from brand to brand. Additionally, herb preparations may contain little or none of the stated ingredient. In some cases, their concentration has exceeded recommended doses, and some have been found to contain foreign substances, including heavy metals, pesticides and other plants. This underscores the need to know as much as you can about the product, the manufacturer and the dose appropriate for your condition.

Evaluating the Claims

This book has been designed to give you the most up-to-date information regarding herbal medicines. But there are times in your search for the right medicine, or while evaluating products on your own, when you come across one that sounds ideal for you. Is it too good to be true? There are some questions you can ask yourself that might help determine the answer:

- What claims are being made for the supplement?
- Who is making these claims?
- Why are the claims being made?
- Where is the product available: a pharmacy, natural foods store, healthcare provider, the Internet?
- Are the ingredients in the supplement generally safe? Will they cause harm at any dose?
- Is the manufacturer a company that is known to use GMPs and quality ingredients?

- Is there support for the claims of efficacy that are made? Will it provide the outcome you want?

Before You Decide

Before deciding which supplement to take, it is necessary to understand why you are taking it, what to expect when taking it and how much to take. Without these key factors, what you take may not provide you with the results you desire. This, of course, assumes that you are currently healthy and are looking at supplements to enhance your health and bodily functions.

That said, if you are taking herbal preparations to treat any condition, it is essential that you determine with the help of your healthcare provider that the signs and symptoms do not represent a major disease. Heartburn can often be confused with a more serious heart condition. A urinary tract infection, if not evaluated, may become a more serious kidney infection. Yes, there are preparations that can help reduce the risk of these in the future, but you must know if there is an actual disease or diagnosis before you begin. It is just like using a prescription medication; you don't use a prescription to treat hayfever if you have a bronchial infection, and you don't use cranberry extract if you are constipated.

If you are treating a disease, be sure that the herbal medicines you use are the ones for the condition and that you are taking the correct dosage. Know how long it should take to get the anticipated results and, if you don't get them, reevaluate what you are doing. Use the herb until the condition is relieved or, if there are no adverse effects, you may continue it for a long-lasting condition if the herb is appropriate for long-term use. If you are using the herb to reduce risk of developing a condition, follow the recommended dosage. Doses for herbal medicines, although they may not be an exact science, are given for a reason—they are what have been observed to be most effective for a particular condition.

Healing Herbs

The following table provides an easy reference to the healing herbs described in this book. (Specific information regarding some of the herbs may be found in Chapter 2. The herbs in Chapter 2 and those listed below are available commercially in many forms. Chapter 4 will give you some suggestions about using these herbs for specific conditions.) This is meant as a guide to help you determine which healing herb might be most useful for you, and what its interactions or adverse reactions and contraindications might be. The information in the second column, "People Use This For," is based on historical use or, when available, effectiveness information based on human studies (unless otherwise noted). Potential side effects and interactions are based, in most cases, on typical doses of the herbs. The last column, "Usage Notes/Comments," gives information, when available, about maximum doses, length of time to take and effects on diseases or conditions. When in doubt about how much to take, read label directions and consult your healthcare provider.

Finding Good Information & Supplements on the Internet

When you are looking for information about supplements on the Internet, it's best to look for sites from government or nonprofit agencies and reputable manufacturers. Use the following checklist to evaluate a site:

✔ Who operates the site? A government, university or reputable medical or health-related association may not always give you the information you want to hear, but in most cases, the information is accurate and honest.

✔ What is the purpose of the site? Is it to educate or sell? Avoid, or at least look skeptically at, the sites of practitioners or organizations that are trying to sell something without reliable information to support its claims.

✔ Does the information provide a source and references? Are studies reviewed in scientific journals? Does the site include information on where the studies are listed so you can check references for accuracy? PubMed (http://www.ncbi.nlm.nih.gov/PubMed/) offers one of the most reliable sources of referenced studies and literature.

✔ Is the information current? The field of herbs, although ancient, has a relatively short history of reliable, documented research. When was the information posted and updated? In general, a Web post more than 6 months old may be outdated. Printed information may not be current if it is more than 3 to 5 years old, depending on the subject. (Some studies that are many years old may be the most recent.)

✔ Can you trust e-mail solicitations? The Internet is ripe with herb and supplement Web sites that do not have reliable information backing them up. Watch out for solicitations and messages that are in UPPERCASE LETTERS, have lots of exclamation points!!! or include phrases like, "This is not a hoax."

✔ Does it sound to good to be true? If it does, it probably is.

✔ Look out for the latest headline. Often, what we hear or see in the news is too brief to include important information that can help you make an informed decision. Also, some articles are sensationalized and leave out important information.

✔ Evaluate your assumptions about herbal medicines:

- It's not wise to assume that even if a product does not help, it also won't hurt.
- Just because an herb is natural does not always mean it is safe.
- If there are no warnings on the labels, do not assume that it's safe to use in any amount. If information is missing from the label—for example, how much to take, a supplement facts label and interaction or adverse information—avoid it.
- If there is a recall of a product, it does not mean that all such harmful products will be immediately and entirely removed from the shelves.

Quick Reference to Healing Herbs

Common Name/Botanical Name

The common name is the name by which the herb is mostly commonly known. Some herbs have very similar names but different actions, so be certain that the herb you choose is the one you want. The most commonly used name is included in the chart.

The botanical name includes only the genus and species, not the family name. Remember that for some individuals, sensitivities to herbs may include all family members. Every effort has been made to include this information, either here or in chapter 2. If in doubt, check it out!

Potential Interactions

Just as with side effects, the interaction information may be based on anecdotal or theoretical information. One difference here is that there are known adverse reactions and interactions based on research and clinical reports. Every effort has been taken to make sure that the most common adverse reactions and/or interactions are listed. If in doubt, please refer to chapter 2 or to one of the references listed on pages 312-313.

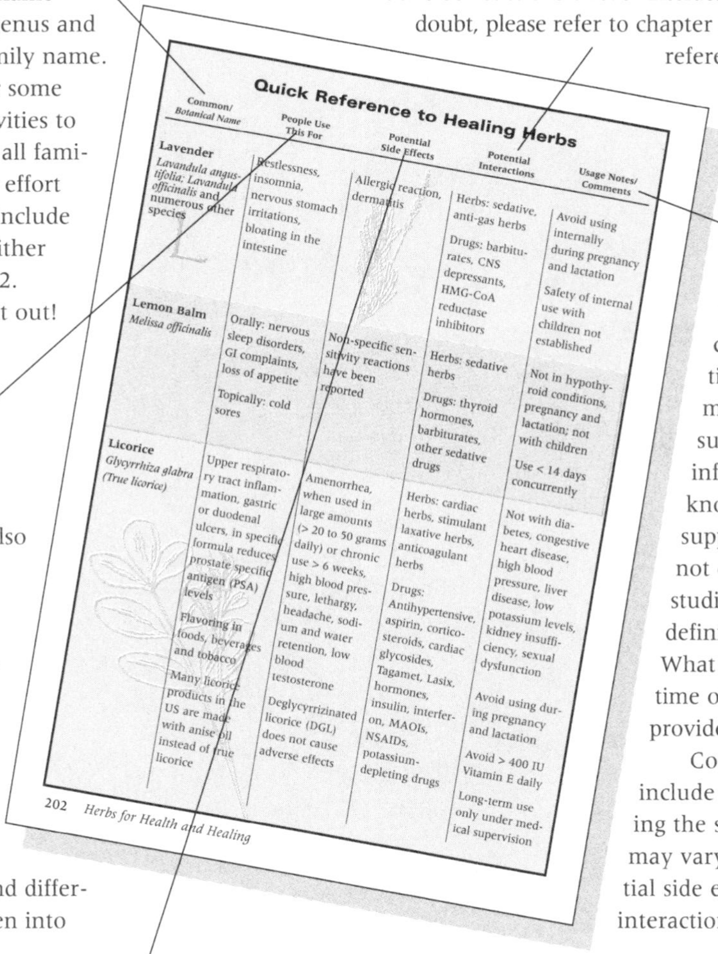

Quick Reference to Healing Herbs

Common/ Botanical Name	People Use This For	Potential Side Effects	Potential Interactions	Usage Notes/ Comments
Lavender *Lavandula angustifolia; Lavandula officinalis* and numerous other species	Restlessness, insomnia, nervous stomach irritations, bloating in the intestine	Allergic reaction, dermatitis	Herbs: sedative, anti-gas herbs Drugs: barbiturates, CNS depressants, HMG-CoA reductase inhibitors	Avoid using internally during pregnancy and lactation Safety of internal use with children not established
Lemon Balm *Melissa officinalis*	Orally: nervous sleep disorders, GI complaints, loss of appetite Topically: cold sores	Non-specific sensitivity reactions have been reported	Herbs: sedative herbs Drugs: thyroid hormones, barbiturates, other sedative drugs	Not in hypothyroid conditions, pregnancy and lactation; not with children Use < 14 days concurrently
Licorice *Glycyrrhiza glabra (True licorice)*	Upper respiratory tract inflammation, gastric or duodenal ulcers, in specific formula reduces prostate specific antigen (PSA) levels Flavoring in foods, beverages and tobacco Many licorice products in the US are made with anise oil instead of true licorice	Amenorrhea, when used in large amounts (> 20 to 50 grams daily) or chronic use > 6 weeks, high blood pressure, lethargy, headache, sodium and water retention, low blood testosterone Deglycyrrizinated licorice (DGL) does not cause adverse effects	Herbs: cardiac herbs, stimulant laxative herbs, anticoagulant herbs Drugs: Antihypertensive, aspirin, corticosteroids, cardiac glycosides, Tagamet, Lasix, hormones, insulin, interferon, MAOIs, NSAIDs, potassium-depleting drugs	Not with diabetes, congestive heart disease, high blood pressure, liver disease, low potassium levels, kidney insufficiency, sexual dysfunction Avoid using during pregnancy and lactation Avoid > 400 IU Vitamin E daily Long-term use only under medical supervision

202 *Herbs for Health and Healing*

People Use This For

This information includes not only current uses, but also historical or folk uses and in some cases, speculative uses. The information may not be research based and is not an endorsement for its use; each person and condition is different, and differences must be taken into consideration.

Usage Notes/ Comments

Usage notes indicate the length of time a supplement may be safely consumed, when that information is known. For some supplements there are not enough long-term studies to provide definitive information. What is known at the time of this writing is provided here.

Comments here may include cautions regarding the supplement that may vary from the potential side effects and possible interactions information.

Potential Side Effects

Here are listed side effects that may occur with use of the herb. The information is based on research, anecdotal and theoretical information. What is listed here is based on the most common and current knowledge about the herb and its effects on humans.

Quick Reference to Healing Herbs*

Common/ *Botanical Name*	People Use This For **	Potential Side Effects	Potential Interactions	Usage Notes/ Comments
Alfalfa *Medicago satvia*	High cholesterol, diuretic, tonic, phytoestrogen	In excess, may increase blood coagulation	Anticoagulant/ antiplatelet drugs, vitamins and herbs	Not in pregnancy
Aloe *Aloe vera*	Wounds, infections, laxative	GI upset, electrolyte imbalance in long-term use	Laxative herbs and drugs	Orally not in pregnancy, lactation. Use less than 7 days
Angelica *Angelica archangelica*	Menopause, respiratory ailments, stimulates bile secretion, antispasmodic	Photosensitivity or photodermatitis Hypotension (low blood pressure)	Anticoagulant/ antiplatelet drugs, vitamins and herbs	Not in pregnancy
Artichoke *Cynara scolymus*	Liver protection, high cholesterol, edema, GI complaints	Allergic reaction if sensitive to related species	None known	Not with bile duct obstruction or gallstones
Ashwaganda *Withania somnifera*	Chronic liver conditions, anti-inflammatory	None reported	Sedative herbs and drugs. Amphetamines	Not in pregnancy or lactation
Astragalus *Astragalus membranaceus*	Colds and respiratory infections, angina	Toxicity is low. Used most commonly with other herbs	Antiviral, immune-suppressing drugs	Not in doses greater than 28 grams
Balsam *Abies balsamea*	Topically: hemorrhoids, antiseptic. Orally: respiratory complaints	No adverse reactions reported	No interactions known	Avoid using in pregnancy and lactation

* Note: This chart is for quick reference. Please refer to chapters 2 and 4 for more information.

** Note: Uses for herbs are based on different levels of evidence for the herb's use. This gives you folk, historical and anecdotal uses. It is not intended to indicate what the herb should or should not be used for. Some herbs are used for purposes for which there is no basis.

For herbs listed in boldface, additional information can be found in chapter 2.

Quick Reference to Healing Herbs

Common/ *Botanical Name*	People Use This For	Potential Side Effects	Potential Interactions	Usage Notes/ Comments
Basil *Ocimum basilicum*	Culinary herb Stomach and GI complaints	Low blood sugar	No interactions known	Long-term use in amounts > than in food may be unsafe
Bergamot *Citrus bergamia*	Psoriasis, vitiligo (loss of skin pigment), fungicide	Occupational allergy. Increased sensitivity in sun-sensitive persons	Drugs that increase sensitivity to the sun	
Bilberry *Fruit and leaf* *Vaccinium myrtillus*	Diarrhea, circulatory problems, vision improvement, particularly with diabetes	Chronic intoxication in animals—leaf No adverse reactions noted with fruit	Anti-diabetic drugs (monitor blood sugar due to potential for decreasing blood sugar) and disulfran	Use with caution in persons with diabetes; leaf extract may lower blood sugar. Not for > 3-4 days w/diarrhea. Leaf: not in pregnancy or lactation.
Black Cohosh *Cimicifuga racemosa*	Menopause, premenstrual discomfort	GI upset Headache, nausea, vomiting, dizziness	Tamoxifen; may have additive effect of preventing the binding of estrogen to breast cancer cells	Not > 6 months without a break. Not in pregnancy or lactation. Not with estrogen-sensitive cancers
Black Currant *Berry* *Ribes nigrum*	Berry: coughs and flavoring component Leaf: arthritis, liver ailments, edema	No adverse reactions reported	No known interactions	Leaf: not for persons with cardiac-related edema or reduced kidney function Avoid leaf in pregnancy

Quick Reference to Healing Herbs

Common/ *Botanical Name*	People Use This For	Potential Side Effects	Potential Interactions	Usage Notes/ Comments
Bladderwrack *Fucus vesiculosis*	Thyroid disorders, obesity, arthritis, GI complaints	Exacerbate hyperthyroidism Long-term use reduces iron absorption	Not with diuretics, anticoagulants/ antiplatelet drugs, lithium or thyroid hormones	Not with sodium restriction, iron deficiency, iodine allergy Not during pregnancy or lactation Not with children
Borage, Borage Oil *Borago officinalis*	Plant: expectorant, menopause, sedative, heart tonic Oil: essential fatty acid deficiency, anti-inflammatory, improved heart function	Plant, orally: constipation, liver damage Oil: may increase bleeding time	Plant: not with eucalyptus, comfrey, groundsel, butterbur, phenothiazine-containing drugs Oil: not with phenothiazines, anesthesia, anticoagulants/ antiplatelet, herbs with anticoagulants/antiplatelet activity, eucalyptus or herbs with pyrrolizidine alkaloids	Plant: not in schizophrenia Oil: not in schizophrenia or liver disease Avoid using either during pregnancy or lactation
Bosweilla (Frankincense) *Boswellia carteri* **Indian Frankincense** *Boswellia serrata*	Colic and gas Hand cream Arthritis, anti-inflammatory, ulcerative colitis Soaps, cosmetics and food	None reported for either herb	None reported for either herb	Not during pregnancy or lactation

Quick Reference to Healing Herbs

Common/ *Botanical Name*	People Use This For	Potential Side Effects	Potential Interactions	Usage Notes/ Comments
Butcher's broom *Ruscus aculeatus*	Hemorrhoids, chronic venous insufficiency, varicose veins	GI upset and nausea	Drugs: MAOIs, alpha-blockers Herbs: diuretics, vasoconstrictors	Not during pregnancy or lactation
Butterbur leaf and root *Petasites hybridus; Petasites officinalis*	Leaf: tension and appetite sedative and appetite stimulant Topically: wound healing Root: urinary tract pain with stones, hayfever	External Use Only Orally: Leaf unsafe Root associated with veno-occlusive disease Do not apply to broken skin Allergic reaction with sensitivity to Asteraceae/ Compositae family	Eucalyptus, comfrey, borage, Joe-Pye weed, Groundsel	Not with allergy to Asteraceae/ Compositae family Not during pregnancy or lactation No more than 1 mcg daily, limited to < 6 weeks
Caraway *Seeds and oil* *Carum carvi*	Seeds: orally for gas, GI complaints, appetite stimulant Oil: digestive problems, gas fullness	Contact dermatitis	No known interactions	Oil: not during pregnancy and lactation Safe in amounts used in foods
Cascara Sagrada *Rhammus purshiana*	Laxative	Stomach cramps, diarrhea Long-term use causes laxative dependence, electrolyte imbalance	Herbs: licorice, digitalis, stimulant laxative herbs, potassium-depleting herbs Drugs: cardiac glycosides, corticosteroids, potassium-depleting diuretics, laxatives. Reduces absorption of any oral drug	Not with GI disease or upset Not during pregnancy or lactation. May be excreted in milk Not > 1 to 2 weeks

Quick Reference to Healing Herbs

Common/ *Botanical Name*	People Use This For	Potential Side Effects	Potential Interactions	Usage Notes/ Comments
Catnip *Nepeta cataria*	Folk uses: headache, colds, flu, fever, GI upset, stimulate menstrual bleeding	Headache and malaise; excess amounts may cause vomiting	Herbs: herbs with sedative properties Drugs: barbiturates, sedatives	Not during pregnancy or lactation Not with excessive menstrual bleeding or pelvic inflammatory disease
Cat's Claw *Uncaria tomentosa; Uncaria guianensis*	Immune system stimulant Contraceptive use reported in folk medicine	Rare: diarrhea with large doses, low blood pressure, bruising or bleeding gums	Drugs: antihypertensive No other interactions known	Not when trying to conceive Avoid during pregnancy and lactation
Cayenne *Capsicum frutescens* and numerous other *Capsicum* species	Topically for rheumatoid arthritis, osteoarthritis, neuralgias Digestive stimulant	Orally: GI irritation, sweating of head and neck; excessive amounts—GI, liver or kidney damage Dermatitis in breast-fed infants whose mothers consume large amounts Skin burns	Herbs: sedative herbs, anticoagulant herbs, Coca Drugs: ACE inhibitors, acid-inhibiting drugs, anti-hypertensive drugs, anticoagulant drugs, aspirin, barbiturates, cocaine, sedatives, drugs metabolized by the liver MAOIs, theophylline	Not with infectious or inflammatory GI conditions Topically < 2 days; 14 days between applications Safe as ingredient in amounts found in food Pregnancy and lactation: avoid amounts larger than found in food

Quick Reference to Healing Herbs

Common/ *Botanical Name*	People Use This For	Potential Side Effects	Potential Interactions	Usage Notes/ Comments
Chamomile *Matricaria recutita*	Orally for GI upsets, sleep Topically: skin and mucous membrane inflammation, bacterial skin disease, mouthwash, bath for genital and anal irritations	Concentrated tea can cause vomiting Allergic skin reactions, severe hypersensitivity and anaphylaxis Allergic reaction in persons allergic to Asteraceae/ Compositae family members	Herbs: herbs with sedative properties, herbs with anticoagulant/Antiplatelet potential Drugs: anticoagulants/ antiplatelets, benzodiazepines, alcohol Indomethacin, sedatives	Not for people with asthma or cross allergy to Asteraceae/ Compositae family Not during pregnancy or lactation
Chaparral *Larrea tridentate; Larrea divaricata*	Arthritis, antimicrobial cancer, TB, bowel cramps, diuretic	Unsafe if taken orally Reactions: nausea, diarrhea, kidney/liver failure, fever, weight loss, anorexia, fatigue and more	MAOIs	Chapparal is unsafe and should not be used by anyone Severe liver damage and liver failure associated with its use
Chaste Tree (chasteberry) *Vitex agnus-castus*	Menstrual irregularities, PMS, breast pain, hot flashes in menopause	Rare GI upset, allergic reactions, heart rhythm irregularities	Drugs: antipsychotic drugs, oral contraceptives and hormone replacement therapy	Not in pregnancy or lactation Avoid > 400 IU Vitamin E
Chervil *Anthriscus cerefolium*	Folk medicine use as a diuretic, expectorant, digestive aid	No adverse reactions reported	No interactions noted	Amounts greater than used in food may be mutagenic during pregnancy and lactation

Quick Reference to Healing Herbs

Common/ *Botanical Name*	People Use This For	Potential Side Effects	Potential Interactions	Usage Notes/ Comments
Chives *Allium schoenoprasum*	Folk remedy uses chives for parasitic worms	Large amounts may lead to GI distress	No interactions known	Avoid large amounts during pregnancy and lactation
Cinnamon *Cinnamomum verum*	Gas, appetite stimulant, premature ejaculation when used as a combination topical therapy	Bark: no known reaction Oil: may irritate mucous membranes and irritate skin	Drugs: acid-inhibiting drugs	Do not use with GI conditions Avoid using amounts greater than in food during pregnancy and lactation
Cocoa *Theobroma cacao*	Contains theobromine, a CNS stimulant Folk use: infectious intestinal diseases, diarrhea, asthma, bronchitis, expectorant Seed coat: liver, bladder and kidney problems, diabetes Cocoa powder for heart disease	Allergic skin reactions, shakiness, diuresis, rapid pulse, constipation, migraine headaches, nausea, GI upset, gas	Herbs: herbs with caffeine, ephedra Drugs: NSAIDs, aspirin, barbiturates, beta-adrenergic agonists, diabetes drugs, Cimetidine, Clozapine, Antabuse, ergotamine, Diflucan, Lithium, MAOIs, Mexitil, OCDs, phenylpropanolamine, quinolones, theophylline, verapamil Foods: grapefruit juice	Not with anxiety disorders, depression, gastric or duodenal ulcers, GERD, heart conditions, irritable bowel syndrome, migraine headaches Safe in amounts used in food

Quick Reference to Healing Herbs

Common/ *Botanical Name*	People Use This For	Potential Side Effects	Potential Interactions	Usage Notes/ Comments
Coffee *Coffee arabica; Coffee canephora* and other *Coffee* species	Stimulant increases mental alertness Athletic performance improvement	Increases the excretion of calcium and magnesium, increase cholesterol levels, LDL cholesterol and triglycerides, may increase risk of pancreatic cancer, heart disease in women, breast and ovarian cancer May cause headaches, high blood pressure, GI upset, irregular heartbeat May increase adverse effect with ephedra	Herbs: herbs and supplements with caffeine, ephedra Drugs: NSAID, antacids, Fosamax, diabetes drugs, aspirin, beta-adrenergic agonists, cimetidine, clozapine, CNS stimulants, Antabuse, ephedrine, estrogen, ergotamine, lithium, Mexitil, MAOIs, OCDs, phenylpropanolamine, quinolones, Rilutek, Lamsil, theophylline	Not with anxiety disorders, cardiovascular disease, cancer, depression, gastric or duodenal ulcers, heart conditions, elevated cholesterol, hyperthyroid disease, kidney disease, osteoporosis, seizure tendency Safe in amounts moderately consumed in foods Avoid with grapefruit juice Tannin content may cause decreased drug absorption
Comfrey *Symphytum officinale*	Topically: anti-inflammatory agent	Liver toxicity in any amount, even tea, venoocclusive disease	Herbs: eucalyptus, borage, butterbur, groundsel	Do not use on broken skin. Not for internal use Not for use during pregnancy or lactation

Quick Reference to Healing Herbs

Common/ *Botanical Name*	People Use This For	Potential Side Effects	Potential Interactions	Usage Notes/ Comments
Cranberry *Vaccinium macrocarpon*	Orally for preventing urinary tract infections, urinary deodorizer, urinary incontinence, antiviral	No adverse reactions More than 3 to 4 L of juice daily may cause diarrhea	Do not use with proton pump inhibitors (drugs for gastric reflux)	Do not use in acute urinary tract infections; seek medical treatment Do not use in people with atrophic gastritis; people with diabetes should avoid sugar-sweetened cranberry juice, low stomach hydrochloric acid
Cumin *Cuminum cyminum*	Culinary spice and flavoring component Used for gas, diuretic, stimulating menstrual flow, diarrhea and colic	Undiluted oil may increase sensitivity to the sun	Drugs: diabetes drugs, barbiturates	Likely safe in amounts commonly found in food Avoid excess during pregnancy and lactation
Dandelion *Taraxacum officinale*	Loss of appetite, bloating, laxative, healthy circulation, rheumatism, arthritic joints and spring tonic	Can increase stomach acid, contact dermatitis, allergic reaction in those allergic to the Asteraceae/ Compositae family	Entire plant—herbs: diuretic herbs, herbs that lower blood sugar Drugs: diuretics, drugs that lower blood sugar, lithium, acid-inhibiting drugs, anti-hypertensives	Caution: in diabetes, gallstones, bile duct obstruction, bleeding disorders Avoid using in amounts larger than is consumed in food Contains more beta-carotene than carrots

Quick Reference to Healing Herbs

Common/ *Botanical Name*	People Use This For	Potential Side Effects	Potential Interactions	Usage Notes/ Comments
Devil's Claw *Harpagophytum procumbens*	Loss of appetite, indigestion, and as supportive therapy for degenerative joint disorders (osteoarthritis)	Rare headache, tinnitis, anorexia, loss of taste, diarrhea	Drugs: acid-inhibiting drugs, drugs that lower blood sugar, Coumadin, cardiac drugs, drugs that lower or raise blood pressure	Not with duodenal or gastric ulcers, caution with gallstones, diabetes, heart disease including high and low blood pressure Avoid using during pregnancy and lactation
Dill *Anetheum graveolens*	Dill seed or oil: stomach upset Historically: gas, hemorrhoids, bronchial asthma, neuralgias, dysuria, genital ulcers and irregular menses	Sensitivity to sun when exposed to juice or plant Allergic reactions in persons with allergies to plants of the carrot family	No known interactions	Not for use in urinary tract infections Safe in amounts commonly used in foods Avoid amounts greater than in foods during pregnancy and lactation
Dong Quai *Angelica sinensis*	Menopause, gynecological complaints Traditionally: high blood pressure, ulcers, anemia, constipation and to prevent allergic reactions	Sensitivity to sun, potentially carcinogenic and mutagenic	Herbs: herbs with anticoagulant/antiplatelet potential Drugs: antiplatelet drugs, Coumadin	Not in pregnancy and lactation

Quick Reference to Healing Herbs

Common/ *Botanical Name*	People Use This For	Potential Side Effects	Potential Interactions	Usage Notes/ Comments
Echinacea *Echinacea angustifolia*	Supportive therapy for flu, shortening length of cold symptoms, urinary tract infections Topically: poorly healing skin wounds	Allergic reactions in persons with allergy to Asteraceae/ Compositae family, fever, nausea and vomiting	Drugs: avoid with immunosuppressant drugs, Spectazole	Avoid in persons with a genetic tendency toward allergic reactions, progressive systemic disorders, HIV or AIDS, diabetes, infertility Not > 8 weeks
Ephedra *Ephedra sinica*	Diseases of the respiratory tract Historically: Colds, fever, chills, headache, edema, diuretic, weight loss	Dizziness, hyperactivity, anxiety, irritability, insomnia, headache, anorexia, irregular heartbeats, high blood pressure, heart failure, seizures, asphyxia, stroke, death Combined with caffeine-containing products increases adverse effects	Herbs: caffeine, coffee, cola nut, guarana, maté, digitalis, Ergot Drugs: Elavil, Decadron, drugs that lower blood sugar, Lanoxin, Migranol, MAOIs, oxytocin, reserpine, theophylline, urinary acidifiers, urinary alkalizers, anticonvulsants, thyroid replacement therapy	Not with: angina, anorexia, anxiety, bulimia, BPH, cerebral insufficiency, essential tremor, glaucoma, heart disease, hyperthyroidism, thyrotoxicosis, high blood pressure, kidney stones, myasthenia gravis, adrenal gland tumor, urinary retention Use < 7 days, < 24 mg daily Discontinue 24 hours before surgery

Quick Reference to Healing Herbs

Common/ *Botanical Name*	People Use This For	Potential Side Effects	Potential Interactions	Usage Notes/ Comments
Eucalyptus *Eucalyptus globulus*	Leaf: respiratory tract mucous membrane inflammation, expectorant Oil: respiratory tract mucous membrane inflammation, topically for rheumatic complaints and respiratory tract inflammation	Leaf: urinary irritant, rarely nausea, vomiting, diarrhea Oil: nausea, vomiting, diarrhea and death	Leaf, drugs: drugs to control blood sugar, drugs metabolized by the liver Oil, herbs: Pyrrolizidine alkaloid-containing plants Oil, drugs: drugs to control blood sugar, drugs metabolized by the liver	Not with diabetes Not in bile duct obstruction, GI inflammation or liver disease Not in pregnancy and lactation Not for children in amounts greater than found in foods
Evening Primrose *Oenothera biennis*	Breast pain during lactation Arthritis, PMS, diabetic peripheral neuropathy	Indigestion, nausea, soft stools and headache	Drugs: anesthesia, phenothiazines, anticoagulants, antiplatelets, Tamoxifen	Not in persons with epilepsy or seizure disorder, schizophrenia, bleeding disorders Not in pregnancy
Fennel *Foeniculum vulgare* Seed and oil.	Spastic GI symptoms, fullness, gas and inflammation of the upper respiratory tract	Allergic cross-sensitivity with celery, carrot, mugwort Dermitìtis Oil: allergic reaction, hallucinations, nausea/vomiting, seizures, pulmonary edema	Seeds, drugs: Cipro, ACE inhibitors, antihypertensives, diuretcs	Not in pregnancy and lactation Use not more than 3 to 4 weeks People with diabetes should use fennel honey with caution

Quick Reference to Healing Herbs

Common/ *Botanical Name*	People Use This For	Potential Side Effects	Potential Interactions	Usage Notes/ Comments
Fenugreek *Trigonella foenum-graecum*	Orally: lowering blood sugar in persons with diabetes, loss of appetite Topically: poultice for local inflammation	Diarrhea and gas. Large amounts can cause low blood sugar, occupational asthma	Herbs: anticoagulant/ antiplatelet drugs Drugs: anticoagulants, corticosteriods, hormone therapy, diabetes drugs, insulin, MAOIs; delay or decrease the absorption of other drugs	Not with fenugreek allergy, kidney stones or diabetes Avoid using during pregnancy and lactation Avoid > 400 IU Vitamin E daily
Feverfew *Tanacetum parthenium*	Leaf: orally for migraine headaches Historical: menstrual irregularities, stomach ache, fever, nausea, vomiting	Orally: mouth ulcers, tongue irritant, stomach pain, indigestion, gas, diarrhea, nausea, vomiting Allergic reaction in persons sensitive to Asteraceae/ Compositae family	Herbs: anticoagulant herbs Drugs: anticoagulant drugs, NSAIDs May decrease absorption of medicinal iron	Not in children under two, pregnant or lactating women Avoid > 400 IU Vitamin E daily
Flax *Linum usitatissimum*	Seed: laxative, high cholesterol, irritable bowel, gastritis Oil: arthritis	Inadequate fluid with flax may cause intestinal blockage Sensitization in occupational exposure	Drugs: may decrease absorption of other drugs Anticoagulant drugs, hormone replacement therapy (HRT), diabetes medication	Seed: not in bowel obstruction, esophageal stricture or acute intestinal inflammation Seed: safe during pregnancy and lactation in food amounts; store in refrigerator or freezer

Quick Reference to Healing Herbs

Common/ *Botanical Name*	People Use This For	Potential Side Effects	Potential Interactions	Usage Notes/ Comments
Garcinia *Garcinia cambogia*	Weight loss	No adverse reactions reported	No interactions reported	Extract containing 50% hydroxycitric acid
Garlic *Allium sativum*	High cholesterol, high triglycerides, increasing HDL cholesterol, high blood pressure, peripheral artery disease, ulcers	Bad breath, GI irritation, heartburn, gas, nausea, vomiting, diarrhea May change intestinal flora Topically may cause dermatitis	Herbs: anticoagulant herbs Supplements: fish oil Drugs: anticoagulants, diabetes drugs	Not with bleeding disorders, diabetes, GI irritation Discontinue 2 weeks prior to surgery Not in pregnancy and lactation in amounts greater than found in foods
Ginger *Zingiber officinale*	Motion sickness, seasickness, morning sickness, dyspepsia, joint pain, postoperative nausea and vomiting	Dermatitis, CNS depression and irregular heartbeats in large doses	Herbs: anticoagulant herbs Drugs: antacids, anticoagulant drugs, barbiturates, blood pressure regulating drugs, cardiac drugs, diabetes drugs, SSRIs	Not in: persons with gallstones, bleeding conditions, diabetes, heart disease treated with drugs, high/low blood pressure Avoid excessive amounts Avoid amounts not found in foods and beverages during pregnancy and lactation

Quick Reference to Healing Herbs

Common/ *Botanical Name*	People Use This For	Potential Side Effects	Potential Interactions	Usage Notes/ Comments
Ginkgo *Ginkgo biloba* *Leaf extract*	Dementia, peripheral vascular disease, vertigo, poor circulation, tinnitis, PMS, heart disease	GI complaints, headache, dizziness, allergic skin reactions, bleeding, seizures	Herbs: anticoagulant herbs Drugs: Coumadin, anticoagulant drugs, cyclosporine, MAOIs, SSRIs, thiazide diuretics, aspirin, diabetic medication	Not with bleeding disorders, epilepsy, infertility; caution with diabetes Effects seen > 6 to 8 weeks use Avoid during pregnancy and lactation Discontinue use 36 hours before surgery
Ginseng *Panax quinquefolius (American)* *Panax ginseng* *(Asian, Chinese)*	American: tonic, stimulant, diuretic, anemia, digestive aid Asian: cognitive function, anxiety, Alzheimer's disease, controlling blood sugar, stress, cancer, athletic performance and stamina	American: diarrhea, headache, insomnia, vertigo Asian: insomnia, Mastalgia, vaginal bleeding, irregular heart rate, liver disease, decreased appetite, edema, diarrhea, skin reactions	Herbs (both ginsengs): coffee, guarana, tea, maté, anticoagulant and immunosuppressant herbs Drugs (both ginsengs): Lasix, anticoagulant drugs, antipsychotic drugs, caffeine, Lanoxin, MAOIs, diabetes drugs, hormones, stimulants, immunosuppressants	Both ginsengs: not in bleeding conditions, cardiac disorders, diabetes, insomnia, schizophrenia, hypertension Not in pregnancy and lactation Not for use with infants and children Take < 3 months Discontinue use at least 7 days before surgery

Quick Reference to Healing Herbs

Common/ *Botanical Name*	People Use This For	Potential Side Effects	Potential Interactions	Usage Notes/ Comments
Ginseng *Eleutherococcus senticosus* *(Siberian)*	Increasing resistance to environmental stress, increasing speed, quality and capacity for physical work, preventing atherosclerosis, normalizing blood pressure, chronic bronchitis, herpes II simple virus, decrease blood coagulation and more	Reactions are rare, but may include insomnia, slight drowsiness, change in heart rhythm, melancholy, anxiety, breast pain in lactating, high blood pressure in persons with rheumatic heart disease Long-term use: inflamed nerves, muscle spasms	Herbs: sedative herbs, coffee Vitamins: B1, B2 and C Drugs: alcohol, anticoagulants, antipsychotic drugs, hormones, barbiturates, diabetes drugs, Lanoxin, lanamycin, insulin Foods: spicy, bitter substances	Not with hypertension, myocardial infarction, psychiatric disorders, fevers, in those who are highly excitable Not in pregnancy and lactation
Goldenseal *Hydrastis canadensis*	Historically: whooping cough, diarrhea, enhancing immunity, bacterial infections, stimulates bile secretion, slows menstrual flow, stimulates uterine contractions	Digestive disorders, constipation, hallucinations, deliriums, anxiety, photosensitivity Overdose can cause nausea, vomiting, low blood pressure, irregular heart rhythm, paralysis, convulsions, death	Herbs: sedative herbs Drugs: antacids, drugs for high blood pressure, barbiturates, heparin, protein bound drugs, sedatives, acetaminophen, anticoagulants Vitamins: B vitamin absorption	Not with heart disease, GI irritation, excess bilirubin (newborns), bleeding disorders, high blood pressure Avoid during pregnancy, lactation Not with newborn infants Dose < 8 mg of root, < 7 days

Quick Reference to Healing Herbs

Common/ *Botanical Name*	People Use This For	Potential Side Effects	Potential Interactions	Usage Notes/ Comments
Gotu Kola *Centella asiatica*	Orally: heart disease, chronic venous insufficiency, memory improvement, edema Topically: skin inflammations, wounds	Whole body itching, sensitivity to the sun, abortion Large amounts elevated blood pressure, nausea Topically: contact dermatitis	Drugs: cholesterol lowering drugs, diabetes drugs, sedatives Herbs: sedative herbs	Not during pregnancy or lactation Not with diabetes or high cholesterol
Grapeseed *Vitis vinifera; vitis coignetiae*	Oil: supplemental essential fatty acids Extract: chronic venous insufficiency, improves vein tone, night vision, anti-inflammatory	No adverse reactions reported	No interactions known to occur	During pregnancy and lactation avoid amounts greater than found in foods
Green Tea *Camellia sinensis*	Improving memory and judgment, lowering cholesterol and triglycerides, reducing risk of some cancers Diuretic, diarrhea, gingivitis, stimulates immune system	GI upset, constipation Large amounts: irregular heartbeat, headache, diuresis, anxiety, insomnia, irritability, dependence Symptoms similar to those in other caffeine-containing herbs Impaired iron metabolism in infants and children	Herbs: caffeine-containing herbs and supplements, ephedra Drugs: NSAIDs, antacids, aspirin, beta-adrenergic agonists, cimetidine, clozapine, CNS stimulants, Antabuse, ephedrine, estrogen, ergotamine, lithium, MAOIs, OCDs, phenylpropanolamine, Mexitil, quinolones, theophylline, verapamil, Coumadin	Not with: diabetes, gastric or duodenal ulcers, heart conditions, depression, anxiety disorders, kidney disease Avoid more than 1 to 2 cups of green tea daily during pregnancy and lactation because of caffeine content Avoid > 400 IU Vitamin E daily

Quick Reference to Healing Herbs

Common/ *Botanical Name*	People Use This For	Potential Side Effects	Potential Interactions	Usage Notes/ Comments
Guarana *Paullinia cupana*	Diuretic, headache, increasing blood pressure in low blood pressure, stimulating the central nervous system, weight loss	Overdose causes: painful urination, abdominal spasms, vomiting, insomnia, nervousness, restlessness, agitation, GI irritation, nausea, vomiting, diuresis, irregular heartbeats, muscle spasms, delirium, convulsions, withdrawal symptoms	Herbs: caffeine containing herbs and supplements, ephedra Drugs: antacids, Fosamax, diabetes drugs, beta-adrenergic agonists, cimetidine, clozapine, CNS stimulants, aspirin, NSAIDs, Antabuse, ephedrine, estrogen, ergotamine, lithium, Mexitil, MAOIs, OCDs, Lamsil, theophylline, phenylpropanolamine, quinolones, Rilutek	Not with gastric or duodenal ulcers, heart conditions, depression, anxiety disorders, kidney disease Not for use in children Not in pregnancy and lactation Not to exceed 3 to 5 grams daily; may cause toxicity > 5 to 10 grams at 1 dose may be fatal
Guggul *Commiphora mukul*	Lowering high cholesterol and triglycerides, some types of acne May stimulate the uterus and menstrual flow	GI upset, headache, mild nausea, belching, hiccups	Drugs: Inderal, Cardizem, thyroid drugs	Monitor use with hyper- or hypothyroid disease and diabetes Not in pregnancy and lactation

Quick Reference to Healing Herbs

Common/ *Botanical Name*	People Use This For	Potential Side Effects	Potential Interactions	Usage Notes/ Comments
Gymnema Leaf *Gymnema sylvestre*	Further blood sugar reduction in persons with type 1 or type 2 diabetes on insulin or oral blood sugar lowering drugs, reducing cholesterol and triglycerides in type 1 diabetics	Decrease in sensitivity to sweet taste	Drugs: insulin and oral blood sugar lowering drugs Vitamins and Foods: may reduce the absorption of iron	Avoid during pregnancy and lactation Insufficient safety information available Typical dose is 400 mg daily
Hawthorn *Crataegus oxyacantha; Crataegus laevigata; Crataegus monogyna* (Leaf with flower extract)	Dilating blood vessels and coronary arteries, congestive heart failure (CHF), improving blood ejected during ventricular contractions, improving exercise tolerance, decreasing breathlessness, fatigue and/or heart palpitations	Nausea, GI complaints, palpitations, headache, dizziness, sleeplessness, agitation and circulatory disturbances when used therapeutically Large doses may cause low blood pressure	Herbs: herbs used for heart conditions, cardiac glycoside coating herbs Drugs: coronary vasodilators, cardiovascular drugs, CNS depressants, digoxin	Not with conventional cardiovascular drug therapy Caution with diabetes Avoid during pregnancy and lactation Greatest benefit usually seen after 6-8 weeks of therapy
Horehound *Marrubium vulgare*	Appetite stimulant, indigestion, bloating, coughs, colds	Large amounts can cause purging Plant juice may cause contact dermatitis	Drugs: may have an additive effect with antihypertensive and diabetes medications	Avoid using in heart conditions, pregnancy and lactation Monitor blood sugar in diabetes and blood pressure in HTN

Quick Reference to Healing Herbs

Common/ *Botanical Name*	People Use This For	Potential Side Effects	Potential Interactions	Usage Notes/ Comments
Horse Chestnut *Aesculus hippocastanum (horse chestnut seed)*	Chronic venous insufficiency including varicose veins, edema, tiredness, leg swelling, itching, high cholesterol	GI irritation, kidney disorders, itching Chestnut poisoning: muscle twitching, weakness, loss of coordination, vomiting, diarrhea, depression, paralysis	Herbs: anticoagulant/ antiplatelet, blood sugar lowering herbs Drugs: anticoagulants, protein-binding drugs, diabetes drugs	Not in infectious or inflammatory GI conditions, kidney impairment, liver impairment, diabetes, bleeding disorders Not in pregnancy and lactation Not with children
Juniper *Juniperus communis*	Traditionally: gas, colic, snakebite, intestinal worms, GI infections, cancer	Excessive oil: kidney irritation Overdose: kidney pain, diuresis, heart irregularities, high blood pressure, uterine bleeding Pollen: allergic reactions	Drugs: diuretics, diabetes drugs, anticoagulants	Not in diabetes, high or low blood pressure, kidney disease, seizure disorders, GI conditions Not in pregnancy and lactation
Kava *Piper methysticum*	Anxiety, stress, restlessness Folk medicine use: sedative, wound healing, headaches, colds, respiratory infections, urinary tract infections, menstrual problems	GI complaints, headache, dizziness, loss of balance, rarely allergic reactions, mouth numbness when herb chewed Long-term use: weight loss, scaly rashes, bloody urine, puffy face	Herbs: sedative herbs Drugs: alprazolam, CNS depressants, barbiturates, sedative drugs, levodopa Foods: alcohol	Not with depression, pregnancy, lactation Worldwide warnings: Kava-containing products linked to liver-related injuries Kava sales banned in several countries

Quick Reference to Healing Herbs

Common/ *Botanical Name*	People Use This For	Potential Side Effects	Potential Interactions	Usage Notes/ Comments
Lavender *Lavandula angustifolia; Lavandula officinalis* and numerous other species	Restlessness, insomnia, nervous stomach irritations, bloating in the intestine	Allergic reaction, dermatitis	Herbs: sedative, anti-gas herbs Drugs: barbiturates, CNS depressants, HMG-CoA reductase inhibitors	Avoid using internally during pregnancy and lactation Safety of internal use with children not established
Lemon Balm *Melissa officinalis*	Orally: nervous sleep disorders, GI complaints, loss of appetite Topically: cold sores	Non-specific sensitivity reactions have been reported	Herbs: sedative herbs Drugs: thyroid hormones, barbiturates, other sedative drugs	Not in hypothyroid conditions, pregnancy and lactation; not with children Use < 14 days concurrently
Licorice *Glycyrrhiza glabra (True licorice)*	Upper respiratory tract inflammation, gastric or duodenal ulcers, in specific formula reduces prostate specific antigen (PSA) levels Flavoring in foods, beverages and tobacco Many licorice products in the US are made with anise oil instead of true licorice	Amenorrhea, when used in large amounts (> 20 to 50 grams daily) or chronic use > 6 weeks, high blood pressure, lethargy, headache, sodium and water retention, low blood testosterone Deglycyrrizinated licorice (DGL) does not cause adverse effects	Herbs: cardiac herbs, stimulant laxative herbs, anticoagulant herbs Drugs: Antihypertensive, aspirin, corticosteroids, cardiac glycosides, Tagamet, Lasix, hormones, insulin, interferon, MAOIs, NSAIDs, potassium-depleting drugs	Not with diabetes, congestive heart disease, high blood pressure, liver disease, low potassium levels, kidney insufficiency, sexual dysfunction Avoid using during pregnancy and lactation Avoid > 400 IU Vitamin E daily Long-term use only under medical supervision

Quick Reference to Healing Herbs

Common/ *Botanical Name*	People Use This For	Potential Side Effects	Potential Interactions	Usage Notes/ Comments
Lobelia *Lobelia inflata*	Smoking cessation Historically: whooping cough, inducing sweating, sedative, apnea in newborns	Nausea, vomiting, diarrhea, coughing, dizziness, tremors Overdose: sweating, irregular heart rate, hypothermia, low blood pressure, convulsions, coma, possibly death	Herbs: tobacco	Not in heart disease, GI conditions, pregnancy, lactation Possible toxic dose: 0.6 to 1 gram; fatal dose may be 4 grams
Milk Thistle *Silybum marianum* **(Fruit, seeds)**	Discomfort after eating, toxic liver damage, supportive treatment of chronic inflammatory liver disease, cirrhosis, hepatitis, loss of appetite	Occasional laxative effect Mild allergic reactions Allergic reactions in persons sensitive to members of the Asteraceae/ Compositae family	Drugs: aspirin; protects the liver from damage caused by drugs, Cisplatin Decreases insulin resistance in diabetes May decrease OCD effectiveness	Not in pregnancy, lactation Monitor blood sugar in diabetes Take 8 to 12 weeks before improvement seen
Mints *Mentha piperita* **(Peppermint leaf)** *Mentha cardiaca* **(Spearmint leaf)**	Digestive complaints, irritable bowel, gallbladder and bile duct spasms	May increase colic in people with gallstones Choking sensation in young children Contact dermititis Temporary infertility in males	No known interactions	Both peppermint and spearmint are popular herbal medicinals, but peppermint is more potent and aromatic Not with gallstones, hiatal hernia; not in medicinal amounts, pregnancy, lactation

Quick Reference to Healing Herbs

Common/ *Botanical Name*	People Use This For	Potential Side Effects	Potential Interactions	Usage Notes/ Comments
Motherwort *Leonurus cardiaca*	Cardiac disorders, combination therapy for hyperthyroidism	Greater than 3 grams: diarrhea, stomach irritation, uterine bleeding Leaves: contact dermatitis Oil: sun sensitivity allergic reactions	Herbs: cardiac glycoside herbs Drugs: CNS depressants, anticoagulants, cardiac glycosides	Not with cardiac disorders, uterine bleeding conditions Not in pregnancy, lactation Not with breast cancer or family history of breast cancer
Mullein *Verbascum densiflorum; Verbascum thapsus*	Respiratory inflammations, cough, sore throat	No adverse reactions reported	No known interactions	Not in pregnancy, lactation
Nettle *Urtica dioica (Stinging nettle)*	Mild diuretic with excess fluid intake to increase urine flow, rheumatic complaints, lower urinary tract inflammation, to prevent urinary stones, allergic inflammation of the nose mucous membranes Topically: rheumatism Root: BPH	Orally: diarrhea Topically: local irritation Root: GI complaints, sweating, allergic skin reactions	Above ground parts only Herbs: sedative herbs, herbs that contain vitamin K Drugs: anticoagulants, diabetes drugs, high and low blood pressure drugs, CNS depressants, anti-inflammatory drugs	Leaf: not in heart or kidney insufficiency, diabetes, low or high blood pressure. Not in pregnancy, lactation Not in BPH or edema without medical supervision

Quick Reference to Healing Herbs

Common/ *Botanical Name*	People Use This For	Potential Side Effects	Potential Interactions	Usage Notes/ Comments
Nutmeg and Mace *Myristica fragrans*	Traditionally: nausea, stomach complaints, kidney problems, cancer, stimulating menstrual flow, insomnia	Five grams or more: thirst, weak pulse, hypothermia, disorientation, giddiness, euphoria, nausea, vomiting, feeling of chest pressure, irregular heart rate and numerous others	Herbs: safrole containing herbs (basil, cinnamon) Drugs: MAOIs, phenobarbital, drugs metabolized by the liver	Avoid larger than amounts found in foods, during pregnancy and lactation
Onion *Allium cepa*	Appetite stimulant, prevent heart disease	Orally: stomach distress Topically, eczema	Herbs: anticoagulant/ antiplatelet herbs Drugs: diabetes drugs, antiplatelet drugs, aspirin	Avoid amounts greater than found in foods in diabetes, pregnancy, lactation
Parsley *Petroselinum crispum*	Preventing and treating kidney stones Traditionally: GI disorders, constipation, jaundice, gas, colic, indigestion, bad breath, edema, promote menstrual flow, prostate disease, low blood pressure, anemia	Allergic skin or mucous membrane reactions More than 5 to 9 grams: liver dysfunction, kidney irritation, hemolytic anemia, decrease in blood platelets, abortion, hypothermia	Drugs: anticoagulant drugs, aspirin, diuretics, MAOIs	Not in amounts greater than found in food with: edema, high blood pressure, kidney disease Not in pregnancy or lactation

Quick Reference to Healing Herbs

Common/ *Botanical Name*	People Use This For	Potential Side Effects	Potential Interactions	Usage Notes/ Comments
Pennyroyal *Mentha pulegium; Hedeoma pulegioides* (Leaf and oil)	Leaf, traditionally: menstrual stimulant, antispasmodic, gas, stimulant, bowel problems Oil: abortion	Abdominal cramps, pain, nausea, vomiting, lethargy alternating with agitation, burning throat, restlessness and more	May decrease absorption of iron from supplements, some foods and herbs Toxic to the liver Large doses may cause abortion	Not with kidney disease Not in pregnancy or lactation Oil: not for oral use
Pine *Pinus sylvestris*	Orally: upper and lower respiratory inflammation Topically: mild muscle pain, neuralgia	No adverse reactions reported	No known interactions	Not with bronchial asthma or whooping cough, as bath additive with skin injury or diseases, pregnancy, lactation
Pokeweed *Phytolacca Americana (berry and root)*	Root, historically: rheumatism, upper and lower respiratory tract inflammations, skin infections and cancers, edema, irregular menstruation, tonsillitis	Berry and root: nausea, vomiting, cramping, abdominal pain, low blood pressure, irregular heartbeats, difficulty breathing, urinary incontinence, and more, including death	No known interactions	Not in children, pregnancy, lactation All parts of the plant are considered toxic except the immature leaves that are sold as "poke salad" Research is investigating ways of safely using pokeweed

Quick Reference to Healing Herbs

Common/ *Botanical Name*	People Use This For	Potential Side Effects	Potential Interactions	Usage Notes/ Comments
Psyllium *Plantago ovata (Blond psyllium)*	Laxative, to decrease high LDL and increase HDL cholesterol, secondary treatment for diarrhea, irritable bowel syndrome, lowers after-meal blood sugar	Gas, abdominal pain, diarrhea, constipation, upset stomach, bowel and esophageal obstruction when taken without adequate fluid Headache, backache, cough, possible kidney disease Occupational sensitization Respiratory allergic reactions	Psyllium interacts by reducing absorption of drugs and nutrients Drugs: Tegretol, diabetes drugs, Lanoxin, Coumadin, Lithium, insulin Foods and nutrients: reduced absorption	Take vitamin mineral supplements 1 hour before or 4 hours after Not with GI conditions, kidney dysfunction, type 2 diabetes (monitor), swallowing problems, sensitivity to psyllium Adequate fluids a must!
Pumpkin *Cucurbita pepo*	Seeds are used for painful urination, secondary to BPH, and bladder irritation, diuretic Insufficient information, but theory that it may also help rid the body of worms	Rare ejaculatory problems when taken as a combination with other herbs used to treat BPH. Pumpkin seeds are high in mono- and polyunsaturated fats that may contribute a significant amount of calories in large amounts	None reported	Not in amounts greater than in food during pregnancy and lactation

Quick Reference to Healing Herbs

Common/ *Botanical Name*	People Use This For	Potential Side Effects	Potential Interactions	Usage Notes/ Comments
Pygeum *Prunus africanas*	Symptoms of benign prostatic hyperplasia (BPH)	Nausea and abdominal pain	No known interactions	Not in pregnancy, lactation Over-harvesting of bark is threatening survival
Red Clover *Trifolium pratense*	Cough, asthma, bronchitis, cancer, menopause May improve pre-peri-menopausal bone density and urinary frequency in BPH	Rash-like reactions, possible estrogen-like activity	Herbs: anticoagulant/ antiplatelet, herbs with estrogen-like activity Drugs: anticoagulant, estrogen, OCDs	Not with blood clotting disorders, estrogen-sensitive conditions; not in pregnancy or lactation Avoid > 400 IU Vitamin E daily
Rhubarb *Rheum officinale*	Constipation in high doses, diarrhea in low doses, diuretic, renal failure, antibacterial, anti-inflammatory	GI cramps, diarrhea, uterine contractions, electrolyte loss, protein in the urine, bloody urine, dehydration, edema, muscular weakness and more	Herbs: cardiac glycosides, cardioactive herbs, stimulant laxative herbs, licorice Drugs: antiarrythmic, corticosteroids, Lanoxin, laxatives, cardiac glycosides; may decrease absorption of other drugs	Not with constipation or diarrhea without medical supervision Not with kidney stones, inflammatory GI conditions Not in amounts greater than in foods during pregnancy, lactation, or for children under 12 Use short term only: < 10 days

Quick Reference to Healing Herbs

Common/ *Botanical Name*	People Use This For	Potential Side Effects	Potential Interactions	Usage Notes/ Comments
Rosemary *Rosmarinus officinalis*	Orally: GI discomfort after eating, bloating, toothache, headache, cough Topically: support therapy for muscle pain and poor circulation, eczema and poultice for wounds	Orally, large amounts: coma, spasm, vomiting, gastric upset, uterine bleeding, kidney irritation, pulmonary edema, death Topically: sun sensitivity, dermatitis, occupational sensitivity	No known interactions in humans	Not with seizure disorders Not in amounts greater than found in foods during pregnancy or lactation Monitor blood sugar in diabetes
Sage *Salvia officinalis*	Orally: gas, bloating, discomfort after eating, excessive perspiration Topically: nose and throat inflammation	Over time, excessive consumption: mouth sores, dry mouth, mental and physical decline, restlessness, irregular heartbeat, kidney damage	Herbs: sedative herbs Drugs: anticonvulsants, drugs to lower blood sugar, sedative drugs	Not with diabetes, seizure disorders Not in amounts greater than in foods during pregnancy or lactation

Quick Reference to Healing Herbs

Common/ *Botanical Name*	People Use This For	Potential Side Effects	Potential Interactions	Usage Notes/ Comments
St. John's Wort *Hypericum perforatum*	Orally: mild to moderate depression, anxiety, physical complaints associated with depression, discomfort after eating Topically: bruises, first degree burns, wounds	Orally: GI symptoms, fatigue, insomnia, restlessness, anxiety, agitation, irritability, sun sensitivity, dizziness, dry mouth Topically: skin irritation and photosensitivity	Herbs: sedative herbs, digitalis Drugs: Triptan, Elavil, antidepressants, barbiturates, immune suppressants, Lanoxin, fenfluramine, narcotics, nortriptyline, OCDs, Paxil, photosensitizing drugs, protease inhibitors, reserpine, Zoloft, theophylline, Coumadin, other drugs metabolized by liver enzymes Food: tyramine containing foods	Not with unipolar depression, thyroid disease, bipolar disorder, male infertility, pregnancy or lactation
Saw Palmetto *Serenoa repens*	Symptoms of BPH, when used in combination with seven other herbs (SP-PCES) in prostate cancer Chronic urinary tract infections	Headaches, rarely GI discomfort, urine retention	Drugs: OCDs, hormone therapy, immune stimulants May decrease absorption of medication	Not during pregnancy, lactation Not with bleeding disorders Not with children

Quick Reference to Healing Herbs

Common/ *Botanical Name*	People Use This For	Potential Side Effects	Potential Interactions	Usage Notes/ Comments
Scotch Broom *Cytisus scoparius*	Heart and circulatory disorders Edema, heart rate irregularities, heavy menstruation, contraction stimulant, bleeding gums, gout and more	Toxicity with > 30 grams of scotch broom: dizziness, headache, palpitations, weak feeling in legs, sweating, sleepiness, pupil dilation, eye paralysis	Drugs: MAOIs, Albuterol, terbutaline, dopamine, epinephrine, norepinephrine, amphetamine	Not in atrial-ventricular block, high blood pressure, pregnancy, lactation
Senna *Senna alexandrine*	Constipation, slimming teas	Abdominal cramping, discomfort, colic Excessive use: potassium depletion, dependence, cachexia, heart irregularities, muscle weakness, hepatitis, neuropathy, asthma, allergy, occupational allergy	Herbs: stimulant laxative herbs, horsetail/licorice Drugs: cardiac glycosides, diuretics, corticosteroids May reduce intestinal absorption of other drugs	Not with GI conditions Caution in heart disease, electrolyte disturbances, fluid depletion, pregnancy, lactation Do not use > 2 weeks or with abdominal pain of unknown origin
Skullcap *Scutellaria lateriflora*	As part of a seven-herb combination for prostate cancer, reduces testosterone, tranquilizer, insomnia, anxiety	Confusion, seizures, liver damage	Herbs: sedative herbs Drugs: sedatives	Not with liver disorders. Not in pregnancy, lactation

Quick Reference to Healing Herbs

Common/ *Botanical Name*	People Use This For	Potential Side Effects	Potential Interactions	Usage Notes/ Comments
Slippery Elm *Ulmus rubra*	Topically: wounds, soothing agent, expectorant Orally: cough, sore throat, GI problems	Orally: whole bark may induce abortion Topically: contact dermatitis	Theoretically may decrease the absorption of other drugs.	Not in pregnancy and lactation
Tea Tree Oil *Melaleuca alternifolia*	Topically: acne, fungal skin infections, vaginal yeast infections	Contact dermatitis, eczema	No known interactions	Likely unsafe if taken orally Not in children, < 5 mL is toxic Not in pregnancy, lactation
Thyme *Thymus vulgaris*	Orally: bronchitis, pertussis Topically: upper respiratory tract inflammations, bad breath	Skin irritation May cause sensitivity if used as a bath for skin injuries, high fever, infectious diseases, cardiac insufficiency	No known interactions	Not in amounts greater than in foods in urinary tract inflammation, GI irritation, allergy to other thyme family members
Turmeric *Curcuma longa*	For discomfort after eating, digestive problems Folk medicine: diarrhea, intermittent fever, edema, colds, worms, leprosy, kidney inflammation, cystitis, cancer prevention and treatment	Overuse or long-term use: GI complaints, distress	Herbs: anticoagulant/ antiplatelet herbs Drugs: antiplatelet drugs, reserpine	Not in amounts greater than found in foods with gallstones, bile duct obstruction, stomach ulcers, hyperacidity, pregnancy or lactation

Quick Reference to Healing Herbs

Common/ *Botanical Name*	People Use This For	Potential Side Effects	Potential Interactions	Usage Notes/ Comments
Uva Ursi *Arctostaphylos uva-ursi*	Orally: urinary tract inflammation In combination with hops and peppermint is used to treat enuresis and painful urination	Nausea, vomiting, GI discomfort, discolored urine, liver toxicity, urinary tract irritation; 6 to 10 grams may cause tinnitis, nausea, vomiting, shortness of breath, convulsions, deliriums, collapse; 30 to 100 grams can cause death	Herbs: urine acidifiers, urine alkalizers Drugs: urine-acidifying drugs, urine-alkalizing drugs Foods: urine-acidifying and -alkalizing foods	Not with kidney disorders, GI irritation, pregnancy, lactation, children under 12 years of age Take no longer than 7 days and no more than 5 times per year
Valerian *Valeriana officinalis*	Hastening onset of sleep, improving sleep quality, restlessness, improving mood, anxiety	Headache, excitability, heart disturbances, insomnia, occasional morning drowsiness Possible withdrawal symptoms with LT use	Herbs: sedative herbs Drugs: alcohol, barbiturates, benzodiazepines, other sedative drugs Foods: alcohol	Not during pregnancy, lactation May take up to 4 weeks before improvement
Wormwood *Artemisia absinthium*	Loss of appetite, indigestion, stimulates bile production, parasites, aphrodisiac, tonic, antispasmodic, stimulates sweating	Long-term use: restlessness, insomnia, vomiting, GI cramps, dizziness, tremors, urine retention, renal damage, convulsions	Herbs: thujone containing herbs (sage, oak moss, tansy, cedar, tree moss) Drugs: antacids, anticonvulsants, acetaminophen, phenobarbital	Not in pregnancy, lactation Oil may act as a convulsant poison

Quick Reference to Healing Herbs

Common/ *Botanical Name*	People Use This For	Potential Side Effects	Potential Interactions	Usage Notes/ Comments
Yohimbe *Pausinystalia yohimbe* 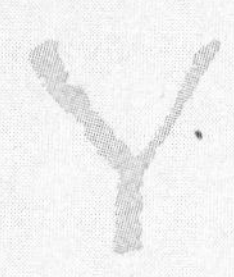	Erectile function, impotence, aphrodisiac, exhaustion, angina, hypertension, neuropathy	Excitation, anorexia, tremor, insomnia, anxiety, high blood pressure, irregular heartbeat, nausea, vomiting, low blood pressure The following are known side effects to the prescription drug Yohimbine: nervousness, anxiety, irritability, headache, high blood pressure, irregular heartbeat	Herbs: caffeine containing herbs, ephedra, herbs with MAOI activity Drugs: alpha 2-adrenergic blocking drugs, diabetes drugs, beta-blocking drugs, Clonidine, guanabenz, MAOIs, Narcan, phenothiazines, sympathomimetic drugs, tricyclic antidepressants Food: tyramine, vasopressor-containing foods	Not with: angina, heart disease, BPH, diabetes, depression, high/low blood pressure, kidney disease, liver disease, post-traumatic stress disorder, inflamed prostate, schizophrenia, yohimbe sensitivity Yohimbine, an alkaloid and active constituent in the plant yohimbe, is available as a prescription drug The amount of yohimbine in yohimbe is unknown due to quality assurance standards Not in pregnancy or lactation Not with children

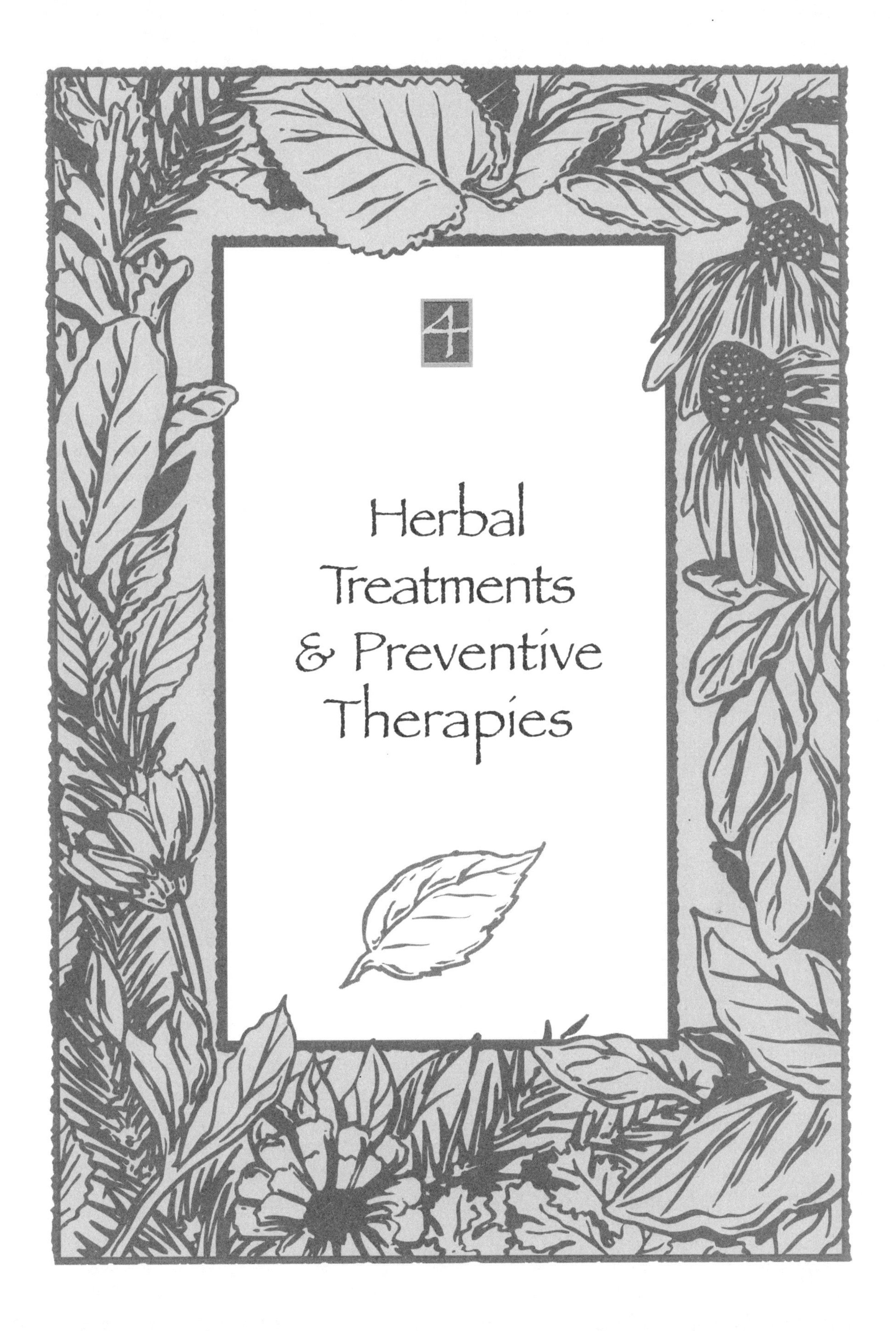

4

Herbal Treatments & Preventive Therapies

4

Herbal Treatments & Preventive Therapies

Herbal medicines are not replacements for conventional diagnosis and treatment, but can be complementary to treatment. Herbal medicines can be preventive by providing essential antioxidants and substances that can enhance health and wellness. Safety is the most important consideration when deciding which herb to use. Some herbs have an excellent record as adjuncts to conventional medical care, yet in many cases it is difficult to sort through the supporting information and know whether an herb is safe and effective or questionable and dangerous. Although the amount of research is increasing, there is still very little concrete information regarding food-herb, drug-herb and herb-herb interactions in humans.

The best defense is caution when trying new herbal therapies. Do not use more than the recommended dose and immediately discontinue if you have any side effects. Know the interactions with any prescription medication, over-the-counter drug or other herb or dietary supplement. Research the herb using reliable sources. Discuss your plans with your healthcare provider, regardless of whether or not you are being treated for a medical condition. If you think you have a medical condition, always discuss your symptoms with your healthcare provider to determine a correct diagnosis. Then decide what helping herbs may be right for you.

This chapter looks at some of the common illnesses and ailments that may benefit from herbal therapy. Wherever possible, this chapter offers as therapy herbs that can be grown in your own garden. Where known and documented, recommendations for specific doses are listed, including expected results and any cautions.

Herbal remedies suggested for use in this chapter are detailed in Chapters 2 and 3. It is important that when you choose an herbal remedy, you choose the correct genus and species to get the desired effect and to avoid potential risks. Also, understand the potential for adverse health reactions if you have heart disease, high blood pressure, diabetes, kidney or liver disease or any other chronic or acute illness. Always consult your healthcare provider if you have a diagnosed illness before beginning herbal therapies.

Heart Disease

In the United States, cardiovascular disease ranks as the leading cause of death. Cardiovascular disease is the number one cause of death for people 65 years old and older, number two for people ages 0-14 and 25-64, and number three for people ages 15-24.

Heart disease includes a number of risk factors that are influenced by lifestyle and heredity. Risk may be reduced by the use of some dietary and herbal supplements.

Angina

Angina is the term for chest pain or discomfort caused by coronary heart disease. Angina happens when the heart muscle doesn't get as much blood (and, therefore, as much oxygen) as it needs. This usually happens because one or more of the heart's arteries, which supply blood to the heart muscle, is narrowed or blocked. Angina is more common during physical exertion because the heart requires more oxygen than it can get, to keep up with demand.

Helping Herbs

Bilberry strengthens the structure of capillaries and blood vessels and, therefore, can help treat angina. *Typical dose:* 1 to 2 (80- to 160-mg) capsules of extract, standardized to contain 25 percent anthocyanosides, daily.

Hawthorn supports the heart by dilating coronary arteries, thus improving the blood supply to the heart. It also dilates blood vessels elsewhere in the body, which allows the blood to circulate more freely with less strain on the heart. Hawthorn strengthens artery walls and is an antioxidant and anti-inflammatory herb. *Typical dose:* 1 cup of tea, made with 2 teaspoons of crushed leaves or fruits, steeped for 20 minutes and strained. Drink up to 2 cups per day. Or, purchase a commercially prepared supplement and follow label directions. Must be used for 4 to 8 weeks for full benefit.

Willow bark is an herbal aspirin that is thought to have the same effect on the

The Importance of Knowing What You Are Taking

For those of us who use herbs as medicines, it is essential that we know what we are planting, purchasing and using in order to avoid adverse reactions or worse. To benefit from herbs, you need to be certain you are using the correct one and in a safe form. For example, the horse chestnut, sometimes referred to as the buckeye, are often either California or Ohio buckeyes. Although these are related species, the *Aesculus hippocastanum*, or common horse chestnut, is the only one that is used for medicinal purposes. All parts of the buckeye tree are toxic if not detoxified, which requires a commercial process. So you must first know the botanical names, then also understand if you can safely prepare the herb at home or use it at all.

heart as low-dose aspirin—preventing heart attack by preventing the formation of blood clots. Blood clots are of major concern to people suffering from angina. *Typical dose:* Drink up to 3 cups of tea per day, made with 1 teaspoon of powdered bark per 8 ounces of cool water that has been allowed to soak for 8 hours and strained. Do not use willow bark if you have gastrointestinal (GI) problems (ulcers, nausea, vomiting or diarrhea) or if you are pregnant or lactating. Use caution with other blood-thinning herbs and drugs.

Arrhythmia

Arrhythmia is irregular beating of the heart. It is common in as many as two million Americans. Arrhythmia can occur in a healthy heart and not be serious, but it may also indicate an acute problem and lead to heart disease, stroke or sudden death.

Helping Herbs

Astragalus has been known as a heart tonic and immune stimulant. *Typical dose:* Try it as a tea, made with 1 to 2 teaspoons of dried herb, steeped in boiling water. Have 2 cups per day—one in the morning, and one in the afternoon or evening.

Scotch broom, according to the German Commission E, is a heart tonic and can help reduce the risk of arrhythmia. *Typical dose:* Make a tea using 1 teaspoon dried herb in 1 cup of boiling water; drink up to 2 cups a day.

High Cholesterol

About 99.5 million American adults have total blood cholesterol levels above the recommended 200 milligrams per deciliter (mg/dL), and about 39.9 million American adults have levels that are considered to be high—240 mg/dL or higher. The risk of heart attack in men and women depends on many variables, not the least of which is the combination of low HDL or good cholesterol and high total cholesterol. The number of risk factors a person has determines their risk category. Not only do the risk factors listed in the sidebar "Risk Factors for Heart Disease" (pages 222-223) play a role in developing coronary heart disease (CHD), additional factors figure into risk categories. The presence of coronary heart disease and/or diabetes automatically places a person at high risk for future events. The more major independent risk factors (listed below) a person has, the greater their risk of developing future CHD. People with 2 or more independent risk factors (high LDL "bad" cholesterol, high total cholesterol, and obesity, for example) should be evaluated for further risk.

Indepndent Risk Factors

- Cigarette smoking
- High blood pressure (B/P > 140/90 mm Hg or taking medication to control blood pressure)
- Low HDL cholesterol (< 40 mg/dL)
- Family history of premature CHD (CHD in male first-degree relative < 55 years; CHD in female first degree relative <65 years)
- Age (men > 45 years; women > 55 years)

Helping Herbs

Artichoke leaves and roots contain a chemical that blocks the absorption of cholesterol and inhibits its production in the liver. The substance cynarin also affects triglycerides. You may choose to eat your artichoke leaves each day (not with butter, please), or you may choose to take a commercially prepared supplement. *Typical dose:* 500 to 3,000 mg daily of prepared supplement divided into three doses. Do not take the supplement if you have gallstones or gallbladder disease.

Fenugreek, with its mucilage, has the ability to lower cholesterol. *Typical dose:* 5 grams of seed, twice daily. May cause gas.

Flaxseed, with its beneficial lignans, has been shown to reduce the risk of heart disease by lowering total and LDL (bad) cholesterol. *Typical dose:* 2 to 4 tablespoons of ground seed daily, in two to three divided doses. Grind the seeds to increase availability of beneficial compounds prior to using. Do not grind too far in advance, as the oil in flaxseed is not stable. May have a laxative effect.

Garlic inhibits two of the enzymes involved in cholesterol production by the liver. This lowers synthesis and the overall amount of cholesterol released into the blood. *Typical dose:* 1 to 3 raw cloves, daily. Briefly cooking garlic may decrease the odor and increase available helping properties. Because heat kills the components that provide its beneficial activity, garlic should not be browned. You may choose to use a prepared supplement that provides a standardized garlic extract containing 1.3 percent allicin content. Follow instructions on label.

Ginger may help lower cholesterol. A bit each day in tea form won't hurt and may even help.

Grapeseed, with its antioxidant potential, may help reduce the risk of atherosclerosis. *Typical dose:* Begin with an initial dose of 25 to 300 mg daily for 3 weeks, then follow with a maintenance dose of 40 to 80 mg daily.

Guggul is a sticky resin from the myrrh tree that is widely used in Ayurvedic healing. The extract gugulipid has been shown to lower LDL cholesterol and triglycerides while raising HDL levels. It also may contain antioxidant properties that help protect the heart from free-radical damage.

Is Your Cholesterol in Check?

This list indicates what your cholesterol numbers mean.

Total Cholesterol

less than 200	desirable
200-239	borderline-high
240 or more	high

LDL ("bad") Cholesterol

This is the primary cholesterol to lower for reduced heart disease risk.

less than 100	optimal
100-129	near optimal/ above optimal
130-159	borderline-high
160-189	high
190 or more	very high

HDL ("good") Cholesterol

less than 40	low
60 or more	high

Risk Factors for Heart Disease

Cardiovascular disease (heart disease) is America's number one killer. Almost 62 million Americans have some form of cardiovascular disease, much of which can be prevented, or at least the severity decreased.

You can't go back and choose your parents, race or sex, so the most important thing to do is to change those things that you do have control over.

Major Risk Factors for Heart Disease that You Can't Change

Age
About four out of five people who die of coronary heart disease are age 65 or older.

Sex
Men have a greater risk of heart attack than women, and they have attacks earlier in life. Even after menopause, when women's death rate from heart disease increases, it's not as great as men's.

Heredity
If your parents have or had heart disease, you are more likely to have it. Most people with a family history of heart disease have one or more other risk factors.

Ethnic Background
African Americans have more severe high blood pressure than Caucasians and a higher risk of heart disease. Mexican Americans, Native Americans, native Hawaiians and some Asian Americans also have higher rates, in part due to higher rates of obesity and diabetes.

Major Risk Factors that You Can Modify

Smoking
Smokers' risk of heart attack is more than twice that of nonsmokers. Cigarette smoking is the biggest risk factor for sudden cardiac death. Cigarette smoking, along with other risk factors, increases the risk for all types of heart disease.

High Cholesterol
As blood cholesterol rises, so does risk of heart disease. Accompanied by other risk factors, like high blood pressure and smoking, the risk increases even more. Cholesterol levels are also affected by age, sex, heredity and diet.

High Blood Pressure
High blood pressure increases the heart's workload, causing the heart to enlarge and weaken. High blood pressure increases your risk of stroke, heart attack, kidney failure and congestive heart failure. High blood pressure, when accompanied by obesity, smoking, high blood cholesterol levels or diabetes, increases the risk of heart attack or stroke several times.

Physical Inactivity
Being inactive is an independent risk factor for heart disease. Thirty minutes of

moderate to vigorous physical activity most days of the week can help prevent heart and blood vessel disease. Exercise can help control blood cholesterol, diabetes and obesity, and help lower blood pressure in some people.

Obesity and Being Overweight

People with a body mass index (BMI) of 25 to 29.9 are considered to be overweight. Those with a BMI over 30 are obese.

Risk is especially high if most of the fat is in the waist. Overweight and obese individuals are more likely to develop heart disease and stroke, even if they have no other risk factors. Excess weight increases the strain on the heart; raises blood pressure, cholesterol and triglyceride levels; and lowers HDL (good) cholesterol levels. Obesity is a risk factor for diabetes as well.

Diabetes

Diabetes significantly increases your risk of developing heart disease and stroke, even when blood sugar is under control. Heart disease kills about two-thirds of people with diabetes.

Other Factors that May Contribute to Heart Disease Risk

Stress

Stress causes people to change their lifestyle, exercise habits and diet, which may affect established risk factors.

Sex Hormones

Estrogen seems to play a role in heart disease. Men have more heart attacks than women do before women reach the age of menopause. The loss of natural estrogen as women age (or due to surgical menopause) may contribute to a higher risk of heart disease after menopause. Estrogen also tends to raise HDL cholesterol and lower total blood cholesterol. Male hormones (testosterone) do the opposite.

Alcohol

The risk of heart disease in people who drink moderately (an average of one drink for women or two drinks for men, per day) is lower than in nondrinkers. One drink is defined as 1½ fl. oz. of 80-proof spirits (such as bourbon, Scotch, vodka, gin and so on), 1 fl. oz. of 100-proof spirits, 4 fl. oz. of wine or 12 fl. oz. of beer. If you don't already use alcohol, don't start; if you do, don't increase the amount you drink. Excess alcohol, over the recommended amounts, increases the risk of stroke and heart attack.

Illegal Drug Use

Using intravenous drugs carries a high risk of stroke. Cocaine use has been linked to fatal strokes and heart attacks, even in first-time users.

Guggul is available commercially in the form of guggulsterone. Extracts should be standardized to contain 2 to 5 percent of guggulsterone. *Typical dose:* 25 mg of guggesterone, 3 times daily, with meals. It may take up to 3 months to notice any real benefits.

Psyllium seed is rich in mucilage. These soluble fibers reduce high cholesterol and triglycerides, apparently by binding with cholesterol and taking it out of the body. *Typical dose:* 2 to 4 teaspoons of powdered psyllium in 8 ounces of water, 2 times per day. Note: Psyllium may cause gas and bloating in the beginning, so adjust your dose accordingly and make sure you drink plenty of water between doses.

Soy protein has been found to be helpful for lowering cholesterol. It is thought that the weak estrogen-like activity of its phytoestrogens contributes to its cholesterol-lowering ability. Its benefit may be most pronounced in women at the age of menopause. Some soy products are also high in soluble fiber (the type of fiber that helps reduce cholesterol). *Typical dose:* 30 to 50 grams of soy protein daily.

High Blood Pressure

Blood pressure measures how the heart pumps blood into the arteries and through the circulatory system and the force of the arteries as they resist the blood flow. High blood pressure (hypertension or HBP) is defined as 140 mm Hg or higher (systolic) and 90 mm Hg or higher (diastolic) for an extended time. HBP is the most significant risk factor for stroke. High blood pressure is referred to as the "silent killer" because people often do not realize they have it. About 50 million Americans, age 6 and older, have high blood pressure. One in five Americans, and one in four adults, has HBP.

Helping Herbs

Dandelion may help relieve fluid retention and, subsequently, blood pressure. Dandelion does not appear to cause potassium loss in the body. If you choose to use it fresh from your yard, you'll get some exercise and a weed-free yard to boot. Do not use dandelion from yards or areas that have been treated with weed killers. *Typical dose:* 2 to 3 cups of tea, made with 1 to 2 teaspoons dried dandelion, steeped in 1 cup of boiling water; 1 to 2 drops of tincture, up to 3 times daily; 4 to 10 grams of leaf or dried aboveground plant divided into three doses daily; or fresh in your salad.

Garlic is also beneficial for lowering blood pressure. *Typical dose:* 1 to 3 cloves, raw or very briefly cooked, daily. You may want to use a prepared supplement that provides a standardized garlic extract containing 1.3 percent allicin content. Follow instructions on label.

Hawthorn supports the heart by dilating coronary arteries, thus improving the blood supply to the heart. It also dilates blood vessels elsewhere in the body, which allows the blood to circulate more freely with less strain on the heart. *Typical dose:* 1 cup of tea, made with 2 teaspoons of crushed leaves or fruits, steeped for 20 minutes and strained. Drink up to 2 cups per day, or purchase a commercially prepared supplement and follow label directions. Must be used for 4 to 8 weeks for full benefit.

Circulatory Problems

Peripheral Vascular Disease (PVD) refers to diseases of blood vessels outside the heart and brain. It's often a narrowing of vessels that carry blood to leg and arm muscles. Raynaud's disease (this page) is one PVD that may respond to herbal therapy. Changes in the blood vessels, such as inflammation, tissue damage and fatty buildups in arteries, result in peripheral artery disease, an example of PVD.

Intermittent claudication occurs in peripheral artery disease when the fatty deposits affect blood circulation, mainly in arteries leading to the legs and feet. Common symptoms in the early stages of the disease are cramping and fatigue in the legs and buttocks. These symptoms occur during activity and disappear when the person stands still.

Helping Herbs for PVD

Garlic benefits circulatory problems by making blood platelets less sticky and preventing blood clots. *Typical dose:* 1 to 3 raw cloves, briefly cooked, daily. You may want to use a prepared supplement that provides a standardized garlic extract containing 1.3 percent allicin content. Follow instructions on label.

Ginkgo is an antioxidant that helps prevent damage to arterial walls. It also dilates the blood vessels in areas that don't seem to be getting enough oxygen and helps prevent the accumulation of platelets that cause clots. *Typical dose:* 40 to 80 milligrams of capsules, standardized to contain 24 percent ginkgo flavone glycosides and 6 percent terpene lactones, 3 times daily. Use caution if you are taking other blood-thinning drugs.

Grapeseed is used for prevention and treatment of circulation problems and for strengthening blood vessels. *Typical dose:* 75 to 300 mg once daily, taken in capsule form. Some sources suggest a maintenance dose of 40 to 80 mg daily. Use caution if you take other blood-thinning drugs.

Raynaud's Phenomenon brings new meaning to the old adage "cold hands, warm heart," especially for those who suffer from this sometimes debilitating condition. Predominantly a circulatory condition in which the small blood vessels constrict. Characterized by extremities that first turn white or blue and then sometimes red, Raynaud's is caused by a constriction of and spasms in the small arteries that take blood to the fingers or toes. Usually, both hands and/or both feet are affected.

The condition usually begins when patients are in their teens or twenties and is more common in women than men, especially in cold, damp climates. Sometimes the disorder is brought on by arthritis, or scleroderma. Raynaud's brought on by mechanical trauma usually occurs later in life and typically affects only one extremity.

Helping Herbs for Raynaud's Phenomenon

Borage contains the beneficial omega-3 fatty acid known as gamma-linolenic acid (GLA). It may help relieve symptoms of Raynaud's when used topically, massaged into the fingers and toes.

Cayenne pepper is a warming spice that may be of benefit if taken internally or used topically. It can be mixed with a bit of evening primrose or borage oil and rubbed on the fingers. Make sure you wash your hands before rubbing your eyes!

Evening primrose oil (EPO), like borage, contains GLA but in slightly higher concentrations. Massaging the oil into the fingers may help relieve symptoms of Raynaud's. The massage itself will benefit circulation.

Garlic thins the blood and works to improve circulation, thus getting more blood to the hands and feet. *Typical dose:* 1 to 3 raw cloves, briefly cooked, daily. You may want to use a prepared supplement that provides a standardized garlic extract containing 1.3 percent allicin content. Follow instructions on label.

Ginger is a warming herb and may help relieve symptoms of Raynaud's as well as reducing platelet stickiness that causes clogging of small blood vessels, thus constricting blood flow. *Typical dose:* 1 to 2 teaspoons of grated fresh root steeped in 1 cup hot water for 10 minutes. Strain and drink 1 cup per day. For specific product dosing, follow instructions on label of commercially prepared supplements. Talk to your physician before taking ginger if you are taking blood-thinning medication.

Ginkgo improves blood flow to the peripheral arteries, heart and brain. It helps prevent microscopic leaking from tiny veins and thus improves overall circulation and provides protection to vessel walls. Ginkgo may also reduce abnormal blood clotting. *Typical dose:* 60 to 80 mg of extract standardized, to 24 percent gingko flavone glycosides and 6 percent terpene lactones 3 times daily.

Gotu kola helps to maintain the health of the skin and its underlying connective tissue. *Typical dose:* Up to 8 (400- to 500-mg) nonstandardized capsules, divided into three doses daily; or 20 mg of standardized product, 3 times daily.

Hawthorn is a tonic for the heart and blood vessels. Hawthorn supports the heart by dilating coronary arteries, thus improving the blood supply to the heart. It also dilates blood vessels elsewhere in the body, which allows the blood to circulate more freely with less strain on the heart. *Typical dose:* 1 cup of tea, made with 2 teaspoons of crushed leaves or fruits, steeped for 20 minutes and strained. Drink up to 2 cups per day. Or, purchase a commercially prepared supplement standardized for oligomeric procyanidins and take 160 mg daily. Must be used for 4 to 8 weeks for full benefit.

Edema refers to the swelling of tissues and accumulation of fluid in the body. Causes of edema include inadequate dietary protein intake, obesity, toxemia during pregnancy and congestive heart failure (CHF), to name a few. Usually resulting from the buildup of fluid between the body's cells, edema can be serious and should not be ignored. Edema may lead to more serious problems, including high blood pressure or kidney or heart failure.

Helping Herbs for Edema

Ephedra's use for treating cardiovascular disease cannot be recommended at this time due to recent information questioning its safety.

Horse chestnut seed encourages strong veins and artery walls, promotes good blood flow and helps prevent the pooling of blood that results in varicose veins. Improved circulation helps reduce edema and swelling. *Typical dose:* 30 to 150 mg per day of a commercially prepared extract standardized to 20 percent aescin (the active component in horse chestnut). Note that crude products may be toxic, so purchase horse chestnut seed from a reputable retailer. Use caution if you are taking other blood-thinning herbs and drugs.

Red clover contains a compound called coumarin that has been linked to protective effects against edema and cancer; it also has antioxidant and blood-thinning properties. (Do not confuse coumarin with the drug Coumadin, which is used to thin the blood.) *Typical dose:* 1 cup of tea, 3 to 4 times daily, or 1 to 2 standardized tablets based on manufacturer's recommendations daily. Do not use with herbs or drugs that have blood-thinning effects.

Varicose veins are twisted, dilated veins with ineffectual valves, found most often in the legs.

Helping Herbs for Varicose Veins

Bilberry strengthens the structure of veins and, therefore, can help treat varicose veins. *Typical dose:* 1 to 2 (80- to 160-mg) capsules of extract, standardized to contain 25 percent anthocyanosides, daily.

Butcher's broom is believed to inhibit inflammation and constrict blood vessels. *Typical dose:* 2 to 3 cups of tea, made with 1 teaspoon dried herb, steeped in 1 cup of water for 15 minutes, daily; or 2 to 3 (200-mg) capsules, with water, 2 to 3 times per day.

Ginkgo improves blood flow to the peripheral arteries, heart and brain. It helps prevent microscopic leaking from tiny veins and thus improves overall circulation and provides protection to vessel walls. Ginkgo may also reduce abnormal blood clotting. *Typical dose:* 60 to 80 mg of extract, standardized, to 24 percent gingko flavone glycosides and 6 percent terpene lactones in capsule form 3 times daily.

Horse chestnut has been shown to reduce varicose veins and the related pain and itching. *Typical dose:* 50 milligrams of commercial extract 2 to 3 times daily. Look for products standardized to 20 percent aescin (the active compound in horse chestnut).

Witch hazel is a soothing external treatment for varicose veins. Simply dip a cotton ball in witch hazel and dab it on the affected area.

Thrombosis is the formation or presence of a blood clot inside a blood vessel or cavity of the heart. The condition is serious and can lead to a heart attack and/or stroke. This condition should not be self-treated. No herbs are known to help at this time.

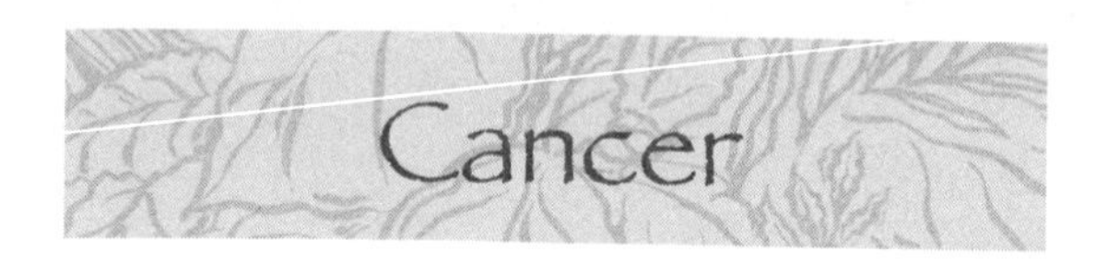

Cancer

Although not the number one cause of death worldwide, cancer is probably the most feared disease. It seems to appear without warning (even though signs may have been there), is persistent in its growth and often carries a poor prognosis. Each one of us has probably had a friend or relative that has developed cancer. Some have lived well, while others have suffered and continue to do so and many have died.

Cancer is a disease in which abnormal cells divide without control. Cancer cells can invade nearby tissues and spread through the bloodstream and lymphatic system to other parts of the body. There is not just one type of cancer, and there is not just one cause of cancer.

The rates for new cancer cases and deaths for all cancers combined have continued to decline in the United States. Four cancer sites—lung, prostate, breast and colorectum—have accounted for about 56 percent of all new cancer cases yearly and have also been the leading causes of cancer deaths.

Breast cancer makes up 16.3 percent of all cancer cases and accounts for 7.8 percent of all deaths due to cancer. Breast cancer death rates have continued to decline because of improvements in early detection and treatment. However, breast cancer incidence rates have increased by more than 40 percent since 1973.

Prostate cancer, which accounts for 14.8 percent of all cases, saw a sharp increase in incidence rates beginning in the late 1980s with the introduction of screening for prostate-specific antigen (PSA). Incidence rates have started to decline. Death rates have also declined in recent years.

Lung cancer accounts for 29 percent of cancer deaths in the United States and 13.2 percent of the cases of cancer. Smoking causes an estimated 30 percent of all cancer deaths, either directly or indirectly.

Colorectal cancer accounts for 11.6 percent of all cancer cases, but varies dramatically among ethnic groups. Death rates have also declined in most populations except black females. Early detection and treatment have significantly altered the outcome of this cancer.

Herbs in Cancer Prevention & Treatment

Even though there is considerable ongoing research on herbs and their role in the treatment of cancer, their use as a possible cure remains questionable. We often hear that these treatments can't hurt but, in fact, they may. The cost of herbal remedies can be excessive and they are not reimbursed by insurance. Some therapies may be toxic; some may actually increase tumor growth by stimulating the immune system and some may even be carcinogenic themselves. Additionally, some people who use nontraditional therapies may forgo traditional therapies that might be lifesaving if used early in treatment.

There are some therapies used in conventional treatments that come from plants. Among these is Taxol, which is used for ovarian and breast cancer; etoposide, from the mayapple, used for testicular and small-cell lung cancer; and vincristine and vinblastine, used for leukemia and lymphoma.

When it comes to cancer, it appears that there are several factors that determine whether a person will or will not get cancer, and possibly determine the type of cancer. This is where herbs—with their antioxidant potential, their fiber content and, possibly, other constituents that have not yet been discovered—can play a role.

Effective and sensitive treatments that incorporate herbal therapies when appropriate are needed, but prevention appears to be the most cost-effective way to treat cancer. Diet appears to be one of the biggest factors in cancer prevention, as are obesity and exercise. Some factors that cannot be controlled include gender, genetics and, to a certain but not definite extent, environment.

The risk of some forms of cancer may double among overweight and obese persons. More than 30 percent of cancer cases could be prevented by controlling calorie intake and exercising a minimum of 30 minutes, 5 days a week. The exercise recommendations include moderate activity, such as brisk walking. These are in line with the Surgeon General's recommendations for overall good health and the American Heart Association's recommendations for cardiovascular health.

Forty-five minutes or more of moderate to vigorous activity, 5 or more days a week, may reduce breast and colon cancer risk. This much exercise may reduce the risk of colon cancer by almost half, and the risk of breast cancer by one-third. Exercise reduces circulating levels of estrogen, which has been linked to higher breast cancer risk in post-menopausal women; reduces other hormones that can increase the risk of colon cancer; and decreases the amount of time cancer-causing agents remain in the intestines. A high-fiber, plant-based diet enhances the effects of exercise in the prevention of colon cancer.

Helping Herbs

Astragalus is an immune stimulant and protects the body by keeping the system at its fighting best. Typical dose: 8 or 9 (400- to 500-mg) capsules daily.

Cat's Claw research has provided the interesting possibility that it may have anti-tumor effects. It is believed to have anti-inflammatory and immune-stimulating properties. *Typical dose:* 2 to 3 grams, 3 times daily, in capsule form. Or try a decoction, made with 2 teaspoons herb to 1 cup of boiling water, steeped for 10 to 20 minutes. Drink up to 3 cups per day.

Echinacea may help persons undergoing chemotherapy or radiation to maintain their immune system. Before using echinacea during therapy, make sure to ask your oncologist. *Typical dose:* Mix 2 teaspoons of root in 1 cup of water; bring to a boil, then simmer for 15 minutes. Drink up to 3 times daily. Or take up to 9 (300- to 400-mg) capsules per day. Take echinacea, in any form, for 2 weeks, then take a 1-week break and repeat.

Grapeseed has been tested for its potential role as an anticancer agent and as an adjunct to reduce the toxicity of chemotherapy. Some promising information is that it helps protect the skin from ultraviolet (UV) light and, thus, may reduce skin cancer risk. *Typical dose:* 75 to 300 mg daily, taken in capsule form, once daily.

Green tea and **black tea** are both rich in antioxidant polyphenols, but green tea seems to be superior for reducing risk of certain types of cancers. Research has noted a lower incidence of cancer among persons who drink green tea daily. There may also be improved prognosis among breast cancer patients who consume green tea, but results are still preliminary. *Typical dose:* Mix 1 teaspoon of tea leaves in 1 cup of hot, not boiling, water. Drink 2 to 5 cups daily.

Milk thistle is a detoxifying herb; it neutralizes free radicals that attack the liver. By protecting the liver, our bodies are better able to deal with potential cancer-causing environmental toxins. *Typical dose:* 140 mg standardized silymarin capsules, 3 times daily; after 6 weeks, decrease to 90 mg, 3 times daily.

Red clover is a rich source of phytoestrogens, including isoflavones—plant chemicals that act as weak estrogens in the human body. Phytoestrogens may be one reason that persons who consume a plant-based diet have a lower incidence of cancers. However, this remains controversial. The protective effect of phytoestrogens depends on a person's diet, race and geographic location. *Typical dose:* Up to 5 (500-mg) capsules daily; or 2 to 3 cups of tea, made with 1 tablespoon flowers to 1 cup hot water.

Saw palmetto appears to play a role in the prevention of prostate cancer, particularly in those taking the seven-herb combination called PC-SPES. PC stands for prostate cancer and SPES is Latin for hope. PC-SPES contains saw palmetto, as well as several Chinese herbs, licorice, reishi mushroom and chrysanthemum. Small clinical trials have shown it can decrease serum prostate-specific antigen (PSA) levels, cause tumor cells to die and cause a decrease in serum testosterone. Availability of PC-SPES is limited at this writing because of an error in manufacturing. In early 2002 the product was found to contain undeclared prescription drug ingredients that could cause serious health problems if not taken under medical supervision. It is worth considering once it becomes available again.

Soy has numerous benefits as a food and for enhancing health. Soy's phytoestrogens, the isoflavones genistein and daidzein, are believed to benefit the body through their ability to act as a weak estrogen. Although we know that soy can help lower elevated cholesterol and decrease menopausal complaints, there is still controversy about whether soy can play a role in cancer prevention. *Typical dose:* 25 to 60 grams of soy protein daily. Do not eat raw soybeans regularly; they may be toxic over time. Isoflavone supplements are not recommended; they may be inconsistent in formulation, and studies show conflicting information regarding their safety and effectiveness.

Turmeric's active ingredient, curcumin, has been shown to decrease the incidence of cell mutations in smokers. It is an anti-inflammatory herb that has several benefits for both cardiovascular and overall health. *Typical dose:* 1 (450-mg) capsule, 3 times daily. Do not take if you are pregnant or lactating, or if you have gallbladder disease or gallstones.

American Cancer Society Guidelines on Diet, Nutrition & Cancer Prevention

These are some of the American Cancer Society's recommendations for nutrition and physical activity. Following these guidelines can help you reduce your overall cancer risk.

Choose most of the foods you eat from plant sources.

- Eat five or more servings of fruits and vegetables each day.
- Regularly eat other foods from plant sources, such as breads, cereals, grain products, rice, pasta or beans.

Limit your intake of high-fat foods, particularly from animal sources.

- Choose foods low in fat.
- Limit consumption of meats, especially high-fat meats.

Be physically active—achieve and maintain a healthy weight.

- Be at least moderately active for 30 minutes or more, 5 to 7 days a week.
- Stay within your healthy weight range and maintain a BMI of 25 or less.

Limit alcoholic beverages, if you drink at all.

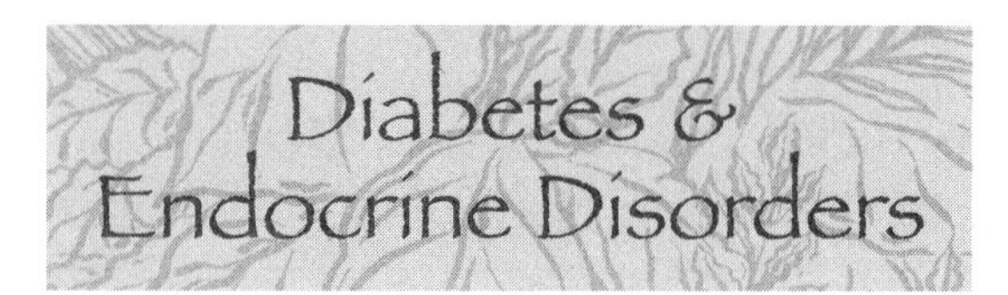

Diabetes

Of the approximately 16 million Americans who have diabetes, an estimated one-third have not yet been diagnosed. The incidence and diagnosis of diabetes is on the rise, especially in children and young adults.

Diabetes is a disorder in the body's ability to use protein, carbohydrate and fat because the pancreas does not produce enough insulin. In people with diabetes, the pancreas either produces little or no insulin, or the cells do not respond normally to the insulin that is produced. Glucose (sugar) builds up in the blood, overflows into the urine and passes out of the body. Even though the blood contains large amounts of sugar, it is not available to the body cells. There are three main types of diabetes:

Type 1 diabetes usually occurs in childhood or early adulthood. The body usually produces no insulin.

Type 2 diabetes has a more gradual onset and does not usually occur until after age 40. The pancreas produces insulin but, for some reason, the body cannot use it. About 80 percent of people with type 2 diabetes are overweight. Type 2 diabetes is often part of a metabolic syndrome that includes obesity, elevated blood pressure and high levels of blood lipids. There is an alarming increase in the number of children with type 2 diabetes, primarily because of an increase in obesity and a decrease in physical activity.

Gestational diabetes develops only during pregnancy. It usually disappears after delivery, but the mother is at increased risk of getting type 2 diabetes later in life.

Diabetes is one of the leading causes of death and disability in the United States. Diabetes is associated with long-term complications that affect almost every part of the body. Blindness, heart and blood vessel disease, strokes, kidney failure, amputations and nerve damage are just a few of the results of uncontrolled diabetes.

Although there is no cure, the symptoms of diabetes can be improved by lifestyle changes, and possibly through the use of some herbal therapies. The role of specific herbs in diabetes is being researched.

Helping Herbs

If you have diabetes and try any of these herbs, inform your healthcare provider and monitor your blood sugar regularly.

Bilberry is used to help prevent the damage that long-term diabetes may cause to the eyes by contributing powerful flavonoids called anthocyanidins and proanthocyanidins. *Typical dose:* 80 to 160 mg of capsules, standardized to contain 25 percent anthocyanidins, daily.

Fenugreek provides a soluble fiber called mucilage that can help regulate blood sugar. It also increases the good cholesterol while lowering the total cholesterol in the blood. *Typical dose:* up to 5 grams of powdered seed. The maximum amount is 6 grams of seed per day, taken in 2-3 divided doses daily. May cause gas.

Garlic is an all-around good-for-you herb that appears to help control blood sugar. Aim for 1 raw clove per day.

Ginseng (American or *Panax quinquefolius*) is reported to have blood sugar-lowering properties. It may enhance the blood sugar-lowering effects of antidiabetes medicines. Monitor blood sugar levels closely. To avoid low blood sugar, take with meals. *Typical dose:* up to one-half gram of root 2 times daily. Some practitioners recommend taking for 15 to 20 days with a 2-week ginseng-free period between courses.

Grapeseed extract is another rich source of anthocyanidins and proanthocyanidins. *Typical dose:* 100 to 300 mg, in capsule form, of proanthocyanidins content daily.

Gymnema sylvestre is an Ayurvedic remedy that is commonly used to treat diabetes. Chew a bit of the herb before meals and it reportedly will help you forego sweets. Gymnema also appears to stimulate the pancreas and enhance insulin use. *Typical dose:* 400 mg in capsule form daily.

Marsh mallow root contains significant amounts of the fiber pectin. Pectin can help keep blood sugar levels down. Follow label directions of a commercial product.

Psyllium is beneficial because of its soluble fiber coating called mucilage. Not only does it act as a powerful laxative, it may help control blood sugar and elevated blood cholesterol. *Typical dose:* 2 to 3 teaspoons, 2 to 3 times daily, with plenty of water. Drink water between doses. Note: Start with small dose, once or twice a day, to decrease the potential for gas.

Graves' Disease

Graves' disease is a disorder in which the thyroid gland produces too much hormone. People with Graves' disease usually have an enlarged thyroid gland and an abnormal protrusion of the eyeballs. Typical symptoms include nervousness, fine tremors of the hands, weight loss, fatigue, heart palpitations, heat intolerance, increased metabolic rate and increased GI motility.

No herbs have been studied for use in treating Graves' disease; however, some practitioners have used lemon balm for treating the disease's symptoms. If you try lemon balm, it is recommended that you do so only under the supervision of your healthcare provider and that you take it for no longer than 14 consecutive days without a break.

Hypo- and Hyperthyroidism

Hypothyroidism is the result of a lowered level of circulating thyroid hormone. Weight gain, mental and physical lethargy, dry skin, constipation, arthritis and slowing of the body's metabolic processes may occur.

Hyperthyroidism, on the other hand, results from an overactive thyroid gland. The gland usually becomes enlarged and secretes much more than normal amounts of thyroid hormones, causing an acceleration in the body's metabolic processes. Weight loss, fatigue, nervousness and constant hunger are a few of the many symptoms.

Helping Herbs

Lemon balm has been found, in animal studies, to interfere with the activity of thyroid-stimulating hormone (TSH) and may prove useful for treating an overactive thyroid gland. *Typical dose:* 2 teaspoons of dried leaves, steeped for 10 minutes, in 1 cup of water. Take up to 3 cups daily. Note: If your thyroid gland is underactive, lemon balm may interfere with TSH; consult with your physician before taking it.

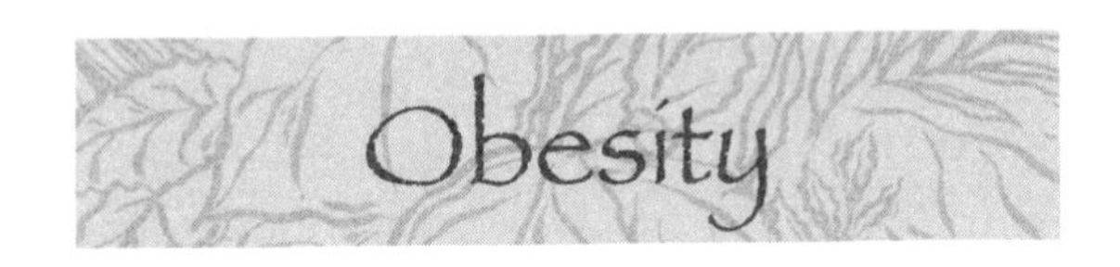

With obesity approaching epidemic proportions in the United States, it is difficult to address all of the considerations regarding this problem in just a few short words. Approximately 97 million adults in the United States are overweight or obese. Being obese or overweight significantly increases the risk of complications from hypertension; high cholesterol and triglycerides; type 2 diabetes; coronary heart disease; stroke; gallbladder disease; osteoarthritis; sleep apnea and respiratory problems; and endometrial, breast, prostate and colon cancers. Higher body weights are also associated with increases in all-cause mortality. Recent studies have shown that the healthcare costs associated with obesity exceed those for smoking-related illnesses by almost $100 per person, per year.

This said, who wouldn't want to lose weight? Many people don't want to, or find it difficult to make the lifestyle changes necessary to make it happen: a lower-fat diet with plenty of healthy whole grains, fruits and vegetables; smaller portions of food; and the most dreaded change, physical activity for at least 30 minutes most, preferably 5, days of the week.

Many people have turned to herbal formulas in order to find a solution, but what they are really seeking is a quick fix, which simply does not exist. Some herbs may be helpful, but some may be harmful, especially if used in combination with other herbs or in health conditions that put a person at risk for adverse effects. Let's take a look at some of the weight-loss herbs and their benefits and risks.

Helping Herbs

Capsicum (red pepper) is sometimes suggested for its ability to raise the metabolic rate, thereby burning more calories. This may be good in theory, but difficult to practice, due to the amounts suggested to raise the metabolic rate. A certain amount of spicy foods in the diet add interest, which is important when you are trying to cut back. It is much easier to eat a small amount of low-calorie flavorful food than low-calorie bland food.

Ephedra may be effective for weight loss when taken in combination with other herbs, such as guarana. However, the safety of this combination is in question because of the stimulating effect of guarana and its possible additive effect to ephedra. The alkaloids ephedrine and pseudoephedrine can directly stimulate the sympathetic nervous system, which may be responsible for part of its effectiveness as an appetite depressant. *Typical dose:* 15 to 30 mg of the total alkaloids calculated as ephedrine. Maximum doses, by some sources, is 300 mg per day. The general consensus at this writing is that the maximum safe dose is not more than 8 mg every 6 hours, not to exceed 24 mg daily. To ensure standard doses, a purchased product is recommended. Do not use if you have heart disease, eating disorder, BPH, diabetes, thyroid conditions, high blood pressure, kidney stones, urinary retention or if you are pregnant or lactating. Consult with your healthcare provider before using any products containing ephedra.

Guarana contains a fair amount of caffeine. It is used in weight-loss formulas to enhance energy and suppress the appetite. *Typical dose:* Make a tea with 1 to 2 grams of crushed seed and 1 cup of boiling water; steep for 10 minutes. Do not use if you have high blood pressure, heart or kidney disease or thyroid or psychiatric disorders. Children and pregnant women should not use guarana.

Psyllium can be an effective appetite suppressant. Taking it 30 minutes before meals can help you eat less and still feel full. To prevent constipation, it is imperative that you drink plenty of fluids, preferably water, when using psyllium. *Typical dose:* Up to 6 (600-mg) capsules daily with 8 ounces of water; or up to 1 teaspoon of husks or 3 teaspoons of powdered psyllium in 8 ounces of water, 2 times daily. For other fiber products, read the label directions. Take psyllium 30 to 60 minutes before or after meals or taking other drugs. Do not take if you have unexplained stomach pain or cramps.

Garcinia is a component of many weight-loss formulas and muscle-building supplements. It is sold as an appetite suppressant. It has been shown to be effective in animal research for reducing food intake, reducing weight gain and body fat and blocking the conversion of carbohydrates to body fat. *Typical dose:* Although its effectiveness in humans is questionable, persons who use it take 1,000 milligrams, 3 times daily, between meals, for the first 4 weeks of a weight-loss plan.

Infants & Children

The use of herbal therapies for treating ailments in infants and children is controversial. Extra care must be taken because of the size and the age of the child. It should be noted that, according to the Poison Control Center, reported poisonings from herbs are more rare than from prescription drugs. According to the American Association of Poison Control Centers, in one year, 704 adverse reactions to dietary supplements involved children 6 to 18 years of age. During the same year, there were more than 475,000 reports of adverse reactions to pharmaceuticals in children older than age 6.

Begin with small doses. Herbs that are questionable for adults should probably be avoided in children without the guidance of an experienced herbalist or physician. You will recall from Chapters 2 and 3 that many herbs are not recommended for children, especially children under the age of 2.

Chamomile and fennel teas have been used for centuries to calm a colicky infant. Some research has been conducted using echinacea but, just as you would with adults, take care in order to avoid adverse effects. Resources are available that offer more guidance for herbal use in infants. Before trying any remedy on a young child, consult different resources, including your healthcare provider.

Women's Health

Women's health issues encompass a number of symptoms and diseases that are of concern to women of all ages. Most are related to hormonal changes that occur during various stages of life. These changes can manifest themselves in physical and psychological symptoms that can be bothersome at least and catastrophic at worst.

Amenorrhea

Amenorrhea is, simply stated, the absence of menstruation. It is normal before sexual maturity and post-menopause, but not in between, except if you're pregnant. Amenorrhea is a sign that something is not right, that stress levels are too high or hormones are out of sync. Before considering herbal therapies, it is best to know that more serious diseases are ruled out. This is the time to discuss herbal remedies with your physician as well.

Herbs that stimulate menstruation have been used for thousands of years before modern medicine. There are dozens of herbal remedies that might prove to be useful, but these appear to be the most effective.

Helping Herbs

Chaste tree (chasteberry or vitex) exhibits hormonal effects that help regulate the menstrual cycle. The chaste tree affects the pituitary gland, which influences the female hormonal balance, resulting in a reduction in estrogen levels and an increase in progesterone. It appears to help in a variety of problems, including erratic cycles, scant or unusually heavy flow, missing ovulation and menstrual cramps. It may take up to 3 months to see the benefit of using chaste tree. *Typical dose:* 40 drops daily of a solution that has been standardized to contain the equivalent of 9 grams of berries per 100 mL.

Black cohosh is another popular herb for most menstrual complaints. It is considered estrogenic and may be beneficial for regulating menstrual cycles. It has the ability to relieve menstrual cramps, pain and swelling. It may take up to 6 weeks to notice any effects. *Typical dose:* 3 to 4 droppers (about 10 to 20 mL or 2 to 4 teaspoons) of tincture, 2 times daily; or up to 3 (500-mg) capsules, standardized to 2 percent triterpene glycosides, daily.

Premenstrual Syndrome

Premenstrual syndrome (PMS) is a compilation of symptoms that usually occur around the time of menstruation. These include: anxiety, bloating, breast tenderness, irritability, moodiness and weight gain primarily due to fluid retention. Severity of symptoms varies from woman to woman and is thought to be related to estrogen levels. There are several herbal preparations that can help relieve the symptoms when used regularly.

Helping Herbs

Chaste tree (chasteberry or vitex) can ease the symptoms of PMS, including fluid retention, mood swings, food cravings, premenstrual acnes, constipation and cold sores. *Typical dose:* 40 drops daily of a solution that has been standardized to contain the equivalent of 9 grams of berries per 100 mL.

Dong quai is thought to relieve menstrual cramps because it relaxes the uterus. It also increases blood circulation to the pelvic area, reducing the feeling of bloating. Dong quai also has mild estrogenic properties and helps relieves constipation. Use dong quai cautiously as it may be carcinogenic/mutagenic. *Typical dose:* Up to 6 (500- to 600-mg) capsules, daily; or 5 to 20 drops of tincture, 3 times daily.

Evening primrose has been used as a treatment for the mood swings, fluid retention and breast tenderness associated with PMS. It is worth a try if you suffer from PMS and nothing else has worked. *Typical dose:* Up to 12 capsules daily, containing 320 to 480 mg of the active constituent gamma linolenic acid (GLA) in 500 mg.

Soy has become popular for the treatment of PMS and other menstrual-related difficulties. It is effective because of its weak estrogenic properties that limit the uptake of estrogen produced by the body. Soy's isoflavones are thought to contribute to soy's effectiveness in treating high cholesterol and possibly osteoporosis. *Typical dose:* 25 to 50 grams of soy protein, obtained from food, daily.

St. John's wort is used to treat mild to moderate depression. It may be effective in treating mild depression in menopause. It may take up to 2 weeks to have any effect. *Typical dose:* 900 mg of capsules in three divided doses daily. Simple teas won't help depression because the active constituents lose their potency when dried. Do not take if you expect to be in direct sunlight as St. John's wort may cause sensitivity to ultraviolet (UV) rays.

Menopause

Menopause means ceasing of menstruation, but actually encompasses the period of life surrounding this change. As hormone production declines between 35 and 60 years of age, menses stop naturally. Menopause may occur earlier in some women because of illness or surgical removal of the ovaries. As hormone levels decrease, ovulation and menstruation become less frequent and eventually stop. Fluctuations in circulating hormones occur as the levels decline, resulting in symptoms such as hot flashes, anxiety, depression, night sweats and vaginal dryness. Hot flashes seem to be the most pronounced complaint among women who are experiencing menopause.

Herbs and other botanicals appear to have a role in helping women get through menopause with fewer symptoms. This is important because many women are choosing not to use the prescription alternative—hormone replacement therapy—because of real and perceived side effects.

Helping Herbs

Black cohosh has been studied most extensively for its effectiveness in treating menopausal symptoms. Studies have shown that black cohosh helps relieve hot flashes, lessens vaginal dryness, improves mood and eases the severity of fatigue. Black cohosh is available commercially in a clinically tested product named Remifemin. *Typical dose:* 10 to 25 drops (½ to 1½ mL) of tincture, up to every 4 hours; or up to 3 (500-mg) capsules, standardized to 2 percent triterpene glycosides, daily. Do not use if you are pregnant. May be used as directed while nursing—it is unsafe in large (more than recommended) doses.

Chaste tree (chasteberry or vitex) is believed to be effective for menopause because of its ability to affect the pituitary gland in stabilizing hormone fluctuations. *Typical dose:* 200 mg, standardized to 0.5 agnuside, 1 to 3 times daily.

Red clover is another herb with weak estrogenic properties. The isoflavones in red clover are similar to those in other plants, including soybeans. Foods that are rich in isoflavones have been shown to reduce hot flashes associated with menopause. A commercially available supplement, Promensil, is available in supermarkets and pharmacies. For purchased supplements, follow instructions on label. *Typical dose:* For a tea, steep 1 to 3 teaspoons of dried flowers in 1 cup of boiling water for 10 to 15 minutes, strain, and drink up to 3 cups daily.

Soy foods and soy isoflavones are being considered as a possible alternative to hormone replacement therapy (HRT) for the symptoms of menopause including hot flashes and night sweats. It is theorized that soy may have the same protective benefits of HRT without the risks. The data are inconclusive regarding soy food's ability to reduce the risk of developing breast cancer. However, soy's estrogenic-like effects may provide some relief for menopausal symptoms. *Typical dose:* 25 to 50 grams of soy protein from soy foods daily. Soy supplements are not recommended due to variability in products and uncertainty regarding isolated isoflavones' effects on breast tissue.

St. John's wort is used to treat mild to moderate depression and may be effective in treating the mild depression associated with menopause. It may take up to 2 weeks to have any effect. *Typical dose:* 900 mg of capsules, in three divided doses, daily. Simple teas won't help depression because the active constituents lose their potency when dried. Do not take if you expect to be in the sun because St. John's wort may cause sensitivity to the ultraviolet (UV) rays.

Yeast Infections

Yeast infections are usually caused by the organism candida, with *Candida albicans* being the most common. This yeast-like fungi may overgrow the lining of the vagina (vaginitis), the mouth (thrush) and even the penis of uncircumcised men. Yeast infections are more common than they were, say, 50 years ago, due in part to over use of antibiotics, steroids, and OCDs (oral contraceptive drugs). In particular, over use of antibiotics destroys the natural beneficial bacteria in the body resulting in the potential for overgrowth of yeast. These infections can be treated using some very effective herbal remedies but, more often than not, are treated with antifungal medication.

Helping Herbs

Echinacea's immune-stimulating properties may help fight vaginal infections. It stimulates white blood cell activity, increases the body's own production of antiviral substances and enhances immunity. It is probably most effective in sudden-onset infections. *Typical dose:* Up to 9 (300- to 400-mg) capsules, taken in 3 divided doses daily. Echinacea is contraindicated in AIDS and other autoimmune diseases. Do not use echinacea if you are allergic to members of the Asteraceae/Compositae family, including daisies and chamomile.

Garlic's antibacterial and antifungal antiviral properties are believed to be the reason for its effectiveness in preventing many conditions. Because garlic may leave you with strong breath and body odor, you may want to try a commercially prepared product. Long-term garlic use bestows the most health benefits. *Typical dose:* 600 to 900 mg of garlic powder, tablets or capsules daily; 4 mL of aged garlic extract; 10 mg of garlic oil "perles" daily; or 1 (or more) medium-sized fresh clove daily.

Goldenseal's active constituent, berberine, is believed to be effective for treating vaginal infections. It is considered antibacterial and yeast-fighting. It may stimulate your liver to help rid itself of toxins and may be especially beneficial if you recently have taken antibiotics to fight infections. *Typical dose:* Up to 6 (500- to 600-mg) capsules daily; or 20 to 50 drops of tincture once daily. Do not use if you are pregnant or nursing.

Vaginal Infections

Anything that disrupts the normal pH or flora of the vaginal tract can cause a vaginal infection. This includes antibiotics, douches, stray feces or even sex. Vaginitis, the inflammation of the lining of the vagina, is a common complaint women take to their healthcare provider, and is often the result of a yeast infection. Vaginitis should not be self-treated unless you have had it before and know what you are dealing with or have discussed the herbal alternatives with your provider.

Helping Herbs

Garlic is the premier antifungal and antibacterial herb, so why shouldn't it work for vaginal infections? To use garlic as a suppository: Wrap a whole peeled clove in sterile gauze and insert it into the vagina. To use garlic as a salve: Insert in the vagina on a tampon or use as a douche by mixing 1 teaspoon garlic juice to a few tablespoons of yogurt.

Tea tree oil is another powerful antifungal and antibiotic for external use only. Mix 2 to 3 drops with 1 tablespoon of yogurt and soak a tampon in the mixture. Insert the tampon and leave overnight. Repeat for 6 nights. If there is no relief, seek medical attention.

Echinacea stimulates the immune system, thus increasing the number of infection-fighting white blood cells. If your infection is not chronic, but appeared suddenly, echinacea might give your immune system the boost it needs. *Typical dose:* Up to 9 (300- to 400-mg) capsules daily until the infection subsides. Do not take echinacea for more than 8 weeks without a break. Do not use echinacea if you have an autoimmune disorder or are allergic to members of the Asteraceae/Compositae family, including marigolds, daisies or chrysanthemums.

Milk thistle can help rid your body of toxins that may be contributing to your ills. *Typical dose:* 140 mg of standardized silymarin extract, 3 times daily.

Infertility

Infertility is the inability to conceive after 6 months to 1 year of trying. The condition may be present in one or both partners and may be temporary and reversible. There are many suspected causes, including psychological or emotional problems and actual physical complaints. Infertility in women is usually not treated by herbal remedies, except chasteberry.

Helping Herbs

Chaste tree (chasteberry or vitex) exhibits hormonal effects that help regulate the menstrual cycle. The chaste tree affects the pituitary gland, which influences the female hormonal balance, resulting in a reduction in estrogen levels and an increase in progesterone. It appears to help in a variety of problems, including erratic cycles, scant or unusually heavy flow, missing ovulation and menstrual cramps. It may take up to 3 months to see the benefit of using chaste tree. *Typical dose:* 40 drops daily of a solution that has been standardized to contain the equivalent of 9 grams of berries per 100 mL.

Men's Health

Issues surrounding men's health are gaining more exposure as the population ages. Some of the same concerns are shared between the sexes: heart health, cancer, weight control and diabetes. However, there are some specific areas of concern that are not shared by the sexes.

Erection Problems

Erection problems were once considered to be psychosomatic. More is now known about this condition and about the physical causes contributing to it, including heart disease, alcohol or drug use, diabetes, sleep deprivation, smoking or prostate surgery. The purpose here is not to discuss the more serious side of erection problems—impotence—but to suggest some herbal remedies that may help with erections.

Helping Herbs

Ashwaganda has been used as the Ayurvedic answer to Chinese ginseng for improving the male libido. It is claimed that ashwaganda treats male impotence and infertility. None of these claims have scientific backing, but trying a cup of the tea occasionally won't hurt. Prepare the tea by steeping 1 to 2 teaspoons in 1 cup hot (not boiling) water for 10 minutes; strain and drink.

Guarana is a known aphrodisiac in Brazil. It contains caffeine, which, like many stimulants, can be a sexual stimulant. This herb may have some negative side effects, such as irritability and inability to sleep, so be careful about when you use it, and how much. To make a tea, steep 1 to 2 teaspoons of the herb in a cup of boiling water, strain and drink. Do not use guarana if you have high blood pressure, heart or kidney disease or a psychiatric disorder.

Ginseng (Panax) has been touted as a sexual stimulant for as long as man has used it—as far back as 3000 B.C.E. It has been shown to be effective for laboratory animals, but the evidence for humans is inconclusive. Documented effects of ginseng include: increased energy, feeling of improved general well-being and improved mental function. *Typical dose:* If you would like to try it, your best bet is to purchase a commercially prepared ginseng standardized to 4 to 5 percent ginsenosides. Take 200 to 500 mg of standardized extract daily.

Saw palmetto, because of its beneficial effect on the prostate gland, may help improve libido. The main effect of saw palmetto is its ability to shrink the prostate gland. An enlarged gland may not actually interfere with sexual function, but relieving the condition can help a man feel better about his sexuality. *Typical dose:* 160 mg of a standardized extract containing 85 to 95 percent fatty acids and sterols, twice daily. Do not use if you have a hormone-sensitive cancer, or other hormone disorder, without consulting your physician.

Yohimbe is a stimulant similar to caffeine, ephedra and guarana. It is considered to be a male aphrodisiac and has centuries of folklore behind its claim. A few clinical studies have shown there may be some promise with yohimbe, but not without significant side effects, including anxiety, high blood pressure, elevated heart rate, flushed appearance, and headaches. It is used in numerous sports-enhancing products as an alternative to metabolic steroids to increase muscle mass. It also promotes weight loss because of its stimulating properties. Yohimbine is a regulated prescription medication used in the treatment of erectile dysfunction. *Typical dose:* Yohimbe products labeled standardized to 15 mg yohimbine are available commercially—follow label directions. Do not use if you have high blood pressure, or if you are taking MAOI (monoamine oxidase inhibitor) antidepressants, over-the-counter medications or supplements with caffeine or ephedra.

Infertility

Infertility is the inability to conceive after 6 months to 1 year of trying. The condition may be present in one or both partners and may be temporary and reversible. There are many suspected causes, including psychological or emotional problems and actual physical complaints. There appear to be several herbal remedies that may help resolve falling sperm counts, although no known clinical studies support these claims.

Helping Herbs

Ashwaganda is as revered in Ayurvedic medicine as ginseng is in Asian medicine. It is considered a tonic for the male libido and sexual function, which certainly can't hurt if you are trying to conceive. *Typical dose:* Use commercially prepared supplements and follow the recommended dose.

Ginger is a stimulating herb, which may account for the theory that it stimulates sperm production and increases sperm count and motility. It is a relatively safe herb, so it may be worth a try. *Typical dose:* 2 to 4 grams of root rhizome daily; or ½ to 3 mL of tincture, 3 times daily; or 1 (250-mg) capsule, 4 times daily. Do not take if you have gallbladder disease or gallstones or if you are taking anticoagulant drugs. Avoid if you are taking more than 400 mg of vitamin E.

Ginseng has long been respected in Asia for its ability to increase male potency. It is another herb that is relatively safe when used as directed. *Typical dose:* 0.4 to 0.8 grams of dried root rhizome daily; or 0.5 to 2 grams of dried root daily; or 200 to 600 mg of extract standardized to 4 percent ginsenosides per day.

Prostate Enlargement

The prostate gland is a walnut-size gland that only men have. The gland surrounds the neck of the bladder, sitting just above the rectum. The prostate gland is the source for a majority of the fluid in semen. As a man ages, the gland grows larger, resulting in what is referred to as benign prostatic hypertrophy (hyperplasia), or BPH.

Reasons for enlargement are uncertain but thought to be related to hormonal changes. As a man ages, the amount of testosterone decreases, while the amount of estrogen increases. With a drop in blood testosterone, the rate of conversion into dihydrotestosterone (DHT) increases, especially in the prostate gland. DHT makes prostate cells grow, resulting in the symptoms associated with BPH: the inability to empty the bladder completely and the hallmark symptom, having to urinate in the middle of the night.

Drugs used to treat BPH keep the prostate cells from multiplying by preventing the conversion of testosterone to DHT. It is believed that the natural herbal alternatives may work just as well.

Helping Herbs

Licorice contains a substance that prevents the conversion of testosterone to dihydrotestosterone. It is a component of some herbal remedies for treatment of BPH. Taking very large doses of licorice long term may cause numerous side effects, including headache, high blood pressure, sodium and water retention and lethargy. *Typical dose:* 1/8 to 1 teaspoon of tincture, up to 3 times daily; or make a tea with 1 heaping teaspoon of chopped, dried licorice root, steeped in 1 cup of water for 15 minutes; strain and drink up to 3 cups daily. Do not use longer than 6 weeks. Do not use if you have heart disease or high blood pressure, or if you take drugs containing digitalis.

Pumpkin seeds have been observed to be effective in treating irritable bladder and painful urination in BPH. The active constituents appear to be the phytosterols and amino acids. They are also rich in minerals and vitamin E. *Typical dose:* 20 to 30 grams, coarsely ground or well-chewed seeds, taken with fluid, 2 times daily.

Pygeum is an evergreen prune tree that is indigenous to Africa and may be beneficial for the treatment of BPH. It has been studied clinically and the results have demonstrated its relative safety. The bark appears to contain active constituents that work together to decrease the swelling and inflammation in the prostate. It may also block testosterone production. It has been demonstrated to improve urinary flow, decrease nighttime urination and enhance the overall quality of life for men with BPH. It may be an option for men with mild symptoms and is certainly worth a try. *Typical dose:* 50 to 100 mg, standardized to contain 14 percent triterpenes and 0.5 percent n-docosanol, 2 times daily. May cause mild GI distress.

Saw palmetto has been used in European countries for many years but has only recently gained popularity in the United States. Saw palmetto is the herb renowned for treating BPH without any serious or significant side effects. It appears to be as effective as the prescription medication finasteride, but there are some differences. Saw palmetto does not lower PSA (prostate-specific atigen) levels, while finasteride does, and saw palmetto does not consistently reduce the overall size of the prostate. Reports of sexual dysfunction are markedly lower in men taking saw palmetto. *Typical dose:* 160 mg of a standardized extract, containing 85 to 95 percent fatty acids and sterols, twice daily. Do not use if you have a hormone-sensitive cancer or other hormone disorder without consulting your physician. Be certain that there is no underlying cause for the problems you are treating with saw palmetto as some symptoms of lower urinary tract problems may be signs of prostate cancer.

Neurological Diseases & Mental Performance

There are numerous diseases that fall under the neurologic classification. To attempt to describe all of them and their potential treatments would fill many more pages than this book can hold. Highlighted here are some of the more common complaints or diseases.

Depression

Depression is that feeling of hopelessness accompanied by other psychological and physical symptoms. Some brief periods of depression are normal—for example, after the loss of a loved one. The problem exists when these symptoms don't go away. The American Psychiatric Association defines depression as a condition in which at least four of the following symptoms persist for more than 30 days:

- Feelings of worthlessness or unfounded guilt
- Recurrent thoughts of death or suicide
- Poor appetite and weight loss, or increased appetite and weight gain
- Insomnia or sleeping more than usual
- Physical inactivity or hyperactivity
- Feeling of fatigue and loss of energy
- Inability to think or concentrate

As these symptoms persist, the body becomes out of balance and more physical symptoms may manifest themselves, including intolerance to cold, change in menstrual cycle and constipation.

Helping Herbs

Ginkgo may be helpful in treating depression, especially in the elderly, by counteracting age-related changes in the receptors for the mood-regulating substance serotonin. The herb has also been shown to be beneficial for memory and other intellectual functions. *Typical dose:* 40 to 60 mg of standardized extract capsules, 3 times daily. Use caution if you are taking blood-thinning medications, as ginkgo may interact.

Kava has been shown to alleviate anxiety that may be part of depression. Because of recent warnings regarding Kava and its safety, it is better to try one of the other remedies.

Lavender is a fragrant herb that calms the nerves and lifts the spirits. The smell of lavender is thought to promote sleep and to be a powerful antidepressant. Its essential oil may be used directly on the body. *Typical dose:* For tea, mix 1 teaspoon flowers with 1 cup of hot water. Steep for 5 minutes, then strain. Drink up to 3 cups daily. Do not use essential oil internally.

St. John's wort is the classic and popular herb used to treat mild to moderate depression. It may take up to 2 weeks to have any noticeable effect. *Typical dose:* 900 mg of capsules, in three divided doses, daily. Simple St. John's wort teas won't help depression because the active constituents lose their potency when dried.

Valerian, in combination with St. John's wort, has been found to be an effective treatment for depression. Valerian by itself may also be beneficial because it helps relieve insomnia and has some sedative properties. *Typical dose:* For the best benefit, use a commercially prepared extract or tincture and follow label directions.

Migraine Headaches

Migraines are recurring vascular headaches. They result in severe pain, sensitivity to light and involuntary disturbances during the acute phase, which may last for days. Nausea, vomiting, facial edema, irritability and extreme fatigue may accompany these disturbances. Persons who suffer from migraine headaches are often incapacitated for days.

Helping Herbs

Feverfew has been studied as a migraine remedy for about 20 years. It appears to work in the majority of patients who try it. Feverfew contains compounds that seem to inhibit the release of serotonin from blood cells in the brain. Serotonin is the brain chemical that controls mood. It is believed that blocking the release of serotonin prevents the constriction of arteries in the brain, which triggers migraine headaches. *Typical dose:* Try chewing 2 average-size fresh leaves daily. (The fresher, the better.) Be careful, however, as they may produce mouth sores. If this happens, try purchasing freeze-dried wholeleaf feverfew standardized to 0.6 to 0.7 percent parthenolide (the active compound in feverfew). Follow instructions on label.

Ginger is considered by Ayurvedic healers to be an excellent treatment for migraine headaches. It's worth a try. Ginger is an anti-inflammatory and helps ease nausea. *Typical dose:* Up to 8 (500- to 600-mg) capsules daily.

Willow (willow bark) is the precursor to today's popular drug aspirin, so it is logical to think that it might provide some relief. *Typical dose:* Up to 6 (400-mg) capsules per day; or as a tea, mix 1/4 to 1/2 teaspoon of powdered bark with 1 cup of hot water and steep for 10 to 15 minutes. Drink up to 3 cups per day. Do not use willow bark if you have GI problems (ulcers, nausea, vomiting or diarrhea) or if you are pregnant or lactating. Use caution if you are taking blood-thinning herbs or drugs.

Stress

Stress is usually a combination of factors in our lives that result in some type of change, either voluntary or involuntary. There can be positive stressors, such as planning a celebration, or negative ones, like losing a job. Either way, stress has an impact on our lives. How we choose to deal with stress may often determine the effect it has on us. However, sometimes there is just too much stress and we need help in order to do something about it.

When there are too many stressors in our lives, stress may lead to anxiety. Anxiety, in turn, may lead to infections, heart disease, a weakened immune system and more.

Anxiety

Anxiety is the result of situations that cause our bodies to produce large amounts of stress hormones, which seem to leave us on edge all the time. When anxiety and stress are allowed to continue, fatigue, decreased ability to handle stress and a decreased immune system result.

Helping Herbs

The chemicals in **catnip** are similar to those in the sedative valerian. Catnip is a mild tranquilizer and sedative. *Typical dose:* Mix 2 teaspoons of dried herb in 1 cup of hot, not boiling, water. Steep for 10 to 20 minutes and strain. Drink up to 3 cups per day.

Chamomile is effective for anxiety. A compound in chamomile binds to the same cell receptors as many tranquilizers and anti-anxiety drugs. Chamomile relaxes and tones the nervous system, relaxes muscles and eases GI complaints that often accompany stress and anxiety. *Typical dose:* 1 cup of tea, made from 2 teaspoons of dried flower steeped in 1 cup of hot water for 10 minutes. Do not use chamomile if you are allergic to members of the Asteraceae/Compositae family (daisies, marigolds).

Kava has been used as a treatment for anxiety and stress for many years. Recent warnings regarding its use and liver toxicity and death prompt this author to not recommend for its use at this time.

Lavender is a fragrant herb that has been used since ancient times as a tranquilizer to treat anxiety and stress. It is calming and enhances the action of other sedatives, so care should be taken when used with herbal or pharmaceutical sedatives. *Typical dose:* Steep 1 to 3 teaspoons of lavender flowers in 1 cup of boiling water for 10 minutes. Strain; drink up to 3 cups daily. For a relaxing bath, add 10 to 12 drops of essential oil to bathwater, or dilute with an equal amount of olive oil and apply to the skin. Do not use the essential oil internally.

Motherwort has mild sedative effects that may be helpful in relieving anxiety and associated insomnia. *Typical dose:* For tea, mix 2 teaspoon dried herb with 1 cup of hot water. Steep for 10 minutes. Drink up to 2 cups daily. Do not use with cardiac drugs or herbs, or during pregnancy and lactation.

Skullcap appears to have a calming, tranquilizing effect. It can be used for all types of anxiety, but is especially beneficial for mood swings associated with hormonal changes in PMS and menopause. *Typical dose:* As a tea made with 1 to 2 teaspoons of dried herb steeped in 1 cup boiling water for 15 minutes, then strained. Drink up to 3 cups daily.

St. John's wort is the classic and popular herb used to treat mild to moderate depression but is helpful in anxiety and stress as well. It's a great overall tonic for the nervous system. It may take up to 2 weeks to have any effect. *Typical dose:* 900 mg of capsules, in three divided doses, daily. Simple St. John's wort teas won't help anxiety as the active constituents lose their potency when dried.

Valerian is a strong anti-anxiety herb that does not cause dependence. Valerian may be beneficial because it helps relieve insomnia and has some sedative properties. *Typical dose:* For the best benefit, use a commercially prepared extract or tincture and follow label directions.

Insomnia

Insomnia is the inability to sleep or to remain asleep throughout the night. One out of two Americans has trouble sleeping at some time in their lives. Insomnia is one condition that may be better treated by herbs than drugs, primarily because of the side effects such as morning drowsiness, dry mouth, constipation and potential for drugs to be habit forming.

Helping Herbs

Catnip has a gentle sedative effect that is useful for inducing sleep. It also helps relieve gas and is antispasmodic, both of which are important if you are trying to sleep. *Typical dose:* Mix 2 teaspoons of dried herb in 1 cup of hot, not boiling, water. Steep for 10 to 20 minutes and strain. Drink up to 3 cups per day.

Chamomile is an age-old sleep-aid remedy. *Typical dose:* As a tea, made from 2 teaspoons of dried flower in 1 cup of hot water, steeped for 10 minutes. Take at bedtime. Use caution if you are allergic to members of the Asteraceae/Compositae family including daisies, marigolds, ragweed and feverfew.

Lemon balm eases insomnia and is effective as a tranquilizer and sedative. Because of its pleasant taste, it can be combined with other herbs that are used for insomnia and don't taste as good. *Typical dose:* As a tea, made with 2 teaspoons of dried leaves in 1 cup of hot water. Steep for 10 minutes and strain; take before bedtime.

Lavender has been used as a sleep aid for centuries. *Typical dose:* Put a handful of lavender flowers in a cloth bag and place under running water for a calming bath; apply a few drops of lavender oil directly to the skin; or make a tea by mixing 1 to 3 teaspoons of lavender flowers and 1 cup of boiling water, steep 10 minutes, strain and drink at bedtime.

Fatigue

Fatigue or tiredness is one of the most common complaints in today's society. This differs from Chronic Fatigue Syndrome, which has a medical diagnosis. Fatigue is often a result of working too hard, not getting enough rest or play and not paying attention to what our bodies need. Sometimes, by making just a few changes in our lives, we can figure out what is dragging us down. If nothing seems obvious, maybe an herbal pick-me-up will help.

Helping Herbs

Astragalus is considered, in Traditional Chinese Medicine, to be beneficial for fatigue. It has been used as a tonic that has positive effects on endurance. It may be worth a try if you are not suffering from an acute illness that is causing the fatigue. *Typical dose:* up to 8 to 14 (400- to 500-mg) capsules of astragalus powder daily.

Ginseng is touted as an overall tonic that is good for just about anything, including fatigue. Chinese (Panax) and Siberian *(Eleutherococcus senticosus)* ginseng appear to have similar properties. Chinese ginseng may be too stimulating for some people; Siberian ginseng may be more tolerable. *Typical dose:* Panax; Up to 600 mg capsules daily; or 100 mg of extract standardized to 4 percent ginsenosides, twice daily. Begin with a low dose and gradually increase the amount. Do not use if you are pregnant or have high blood pressure. *Typical dose:* Siberian; up to 3 grams of dry root daily in one to three doses for up to 1 month, with a 2- to 3-week ginseng-free period every 30 to 60 days of treatment.

Peppermint, by virtue of its flavor, may pick you up. It eases anxiety, tension and the gastrointestinal stress that may accompany fatigue. *Typical dose:* As a tea, 2 to 4 teaspoons of dried peppermint leaf, steeped in 2 to 3 cups of hot water for 15 minutes. Take as often as needed. Do not use if you have heartburn or esophageal reflux.

Rosemary is a multipurpose herb that is soothing but stimulating. Its antioxidants are reported to help improve memory while it boosts the spirits. *Typical dose:* Tea made by steeping 1 teaspoon of dried leaves in 1 cup of hot water for 15 minutes. Take up to 3 cups daily.

Chronic Fatigue Syndrome

Chronic Fatigue Syndrome (CFS) is an illness that often begins with a cold or flu-like symptoms followed by unending fatigue that cannot be relieved by rest. It is a confusing illness, one that often is overlooked or believed to actually be nonexistent. And it is relentless, often disappearing for a while, then mysteriously and unwelcomely returning. Herbal therapies may not be the cure, but they certainly may help relieve some of the symptoms.

Helping Herbs

Ginseng is touted as an overall tonic that is good for just about anything. Ginseng has been considered an adaptogen or a substance that increases general resistance to all types of stress. Chinese (Panax) and Siberian *(Eleutherococcus senticosus)* ginseng appear to have similar properties. Chinese ginseng may be too stimulating for some people; Siberian ginseng may be more tolerable. *Typical dose:* Panax; Up to 600 mg daily; or 100 mg of extract standardized to 4 percent ginsenosides, 2 times daily. *Typical dose:* Siberian; Up to 3 grams dried root daily in one to three doses for up to 1 month with a 2- to 3-week ginseng-free period between consecutive courses. Begin with the lower dose and gradually increase the amount. Do not use if you are pregnant or have high blood pressure.

Echinacea may help enhance a depressed immune system, which is common in persons suffering from CFS. *Typical dose:* Up to 9 (300- to 400-mg) capsules daily. Take for 2 weeks, then take a break for 1 week and repeat the cycle. Do not take if you are allergic to other members in the Asteraceae/Compositae family, including chrysanthemums, chamomile, daisies and marigolds. Echinacea is contraindicated in persons with AIDS or HIV infections.

Astragalus is considered, in Traditional Chinese Medicine, to be beneficial for general fatigue and possibly for CFS. It has been used as a tonic that has positive effects on endurance. It may be worth a try if you are not suffering from an acute illness that is causing the fatigue. *Typical dose:* up to 8 to 14 (400- to 500-mg) capsules of astragalus powder daily.

Licorice may be beneficial if you are low in the adrenal hormone cortisol. This is common in those with CFS. Up to 3,000 mg of licorice root, twice daily, has been shown to be beneficial, but may have adverse side effects. Do not use longer than 6 weeks without medical supervision. Do not take if you have high blood pressure, diabetes, thyroid disease or kidney, liver or heart disease. Do not use if you are taking diuretics or if you are pregnant.

St. John's wort can boost energy by relieving mild to moderate depression. It's a great overall tonic for the nervous system. It may take up to 2 weeks to have any effect. *Typical dose:* 900 mg of capsules, in three divided doses, daily. Simple St. John's wort teas won't help depression because the active constituents lose their potency when dried.

Valerian may help if you lose sleep because of CFS. *Typical dose:* For the best benefit, use a commercially prepared extract or tincture and follow label directions.

Altitude Sickness

Altitude sickness includes a myriad of symptoms that most often occur at altitudes above 8,000 feet. They usually occur when a person is not accustomed to the altitude and subside after about 5 days. Symptoms are generally not serious for people who spend just a few days at a new altitude, but can be for those who scale the world's highest peaks. If symptoms persist or worsen, they might be a sign of something more serious, such as a heart attack or stroke.

Symptoms include headache, insomnia, weakness, poor appetite, nausea, shortness of breath upon exertion and overall feeling of being ill.

Helping Herbs

Garlic helps thin the blood and keep it from clotting, which is a benefit at higher altitude where the air is thin. *Typical dose:* 1 to 3 raw or briefly cooked cloves daily. You may want to use a prepared supplement that provides a standardized garlic extract containing 1.3 percent allicin content.

Ginkgo improves blood flow to the peripheral arteries, heart and brain: Gingko improves the body's ability to tolerate lower levels of oxygen. It helps prevent microscopic leaking of blood and fluid from tiny veins, thus improving overall circulation and providing protection to vessel walls. It reduces brain swelling due to trauma or toxins and neutralizes free radicals. Ginkgo may also reduce abnormal blood clotting. *Typical dose:* 60 to 80 mg of extract standardized to 24 percent ginkgo flavone glycosides and 6 percent terpene lactones 3 times daily.

Ginseng is touted as an overall tonic that is good for just about anything, and it may help soothe and lessen the symptoms of altitude sickness. Chinese (Panax) ginseng may improve respiration and blood oxygenation, which can help relieve some symptoms. Some research indicates that Siberian *(Eleutherococcus senticosus)* ginseng helps reduce altitude sickness if it is taken for at least 2 days prior to ascending. Chinese ginseng may be too stimulating for some people; Siberian ginseng may be more tolerable. *Typical dose:* Panax: Up to 4 (500- to 600-mg) capsules daily; or 100 mg of extract, standardized to 4 percent total ginsenosides 2 times daily. Siberian: Up to 3 grams dried root daily, taken in one to three doses. Begin with the lower dose and gradually increase the amount. Do not use if you are pregnant or have high blood pressure. Some practitioners recommend taking it daily for 1 month, stopping for 1 month, then resume for 1 month; take it only every other month for long-term use.

Ginger helps relieve the nausea that may accompany altitude sickness. *Typical dose:* Up to 8 (500- to 600-mg) capsules daily. You may also choose to use raw or crystallized ginger, or ginger ale that contains real ginger (not just the flavoring). Don't take ginger if you have gallbladder disease.

Dizziness & Vertigo

Dizziness is a feeling of unsteadiness, while vertigo is a feeling that everything around you is spinning uncontrollably. Both can be signs of something more serious; if they continue, consult a physician or healthcare provider.

Helping Herbs

Ginger helps relieve the nausea that may accompany dizziness. *Typical dose:* Up to 8 (500- to 600-mg) capsules daily. Don't take ginger if you have gallbladder disease.

Ginkgo improves blood and oxygen flow to the peripheral arteries, heart and brain. It helps prevent microscopic leaking of blood and fluid from tiny veins and thus improves overall circulation and provides protection to vessel walls. Ginkgo may also reduce abnormal blood clotting. *Typical dose:* 60 to 80 mg of extract standardized to 24 percent ginkgo flavone glycosides and 6 percent terpene lactones 3 times daily.

Parkinson's Disease

Parkinson's disease (PD) is a slowly progressing disease of the nervous system. Although it is thought that PD affects only older people (1 percent of those age 60 or more, 2 percent of people age 70 or more), it affects the young as well: 15 percent of PD patients are age 50 or younger and 10 percent are 40 or younger. PD also appears in teenagers (juvenile PD). More men are affected than women.

PD progresses from diagnosis to major disability over 10 to 20 years and is characterized by four principal symptoms:

- Rigidity of the limbs.
- Tremor of the limbs. This is more prominent in the hands and may be worse on one side than the other.
- Bradykinesia, which is difficulty initiating movement, slowness in movement and lack or incompleteness of movement. Bradykinesia is the most prominent and disabling symptom of PD.
- Postural reflexes are impaired, so when a person trips, they are unable to stop falling or ease their fall, resulting in injury. This may be perceived as unsteadiness or lack of balance.

If you think you or anyone you know has Parkinson's, or the symptoms of the disease, seek medical treatment. Herbal remedies may help, but Parkinson's is a serious disease. Some herbs may interact with drugs used in treating the disease.

Helping Herbs

Ginkgo is an antioxidant that helps prevent damage to arterial walls. It also dilates the blood vessels in areas that don't seem to be getting enough oxygen and helps prevent the accumulation of platelets that cause clots. This can stall the progress of dementia, a problem that often plagues persons in the later stages of Parkinson's disease. *Typical dose:* 60 to 80 milligrams of capsules, standardized to 24 percent ginkgo flavone glycosides and

6 percent terpene lactone, 3 times daily. Use caution if you are taking other blood-thinning drugs.

Evening primrose oil has small amounts of the amino acid tryptophan, which boosts the effectiveness of levodopa, the drug most commonly used for treating Parkinson's. It also contains unsaturated fatty acids, which appear to have beneficial effects on brain chemistry. *Typical dose:* 2 tablespoons of EPO daily; or 1,500 to 2,400 mg in capsules daily.

Alzheimer's Disease

Alzheimer's disease is a progressive, neurodegenerative disease characterized by loss of function and the death of nerve cells in several areas of the brain, leading to loss of mental functions, including memory and learning. Alzheimer's disease is the most common cause of dementia. It is most often seen in persons over age 65, but can occur in younger individuals. The best way to keep the brain working is to keep the body active and healthy through regular exercise, a healthy diet and activities that are mentally challenging.

Helping Herbs

Ginkgo helps prevent damage to arterial walls and dilates the blood vessels in areas that don't seem to get enough oxygen. This can stall the progress of dementia. *Typical dose:* 60 to 80 mg of capsules, standardized to 24 percent gingko flavone glycosides and 6 percent terpene lactone, 3 times daily. Use caution if you are taking other blood-thinning drugs.

Ginseng is touted as an overall tonic that is good for just about anything. Chinese (Panax) and Siberian *(Eleutherococcus senticosus)* ginseng appear to have similar properties. Chinese ginseng may be too stimulating for some people. *Typical dose:* Panax: Up to 600 mg daily taken in 100- to 500-mg capsules; or 100 mg of extract standardized to 4 percent ginsenosides, 2 times daily. Begin with low dose and gradually increase the amount. Do not use if you are pregnant or have high blood pressure.

Siberian ginseng's history includes its use as a tonic to help people get through harsh winters. Ginseng is an adaptogen; it helps normalize the functions of many body processes. Siberian ginseng is purported to restore memory, increase stamina, stabilize the blood sugar and enhance the immune system. Typical dose: Siberian: Up to 3 grams of dry root daily in one to three doses for up to one month with a 2- to 3-week ginseng-free period after every 30 to 60 days of a treatment.

Rosemary has a long history as an herb that improves memory and cognition. It contains many antioxidants that help neutralize free radicals that may be implicated in the development and progression of Alzheimer's disease. *Typical dose:* 2 drops (1 mL) of rosemary oil in 4 ounces water daily, or 4-6 grams of herb or its equivalent.

Gastrointestinal Tract or Digestive System

The gastrointestinal (GI) tract is a series of organs and structures used for digesting the food we eat. It is where the nutrients from our food are absorbed. The gastrointestinal tract includes the mouth, esophagus, stomach, small intestine, large intestine, rectum and anus. Organs that help with digestion but are not part of the digestive tract include the tongue, glands in the mouth that make saliva, the pancreas, liver and gallbladder. All of these systems are ready and waiting to take the food you eat and fuel your body, repair tissue and, hopefully, help prevent or at least reduce the risk of disease.

Listed here are some of the more common conditions that may benefit from an herbal remedy. If you experience unusual or prolonged symptoms including, but not limited to, nausea, vomiting, diarrhea, abdominal pain, constipation, loss of appetite or unusual bleeding, seek medical treatment before using herbal remedies. Herbs may help reduce mild symptoms, but if symptoms persist, it may be a sign of something that needs medical attention.

Bad Breath

Bacteria in the mouth cause most bad breath. Bacteria produce waste products that give off an unpleasant odor. Persons with gum disease tend to have chronic bad breath. If not treated, gum disease can result in tooth loss. For most people, simple hygiene, including brushing their teeth and flossing daily, will help keep bad breath and gum disease at bay. If these don't work, herbs might help.

Chronic bad breath may be a sign of a bigger problem, however. Sometimes, liver disease, diabetes, cancer of the upper respiratory system and kidney failure will cause bad breath. If your bad breath does not go away with proper care, it's a good idea to seek a medical opinion.

Helping Herbs

Eucalyptus is an ingredient found in many commercial mouthwashes. You can make your own mouthwash by steeping 3 ounces dried (or 6 ounces fresh) eucalyptus in 2 cups of vodka. Allow to steep several weeks. Strain if desired. Use as you would any purchased mouthwash. You can combine several breath-freshening herbs in this concoction if you like.

Parsley is a nutritious and effective breath freshener with many added benefits. Regular use may help reduce your risk of high blood pressure and congestive heart failure, or help treat allergies and fever. Try chewing a bit of parsley if you feel your breath may be offensive.

Dill is considered a digestive aid. It inhibits the growth of bacteria in the intestinal tract and may do the same for bacteria in your mouth. To benefit from dill as a breath freshener, chew ½ to 1 teaspoon after meals.

Peppermint's aromatic oil is a potent antiseptic that can soothe even the worst breath when taken as a tea. *Typical dose:* Take 6 to 12 drops diluted in 150 mL hot (not boiling) water or 1 to 2 teaspoons dried herb in 1 cup boiling water 3 to 4 times daily. May help sooth an upset stomach as well.

Sage tea may cure bad breath and mouth sores. *Typical dose:* 1 to 2 teaspoons steeped in 1 cup of hot water for 10 to 15 minutes. Strain and drink when you think you need it, up to 3 times daily.

Toothache

A toothache is your body's way of telling you something is not quite right in your mouth. Toothaches usually occur when the nerve of the tooth is dead or dying. Toothaches need professional treatment because the bacteria that are attacking the teeth can travel through the blood and infect other parts of the body. Herbal remedies may provide relief, but if pain continues, it may be signaling a bigger problem that needs immediate attention. Even if pain subsides, that may mean the tooth is dead and the bacteria are still marching on.

Helping Herbs

Chamomile is popular in Europe for the treatment of mouth sores. It is gentle on irritated gums and on your nerves as well. *Typical dose:* Drink 3 cups of tea daily, made with 1 teaspoon of dried flowers to 1 cup of hot water, steeped for 10 minutes, strained and cooled.

Clove oil is a local anesthetic and antiseptic for toothache. It is not intended for ingestion and is not recommended for application without the guidance of a dental professional. There are some products on the market that contain clove oil and are effective for toothache. Read label instructions before using.

Garlic is an antibacterial herb and is not just for cooking. If you have a toothache, bruise a garlic clove and place it next to the infected tooth. If it stings too much, remove it.

Turmeric is found in many dental products because of its antibacterial and anti-inflammatory properties. It gives the yellow tint to mouthwashes and stimulates circulation, bringing immune cells to the infected site. Mix 1 teaspoon of turmeric with enough water to make a paste; place it on the infected tooth.

Gingivitis

Gingivitis is an inflammation of the gums with tenderness, swelling, redness and a watery discharge. If allowed to progress, the gum tissue supporting the teeth deteriorates and may result in tooth loss. Herbal remedies may help rid the mouth of the bacteria that brushing and flossing could not reach.

Helping Herbs

Bloodroot may reduce dental plaque, which is a major cause of gum disease and tooth loss. The active component of bloodroot is Sanguinarine. It is thought to bind with plaque and keep it from adhering to teeth. Look for commercial products that contain bloodroot.

Chamomile, when used as a mouthwash, has been shown to soothe irritated gums and has antibacterial properties that may help fight gingivitis. *Typical dose:* As a tea, steep 1 to 2 teaspoons of flowers in 1 cup of hot water steeped for 10 minutes and strain. Have up to 4 cups per day.

Peppermint can lend its antibacterial power to fighting the pesky germs that cause tooth decay and, subsequently, gingivitis. *Typical dose:* Make a tea with 2 teaspoons of crushed leaves in 1 cup boiling water and steep for 10 minutes. Drink the tea or use as a mouthwash.

Tea tree oil is a powerful antiseptic that can be used to treat mouth sores and gingivitis. Do not swallow tea tree oil. When taken internally by children, tea tree oil can lead to weakness, confusion and coma. Adults who ingest tea tree oil may experience a rash of tiny red or purple spots and an increase in white blood cells. These conditions will reverse themselves when ingestion is discontinued. If you want to try it, add a few drops of tea tree oil to a glass of water, swish some in your mouth and spit it out. Do not use undiluted.

Canker Sores

Canker sores are nothing more than pesky mouth ulcers of questionable origin. Causes are linked to poor diet, stress, food allergies, viruses and immune system dysfunction. In most cases, they go away by themselves, but a little help never hurts.

Helping Herbs

Gotu kola is a healing herb that promotes the growth of connective tissue. *Typical dose:* 1 cup of tea daily, made by steeping 1 teaspoon of dried herb in 1 cup of hot water for 10 minutes. This may also be used as a soothing rinse.

Echinacea tinctures may numb canker sores, thereby relieving the pain. Use the tincture cautiously, because it contains alcohol that may sting. *Typical dose:* 20 to 40 drops in 2 to 3 ounces of water, up to 4 times per day.

Goldenseal was a favorite herb of Native Americans, used for all kinds of wounds and sores. It is an antiseptic and anti-inflammatory, so it may fight infection and swelling. *Typical dose:* 20 to 50 drops of tincture in about 2 ounces of water, swished in the mouth. Do not use if you are pregnant or nursing.

Licorice can help heal canker sores in a relatively short period of time. Open a capsule of licorice powder and dab a bit on the sore.

Chamomile, when used as a mouthwash, has been shown to be effective for canker sores and mouth ulcers. It may be beneficial for mouth sores that are a result of chemotherapy. *Typical dose:* As a tea, steep 1 to 2 teaspoons of flowers in 1 cup of hot water for 10 minutes and strain. Have up to 4 cups per day. Tea may be also used as a mouthwash.

Cold Sores, Fever Blisters & Herpes

Cold sores and fever blisters are not unlike canker sores except they are out there for everybody to see! Cold sores come from the same virus that gives us genital herpes—herpes simplex, which is a cousin to the virus that causes shingles and chicken pox. Cold sores generally develop around the mouth and lips. Stress is a known cause, and exposure to intense sunlight might be another.

Genital herpes occur in and around the vagina and cervix in women and on the penis in men. When they first occur, genital herpes are generally sexually transmitted, thereafter they are a recurrence from the virus which has laid dormant in the body.

Helping Herbs

Echinacea has antiviral and immune-stimulating properties. Using echinacea may help reduce the severity of cold sores or genital herpes while preventing recurrence. A bit of tincture applied to the sore will help relieve some of the pain as well. *Typical dose:* Up to 9 (300- to 400-mg) capsules per day; or 60 drops of tincture, 3 times daily. Do not exceed 8 weeks of use.

Lemon balm has antiviral activity that may be beneficial in all types of herpes virus sores. *Typical dose:* As a tea, made from 2 teaspoons of dried leaves in 1 cup of hot water, steeped for 10 minutes and taken up to 4 times daily.

Licorice is effective against herpes virus through its ability to inactivate the virus and to relieve the inflammation. At the first sign of an outbreak, take a tea made of licorice. For topical relief, apply a bit of a commercially prepared product (follow label directions) or break open a capsule containing 1 to 4 grams of powdered root and apply directly to the sore. *Typical dose:* Steep 2 teaspoons of powdered root in 1 cup of hot water for 15 minutes and strain. Drink up to 3 cups daily. Do not use licorice internally longer than 6 weeks. Do not use if you are pregnant or lactating; if you are suffering from heart disease, high blood pressure or liver disease; or if you are taking diuretics.

Mints other than lemon balm can provide relief for herpes virus sores. Tea made with peppermint or other members of the mint family will soothe the sores and provide added important antioxidants.

Mullein helps fight the herpes virus and soothes irritated skin. *Typical dose:* 6 to 8 cups of tea daily, made from dried mullein flowers; steep 2 teaspoons in 1 cup of hot water for 10 minutes, strain and enjoy.

St. John's wort fights the herpes virus from the inside and out. *Typical dose:* 300 mg in capsule form, 3 times daily; or make a tea with 1 teaspoon of dried herb to 1 cup of hot water, steeped for 10 minutes. The tea can be taken internally or used as a compress. If you are using St. John's wort, avoid exposure to direct sunlight; it may cause photosensitivity.

Shingles

Shingles is the adult version of chicken pox. If we had chicken pox as a child, the herpes zoster virus that causes it remains in the body, only to rear its ugly welts once again. Shingles symptoms include a painful rash that appears most often on the torso and is made up of painful blisters that usually dry up in a few weeks. But, unlike chicken pox, the pain of shingles remains even after visible signs are gone.

The cause is uncertain, but most fingers point to a compromised immune system. This means that persons with AIDS, illnesses that attack the immune system, some kinds of cancers and some medications that suppress the immune system, like steroids, can trigger shingles. Fortunately, there are some herbal remedies that can ease some of the pain and symptoms.

Helping Herbs

Bergamot is an essential oil that may be beneficial in treating shingles. *Typical dose:* Dilute the oil by adding 5 to 10 drops to 2 tablespoons of olive oil and apply directly to the painful area, several times daily.

Capsicum (red pepper) may help shingles when applied topically. It is available commercially as creams called Capzasin-P and Zostrix, which relieve pain and clear up red, scaly skin. Some burning may occur with their use. Wash your hands thoroughly after applying, and avoid touching your eyes. These products are made from hot peppers.

Lemon balm has antiviral activity that may be beneficial for all types of herpes virus sores. *Typical dose:* As a tea, made from 2 teaspoons of dried leaves in 1 cup of hot water, steeped for 10 minutes. Take up to 4 times daily.

Licorice contains virus-fighting and immune-boosting ingredients that inhibit the herpes simplex virus that causes shingles. Licorice tea can be taken alone or in combination with other herbs that fight the herpes virus. These include peppermint and lemon balm. *Typical dose:* Steep 2 teaspoons of powdered root in 1 cup of hot water for 15 minutes and strain. Drink up to 3 cups daily. Do not use licorice internally longer than 6 weeks. Do not use if you are pregnant or lactating; if you are suffering from heart disease, high blood pressure or liver disease; or if you are taking diuretics.

Mullein helps fight the herpes virus and soothes irritated skin. *Typical dose:* 6 to 8 cups of tea daily, made from dried mullein flowers; steep 2 teaspoons in 1 cup of hot water for 10 minutes, strain and enjoy.

Stomach Ache

Stomach ache is a non-specific pain in the stomach. It may be caused by eating too much, stress, constipation, gas and more. Because stomach ache is non-specific, the best herbal remedies are listed under specific conditions or treated by what we already know as stomach-soothing herbs. Seek medical treatment if you experience severe cramping, nausea or vomiting, or if symptoms do not resolve in 24 hours.

Helping Herbs

Ginger is an effective antispasmodic for GI complaints. It prevents indigestion and abdominal cramping by soothing the muscles that line the intestine. *Typical dose:* Make a ginger tea by steeping 2 teaspoons of powdered or fresh grated root in 1 cup of boiling water for 10 minutes. Drink up to 2 cups per day.

Lemon balm acts as a digestive aid by relaxing the smooth muscle of the digestive tract. *Typical dose:* As a tea, made from 2 teaspoons of dried leaves in 1 cup of hot water, steeped for 10 minutes. Take up to 4 times daily.

Peppermint soothes the smooth muscle lining of the digestive tract, thus calming an achy tummy. *Typical dose:* Steep 1 to 2 teaspoons of dried peppermint in 1 cup of boiling water for 10 minutes. Drink up to 3 cups per day. Do not use if you have GERD.

Heartburn

Heartburn is a painful, burning feeling in the chest. Heartburn is caused by stomach acid flowing back into the esophagus.

Heartburn may be a symptom of esophageal reflux or GERD. GERD is the flow of the stomach's contents back up into the esophagus. This happens when the muscle between the esophagus and the stomach (the lower esophageal sphincter) is weak, or relaxes when it shouldn't.

Helping Herbs

Aloe gel (not the irritating latex) has soothing properties and has been shown to be effective for healing ulcers, burns and inflamed intestinal walls. It is important to get a pure source of aloe pulp if you want to try it. The best for heartburn is a food-grade freeze-dried product. Follow label directions if you choose to try it.

Chamomile is a soothing tea for heartburn and stomach distress. *Typical dose:* As a tea, steep 1 to 2 teaspoons of flowers in 1 cup of hot water for 10 minutes and strain. Have up to 4 cups per day. Do not use chamomile if you are allergic to members of the Asteraceae/Compositae family, including daisies, marigolds and feverfew.

Licorice has been shown to be anti-inflammatory and soothing to the mucous membranes. For heartburn, the deglycyrrhizinated (DGL) licorice is the best choice, as it does not have the negative side effects that true licorice has. You may use true licorice if you like, but do not take more than 3 cups per day for more than 6 weeks. True licorice may increase blood pressure, interfere with blood sugar, decreases potassium in the blood and interacts with many prescription drugs. *Typical dose:* For mild heartburn, use 1 to 2 teaspoons of dried chopped root in 1 cup of hot water and steep for 10 to 15 minutes; for more severe heartburn, use 1/4 teaspoon of powdered root or liquid extract in 1/4 cup of water. Take 1 cup of tea or 1/4 cup of the stronger concoction after meals and at bedtime.

Ulcers

Simply stated, an ulcer is a sore on the stomach lining or in the duodenum, where the stomach connects with the small intestine. People with allergies tend to have more ulcers. We used to think that stress caused ulcers, but we now know that the real cause is usually an infection caused by the bacteria Helicobacter pylori. Poor diet, heredity, lack of fiber in the diet and deficiencies of vitamins A and E may contribute to ulcers. Drugs have adverse side effects, so herbs may offer a safe alternative for treatment. If you think you have an ulcer, it is best to get a medical examination to confirm the fact before beginning herbal treatment. That way, you know what you are up against and what to use to treat it.

Helping Herbs

Calendula has antibacterial and antiviral properties that may be effective against the virus that causes ulcers. It appears to alleviate the symptoms of chronic inflammation and reduces bleeding through its astringent properties. *Typical dose:* Make a tea of 1 to 2 teaspoons of dried flowers steeped in 1 cup of hot water for 10 minutes. Drink up to 3 cups per day.

European medical herbalists consider **chamomile** to be the remedy of choice as a digestive aid and for ulcers. *Typical dose:* As a tea, steep 1 to 2 teaspoons of flowers in 1 cup of hot water for 10 minutes and strain. Have up to 4 cups per day. Do not use chamomile if you are allergic to members of the Asteraceae/Compositae family, including daisies, marigolds and feverfew.

Licorice has been shown to accelerate the healing of stomach ulcers. It is anti-inflammatory and soothing to the mucous membranes. For ulcers, choose deglycyrrhizinated (DGL) licorice because it does not have true licorice's negative side effects. You may use true licorice if you like, but do not take more than 3 cups per day for more than 6 weeks. If you are taking diabetes, heart or blood pressure medicines, avoid using licorice. *Typical dose:* For mild heartburn, use 1 to 2 teaspoons of dried chopped root in 1 cup of hot water and steep for 10 to 15 minutes; for more severe heartburn, use 1/8 to 1/2 teaspoon of powdered root or liquid extract in 1/4 cup of water. Take 1 cup of tea or 1/4 cup of the stronger concoction after meals and at bedtime.

Slippery elm forms protective mucilage that is beneficial for the stomach. When taken as a tea or decoction, it soothes the digestive tract. *Typical dose:* Make a decoction blending 3 teaspoons of powdered herb in 1 cup of water; bring it to a boil and simmer for 15 minutes. Drink up to 3 cups per day.

Gallstones

Gallstones are solid masses or stones made of cholesterol, or bilirubin, that form in the gallbladder or bile ducts. Gallstones don't cause problems if they stay in the gallbladder; when they move to the ducts, they cause trouble. Symptoms include intense sudden-onset pain, usually in the upper right abdomen. Fever, nausea and sometimes vomiting accompany gallstones. The best way to prevent gallstones is to eat a low-fat, low-cholesterol diet. There are some herbs that may help relieve some of the discomfort of gallstones, but ultimately, treatment may need to be removal.

Helping Herbs

Dandelion root stimulates the flow of bile and may help prevent gallstones. *Typical dose:* Make a tea using 1 ounce of dried leaves steeped in 1 cup of boiling water for 10 minutes, then strained. Drink up to 3 cups per day.

Peppermint is a traditional treatment for gallstones. It is soothing to the stomach and reduces spasms that may be associated with a gallbladder attack. It is thought that enteric-coated peppermint capsules may actually dissolve gallstones. *Typical dose:* 0.2 to 0.4 mL enteric-coated capsules, 2 times daily, between meals.

Turmeric contains a compound, curcumin, that is effective in treating gallstones. It stimulates the production and solubility of bile, which helps prevent the formation of stones and eliminate those that have formed. *Typical dose:* Use 1 teaspoon of turmeric powder in 1 cup of hot water (not boiling) and drink up to 3 cups daily. Juice of the active constituents in turmeric are not water soluble. Powdered root taken in or 1/2- to 1-gram capsules up to 3 times daily, may prove more effective.

Motion Sickness

Motion sickness occurs when a person's eyes see one type of movement while their brain is processing another. This results in nausea, dizziness and, sometimes, vomiting. Motion sickness can be effectively treated using herbs.

Helping Herbs

Ginger is renowned for its ability to ease the discomfort of motion sickness. It has been used for thousands of years for seasickness and to relieve morning sickness. It is an antispasmodic, meaning it is effective against spasms of the smooth muscle of the gastrointestinal tract. Use whatever remedy sounds good. *Typical dose:* Up to 8 (500- to 600-mg) capsules daily. You can also chew raw or crystallized ginger or ginger ale that contains real ginger (not just the flavoring). Don't take ginger if you have gallbladder disease.

Fennel is like many other aromatic herbs as it relaxes the smooth muscle lining of the digestive tract. It also helps to relieve gas and promotes the secretion of bile, so it is very effective in treating the symptoms of motion sickness. *Typical dose:* Try a tea made with 2 to 3 teaspoons of crushed seeds steeped in 1 cup hot water for 10 to 15 minutes; strain and drink up to 3 cups daily. Or try chewing about 20 seeds, as needed.

Peppermint soothes the smooth muscle lining the GI tract and reduces the nausea and vomiting associated with motion sickness. Strong peppermint candies can bring relief to a stressed stomach, which is why they are often offered at the end of a meal. *Typical dose:* 10 to 20 drops of tincture before trips either in a small amount of water or undiluted. Or 1 cup of tea made by steeping 3 to 4 teaspoons of dried peppermint in 1½ to 3 cups of hot water for 15 minutes; strain and drink warm or cold. Note: Undiluted essential peppermint oil may be irritating. Use cautiously, if at all, during pregnancy and lactation. Do not use if you have GERD.

Nausea & Vomiting

Nausea, the feeling of wanting to throw up (vomit), can be caused by many factors. Too much celebrating, chemotherapy, the "stomach flu," morning sickness in pregnancy, emotional stress, headache and more may make us nauseated. Regardless of the cause, relief is the desired outcome. Vomiting is often the result of prolonged nausea. Assuming there are no underlying physical problems, nausea and vomiting may be treated using herbal remedies.

No matter what has caused the vomiting, it is essential to replace lost fluids. Some teas, water and sports drinks will help replace lost fluids and electrolytes. If you can't keep fluid down and have not urinated for 8 hours, or if nausea and vomiting continue for more than 24 hours, medical attention is needed.

Helping Herbs

Ginger is an antispasmodic, meaning it is effective against spasms of the smooth muscle of the GI tract. This helps to reduce nausea. Use whatever remedy sounds good. Ginger may be used cautiously for morning sickness in pregnancy. Consult with your healthcare provider before trying ginger for morning sickness. *Typical dose:* Up to 8 (500- to 600-mg) capsules daily. You may also choose to use raw or crystallized ginger or ginger ale that contains real ginger (not just the flavoring). Don't take ginger if you have gallbladder disease.

Peppermint, like other antispasmodic aromatic herbs, soothes the smooth muscle lining the GI tract and reduces nausea and vomiting. *Typical dose:* 10 to 20 drops of tincture either undiluted or in a small amount of water. Or 1 cup of tea, made by steeping 3 to 4 teaspoons of dried peppermint in 1½ to 3 cups of hot water for 15 minutes; strain and drink warm or cold. Note: Do not use undiluted essential peppermint oil because it may irritate. Use cautiously, if at all, during pregnancy and lactation. Do not use if you have GERD.

Lemon balm acts as an antispasmodic herb that calms nausea by relaxing the smooth muscle of the digestive tract. *Typical dose:* As a tea, made from 2 teaspoons of dried leaves in 1 cup of hot water, steeped for 10 minutes. Take up to 4 times daily.

Flatulence

Flatulence is excessive gas in the stomach or intestine. The production of gas is normal in digestion, but too much can be uncomfortable and embarrassing. If it builds up, it may cause bloating. Intestinal bacteria that ferment food in the colon produce gas. Some foods have a bad reputation for causing gas—cruciferous vegetables, beans, dairy products and some other high fiber foods. If you follow a healthy diet plan, you may notice a bit more gas, because complex carbohydrates, fruits and vegetables are more likely to produce gas. Herbal remedies can help relieve some of the physical (and other) discomforts caused by flatulence.

Helping Herbs

Peppermint can bring relief to a stressed stomach and naturally reduces gas. *Typical dose:* 10 to 20 drops of tincture either undiluted or in a small amount of water. Or 1 cup of tea, made by steeping 3 to 4 teaspoons of dried peppermint in 1½ to 3 cups of hot water for 15 minutes; strain and drink warm or cold. Note: Do not use undiluted essential peppermint oil, because it may irritate. Use cautiously, if at all, during pregnancy and lactation. Do not use if you have GERD.

Chamomile relaxes smooth muscles and eases GI complaints, such as gas and poor bile flow. *Typical dose:* 1 cup of tea, made from 2 teaspoons of dried flowers. Steep in 1 cup of hot water for 10 minutes. Take 1 cup every 2 hours or as needed.

Ginger is renowned for its ability to ease the discomfort of an upset stomach and excess gas. *Typical dose:* Up to 8 (500- to 600-mg) capsules daily. Or, use raw or crystallized ginger or ginger ale that contains real ginger (not just the flavoring). Don't take ginger if you have gallbladder disease.

Fennel is like many other aromatic herbs in that it relaxes the smooth muscle lining of the digestive tract. It also helps to relieve gas. *Typical dose:* Try a tea made with 2 to 3 teaspoons of crushed seeds steeped in 1 cup hot water for 10 to 15 minutes; strain and drink up to 3 cups daily. Or try chewing about 20 seeds, as needed.

Inflammatory Bowel Disease

Inflammatory bowel disease (IBD) includes several long-lasting problems that cause irritation and ulcers in the GI tract. The most common disorders are ulcerative colitis and Crohn's disease. Conventional treatment of IBD often includes the use of corticosteroids, especially during acute attacks. This treatment can result in additional stress to the body because corticosteroids can cause numerous side effects. These side effects including acne, weight gain and GI symptoms that may be difficult to distinguish from IBD.

The anxiety of IBD worsens the symptoms. Although the actual cause of IBD is unknown, food sensitivities may be associated with IBD in some people. Some people experience food sensitivities including intolerance to gluten, which is the protein found in wheat, oats and rye, and intolerance to milk. A physician should treat IBD, but some herbal remedies can be used with your therapy to help ease side effects. Make sure you talk with your physician about using these therapies.

Helping Herbs

Psyllium husks and seeds absorb water and swell in the intestines to many times their original size. It is very useful for adding bulk to the stools and stimulating the bowels. Its bulking ability helps to relieve the diarrhea that accompanies IBD. Because psyllium is a mucilage-containing herb, it has a soothing effect on the intestines, thus easing intestinal cramping. *Typical dose:* 2 to 3 teaspoons of husks or powdered seed stirred into 8 ounces of water daily. Take 30 to 60 minutes prior to or after taking any other drugs or eating; psyllium can decrease the absorbtion of drugs and nutrients. Drink the mixture immediately as it thickens. Drink plenty of water throughout the day. Do not use if you have a psyllium seed husk allergy.

Valerian may be a useful addition to other herbs and medications that relieve smooth muscle spasms. Valerian is a strong anti-anxiety herb that may help to relieve the stress that may contribute to IBD. *Typical dose:* For the best benefit, use a commercially prepared extract or tincture and follow label directions.

Irritable Bowel Syndrome

Unlike IBD, which presents with inflammation and ulceration in the GI tract, Irritable Bowel Syndrome (IBS) results from changes in muscle contractions in the GI tract. The symptoms of IBS come and go in cycles. Nerves that control the muscles in the GI tract are overactive, and the GI tract becomes sensitive to food, stool, gas and stress. IBS results in abdominal pain, bloating and constipation or diarrhea. It may also be called spastic colon or mucous colitis. Diet, stress, parasites and overuse of antibiotics may all contribute to IBS.

Helping Herbs

Peppermint soothes the smooth muscle lining the GI tract and allows gas trapped in the stomach to be expelled. Mint tea can have a calming effect, but for irritable bowel, the essential oil appears to work better. It seems to decrease the erratic contractions and spasms that are typical with the condition. *Typical dose:* Enteric-coated capsules containing 0.2 mL of peppermint oil, 2 or 3 times daily, as needed. Or 1 cup of tea made by steeping 3 to 4 teaspoons of dried peppermint in 1½ to 3 cups of hot water for 15 minutes; strain and drink warm or cold. Note: Do not use undiluted essential peppermint oil, because it may irritate the GI tract. Use cautiously, if at all, during pregnancy and lactation. Do not use peppermint internally if you have heartburn or esophageal reflux.

Psyllium husks and seeds absorb water and swell in the intestine to many times their original size. This bulking ability helps to relieve diarrhea that accompanies IBS. Because psyllium is a mucilage-containing herb, it has a soothing effect on the intestines, thus easing intestinal cramping. *Typical dose:* 2 to 3 teaspoons of husks or powdered seed stirred into 8 ounces of water daily. Take 30 to 60 minutes prior to or after taking any other drugs or eating; psyllium can decrease the absorbtion of drugs and nutrients. Drink the mixture immediately because it thickens quickly upon standing. Drink plenty of water throughout the day. Do not use if you have a psyllium seed husk allergy.

Chamomile relaxes and tones the nervous system, relaxes muscles and eases GI complaints, including spasms and excess gas. *Typical dose:* 1 cup of tea, made from 2 teaspoons of dried flowers, steeped in 1 cup of hot water for 10 minutes. Take 1 cup of tea 3 to 4 times daily between meals. Avoid chamomile if you are allergic to members of the Asteraceae/Compositae family, including marigolds, daisies and chrysanthemums.

Parasites

Parasites infect persons throughout the world and cause thousands of deaths each year. They are tiny microorganisms known as amoebas. The most well-known parasites in the United States cause giardiasis and amebiasis. Giardia is widespread in American wildlife and has been passed to humans. Effects of these parasites include diarrhea, gas and severe abdominal pain. While the standard treatment is drug therapy, it often has its own side effects. Some herbal therapies can get rid of parasites, but only when using large and sometimes toxic amounts. Use of herbs or medications should be done under medical supervision.

Helping Herbs

Goldenseal contains the substance berberine, which is thought to be beneficial for ridding the body of parasites. The dose required to get rid of intestinal parasites may be toxic for some people, so it is wise to discuss its use with your physician. The recommended dose is ⅓ to ½ ounce of dried herb divided into three doses and taken over a 24-hour period. Do not use goldenseal if you are pregnant or lactating. Do not use in young children.

Worms

Many people, physicians included, think that intestinal worms are a thing of the past in the United States. This is far from true. Young children from all social classes have been identified as having worms. The worms we are talking about here are intestinal parasites that occupy the intestinal tract and occasionally move into other parts of the body. These include fluke-worms, hookworms, pinworms, roundworms, tapeworms and whipworms.

Although there are herbal treatments for worms, diagnosis should be made by a physician and the treatment, including use of herbs, discussed with her or him. The following herbs may prove useful in helping to rid the body of worms and parasites.

Helping Herbs

Ginger is served in Japan with raw fish because it appears to be effective against parasites, including worms that may be in the fish. Two grams of fresh root, either powdered and taken in a small amount of water (1/4 to 1/2 cup) or as a fresh condiment with meals 1 to 2 times daily. Maximum dose per day is 4 grams.

Garlic may be effective against a number of parasites, including pinworms, roundworms and the amoeba giardia. Try one fresh garlic clove, raw, in salads or by itself, daily.

Cloves are believed to be effective for parasites and intestinal worms. Make a tea of 1 teaspoon powdered herb in 1 cup boiling water; steep for 10 to 20 minutes, strain if desired. Drink up to 3 cups daily.

Pumpkin seeds were used by Native Americans to eliminate both tapeworms and roundworms. *Typical dose:* 20 to 170 grams of ground, unpeeled seeds 3 times daily with milk and honey to sweeten the taste.

Constipation

Constipation is a condition in which the stool becomes hard and dry. A person who is constipated usually has fewer than three bowel movements in a week. If you experience constipation, the first thing you should change is your diet, because constipation is usually a result of not getting enough fiber and fluids. Some drugs can cause constipation and can also be a contributor to IBS and bowel obstruction.

Helping Herbs

Cascara sagrada is considered a safe, effective laxative. Cascara contains anthraquinones that stimulate the intestine and result in the urge to defecate. It is available in commercially prepared products that are effective and safe to use. Read the label directions carefully before using. Do not use if you have a history of intestinal obstruction, Crohn's disease, ulcerative colitus, ulcers or stomach pain of unknown origin. Stimulant laxitives should not be used long term, to avoid laxative dependence. Do not give to children under 2 years of age.

Common Causes of Constipation

- Not enough fiber in diet
- Not enough liquids
- Lack of exercise
- Changes in life or routine, such as travel
- Pregnancy
- Older age
- Ignoring the urge to have a bowel movement
- Problems with the colon and rectum
- Problems with intestinal function
- Irritable Bowl Syndrome
- Medications

Flax is beneficial for numerous conditions, including relief of constipation. Flax contains heart-healthy and bowel-friendly fibers called lignans. It is best to grind seeds right before using to make them easier for the body to use. The oil in flaxseeds is very unstable, so keep the seeds in the freezer or refrigerator to maintain maximum freshness. *Typical dose:* Grind 1 tablespoon of seeds and take in 1 cup of water, or sprinkle on your food up to 3 times daily. Drink adequate fluid throughout the day.

Psyllium husks and seeds are an excellent natural source of fiber. They absorb water and swell in the intestines to many times their original size. Psyllium's ability to form bulk helps to relieve constipation. Since psyllium is a mucilage-containing herb, it has a soothing effect on the intestines, thus easing intestinal cramping. *Typical dose:* 2 to 3 teaspoons of husks or powdered seed stirred into 8 ounces of water daily. Take 30 to 60 minutes prior to or after taking any other drugs or eating; psyllium can decrease the absorbtion of drugs and nutrients. Drink the mixture immediately because it thickens quickly upon standing. Drink plenty of water throughout the day. Do not use if you have a psyllium seed husk allergy.

Rhubarb is a powerful natural laxative that contains anthraquinones, which are compounds similar to those found in other laxative herbs. Rhubarb and other anthraquinone-containing herbs should be used only as a last resort to treat constipation. Rhubarb is not for long-term use. *Typical dose:* Try a decoction made by gently boiling ½ teaspoon of powdered root in 1 cup of water for 10 minutes; take 1 tablespoon at a time, up to 1 cup daily. Fresh stewed rhubarb may not be as effective, but it is worth a tasty try.

Diarrhea

The symptoms of diarrhea include frequent, loose and watery bowel movements. Common causes include gastrointestinal infections, irritable bowel syndrome, medicines, food-borne illness and malabsorption. Excess doses of vitamin C can also contribute to diarrhea. The main risk of diarrhea is dehydration, caused by a reduction in fluid intake along with an increase in the amount of fluid excreted in the stool.

Using herbs that contain bulk-forming agents, as well as soft-cooked fruits and vegetables, can help keep diarrhea at bay by absorbing excess fluid in the GI tract. If diarrhea lasts longer than a week or is persistent, if you have a fever, bad stomach cramps, blood, mucus or pus in your stools, seek immediate medical attention. Make sure you tell your physician what you are taking and if you have been out of the country or drank water from a stream, either of which may indicate parasites.

Helping Herbs

Bilberry or its family member, blueberry, may be an effective treatment for diarrhea. These berries contain tannins, which are binding, and pectins, which are mucilages that are fluid-absorbing. *Typical dose:* 2 to 3 capsules or tablets, standardized to 25 percent anthocyanosides, daily.

Peppermint has an antispasmodic action that relieves the intestinal cramping associated with diarrhea. *Typical dose:* Steep 1 to 2 teaspoons of dried peppermint in 1 cup of boiling water for 10 minutes. Drink up to 3 cups per day.

Psyllium husks and seeds are an excellent natural source of fiber. They absorb water and swell in the intestine to many times their original size. Psyllium's bulking ability helps to absorb excess fluid that contributes to diarrhea. Because psyllium is a mucilage-containing herb, it has a soothing effect on the intestines, thus easing intestinal cramping. *Typical dose:* 2 to 3 teaspoons of husks or powdered seed stirred into 8 ounces of water daily. Take 30 to 60 minutes before or after taking any other drugs or eating to prevent interference with absorbtion of other drugs or nutrients. Drink the mixture immediately because it thickens quickly upon standing. Drink plenty of water throughout the day. Do not use if you have a psyllium seed husk allergy.

Diverticulosis & Diverticulitis

Diverticulosis is a condition that happens when small pouches (diverticula) push outward through weak spots in the colon. Diverticulitis occurs when the diverticula become irritated or infected. In the past, the treatment was a diet that was low in fiber and limited fruits, vegetables and whole grains. What is now known is that the foods that were once avoided are those that should be included, along with regular exercise. Plenty of fluids should also be consumed to help move the fibers through your system. If you do not already have either condition, remember that the best treatment for both is prevention using the same recommendations—a high-fiber diet with plenty of fluid and exercise. Some herbal remedies may be helpful for prevention and treatment of diverticulosis and diverticulitis.

Helping Herbs

Flax contains heart-healthy and bowel-friendly fibers called lignans. These help decrease the amount of time that waste stays in the intestinal tract and reduce pressure that increases the potential for diverticula to develop. It is best to grind seeds right before using to make them easier for the body to use. The oil in flaxseeds is very unstable, so keep the seeds in the freezer or refrigerator to maintain maximum freshness. *Typical dose:* Grind 1 tablespoon of seeds and take in 1 cup of water, or sprinkle on your food up to 3 times daily. Keep well hydrated throughout the day.

Psyllium husks and seeds are an excellent natural source of fiber. They absorb water and swell in the intestine to many times their original size. Psyllium's bulking ability helps to relieve constipation. Constipation and the resulting straining to achieve a bowel movement may increase intestinal pressure, which is believed to contribute to the development of diverticula. *Typical dose:* 2 to 3 teaspoons of husks or powdered seed stirred into 8 ounces of water daily. Take 30 to 60 minutes before or after taking any other drugs or eating to avoid interference with absorbtion of other drugs or nutrients. May cause gas and bloating, so begin with a lower dose. Drink the mixture immediately because it thickens quickly upon standing. Drink plenty of water throughout the day. Do not use if you have a psyllium seed husk allergy.

Slippery elm may provide relief for diverticulitis by helping to calm the GI tract. The bark is quite fibrous and is the main source of a gentle laxative that keeps things moving while being soothing. *Typical dose:* 2 teaspoons inner bark in 2 cups of boiling water. Take up to 2 cups, up to 3 times daily.

Hemorrhoids

Hemorrhoids are swollen blood vessels (varicose veins) in and around the anus and lower rectum. Straining to have a bowel movement as a common result of constipation causes the veins to stretch and swell. They cause itching, pain and sometimes bleeding.

The causes of hemorrhoids include a genetic predisposition to them, sitting or standing for long periods of time and anything that increases pressure in the veins, such as pregnancy, heavy lifting and obesity.

Prevention, once again, is the best medicine. If you already have them, there are some herbs you might be able to use to ease the symptoms. As with other conditions, it is important to know that the diagnosis is correct before you take any medication.

Helping Herbs

Butcher's broom is believed to inhibit inflammation and constrict blood vessels. *Typical dose:* 2 to 3 cups of tea, made with 1 teaspoon dried herb steeped in 1 cup of water for 15 minutes, or 2 to 3 (200-mg) capsules with water, 2 to 3 times per day.

Comfrey contains a substance called allantoin, which speeds healing, and tannins that act as an astringent. Apply comfrey externally as a poultice by wrapping fresh leaves in a clean, wet cloth. Commercial preparations may also be purchased and used according to directions. Do not take comfrey internally.

Ginkgo is a blood vessel–strengthening and blood-thinning herb. Its anti-inflammatory properties help relieve the itching associated with hemorrhoids. *Typical dose:* 40 to 60 mg of capsules, standardized to 24 percent flavone glycosides and 6 percent ginkgolides, 2 to 3 times daily.

Horse chestnut has been shown to reduce hemorrhoids and the related pain and itching. *Typical dose:* 250 milligrams of commercial horse chestnut seed extract capsules standardized to 20 percent aescins, 3 times daily.

Horse chestnut and **witch hazel** combined as an astringent salve appear to have some promise. The witch hazel is an astringent, which tones the skin, and both contain powerful antioxidants. Look for salves with these herbs, combined with rosemary and sage, if available and if you like, in natural foods stores. Use as directed.

Plantain, with its allantoin and other healing properties, works well for soothing and reducing inflammation in hemorrhoids when the juice of the leaves is applied directly.

Psyllium helps to relieve constipation. Constipation and its associated straining to defecate may contribute to hemorrhoids. *Typical dose:* 2 to 3 teaspoons of psyllium seed husk or powdered psyllium in 8 ounces of water, 2 times daily. To relieve potential symptoms of gas and bloating, start with a small dose and make sure you drink plenty of water. Take 30 to 60 minutes before or after taking other drugs or eating to avoid interference with absorption of other drugs or nutrients.

Witch hazel has potent astringents in the form of tannins that are helpful in toning and relieving inflammation of hemorrhoids. Apply a commercially prepared solution, as directed, with a cotton ball.

Liver Disease

The liver is the body's largest internal organ. The liver has many important functions, including making bile, changing food into energy and cleaning alcohol and poisons from the blood. Many things affect how well the liver functions, including its exposure to toxins, pollutants and viruses.

Sometimes, subclinical conditions (conditions that are so mild they produce no symptoms) exist. We know that something is not right, but can't put our finger on it. These subclinical conditions may be a result of cholestasis, often referred to as sluggish liver. What this means is that the bile the liver produces is not efficiently digesting fats and detoxifying some potentially harmful substances. When this happens, we get bloated, constipated and fatigued, and we suffer from more allergies and PMS. To counteract this and to help keep our liver healthy, we can use some herbal remedies. These remedies may play a role in protecting the liver from toxins, or to help heal a liver that has been exposed to hepatitis or cirrhosis.

Helping Herbs

Before treating any liver condition with herbs, discuss plans with your healthcare provider.

Chicory may help protect the liver by providing the antioxidant beta-carotene which neutralizes free radicals and by stimulating bile production. Chicory roots have long been used as a coffee substitute when dried, roasted and ground. Purchase chicory already roasted or purchase standardized root extracts and use according to label directions. *Typical dose:* One cup of tea prepared by steeping 1 to 2 teaspoons of root in 3/4 cup of boiling water for 10 minutes. Strain and have 2 3/4 cups of tea per day.

Dandelion root has been used as a liver tonic for thousands of years. It is a diuretic that helps flush excess fluid from the body. It enhances the production of bile and improves gallbladder function. The leaves may be used as a vegetable in the spring when they are fresh and tender. *Typical dose:* 2 to 4 teaspoons of dried leaf in 3/4 cup boiling water, steeped for 10 minutes, strained or 1 to 3 teaspoons of powdered root in 3/4 cup boiling water, steeped for 10 minutes, strained. Take up to 3 3/4 cups daily.

Licorice may inhibit damage to the liver with the antioxidant compound glycyrrhetic acid. Licorice's antiviral properties may be especially beneficial in treating liver disease if the cause is viral hepatitis. *Typical dose:* 1/8 to 1 teaspoon of tincture, up to 3 times daily; or make a tea with 1 heaping teaspoon of chopped, dried licorice root steeped in 1 cup of water for 15 minutes, strain and drink up to 3 cups daily. Do not use longer than 6 weeks. Do not use if you have heart disease or high blood pressure, or if you are pregnant or taking drugs containing digitalis.

Milk thistle is a detoxifying herb that neutralizes free radicals that attack the liver. It protects the liver cells from inflammatory compounds that are responsible for some types of liver damage. Milk thistle actually alters liver cell membranes and makes it hard for the toxins to invade them. *Typical dose:* 140 mg of standardized silymarin capsules, 3 times daily; after 6 weeks, decrease to 90 mg, 3 times daily.

Respiratory Tract

The respiratory tract is made up of organs and structures that enable us to take in oxygen and expel carbon dioxide—in other words, breathe. The oxygen is exchanged between the lungs and the circulating blood and is carried to all parts of the body. It also warms the air passing into the body and assists in speech by providing air for the larynx and vocal cords.

Getting a cold or the flu seems to upset everything because it interferes with our breathing, talking and overall well-being. Respiratory allergies and asthma have much the same effect, but they are more functional rather than being caused by a "bug" we got from someone.

No matter what causes our respiratory distress, the preparations we use to soothe the symptoms often have herbal ingredients. Many of these ingredients are available to us in our home garden or a natural foods store.

Asthma

Asthma is a chronic lung disease that does not go away. It causes breathing problems, including tightness in the chest, shortness of breath and a wheezing sound when breathing. When these symptoms happen, it is usually called an asthma attack.

Usually, symptoms are started or "triggered" by something that irritates your lungs. There are many kinds of triggers, ranging from viruses (such as colds) and allergies, to gases and particles in the air. Unfortunately, many people suffering from asthma may be sensitive to herbal preparations. Flowers and plants often trigger an attack. It is very important to know if these may be triggers before you try any herbal preparations for asthma.

Helping Herbs

Coffee is a bronchial dilator, meaning it opens up the bronchial tubes that lead to the lungs, which improves breathing. The drug caffeine that is in coffee is a chemical cousin to the drug used to treat asthma—theophylline. If you have an asthma attack and have nothing to treat it, try a strong cup of caffeinated coffee and seek immediate medical attention if symptoms worsen.

Ephedra is effective for short-term treatment of diseases of the respiratory tract, including asthma, bronchitis and bronchospasms. However, doses for these ailments often exceed the safe limit. The active ingredient, ephedrine, helps relieve coughs, may control the reproduction of bacteria and is anti-inflammatory. *Typical dose:* 15 to 30 mg of the total alkaloids calculated as ephedrine. Maximum dose, according to some sources, is 300 mg per day. The general consensus at this writing is that the maximum safe dose is not more than 8 mg every 6 hours, not to exceed 24 mg daily. To ensure standard doses, a purchased product is recommended. Do not use if you have heart disease, an eating disorder, BPH (Benign Prostatic Hypeaplasia), diabetes, thyroid conditions, high blood pressure, kidney stones or urinary retention, or if you are pregnant or lactating.

Licorice has been prescribed for hundreds of years for the relief of asthma. The herb acts as an expectorant, mucus inhibitor and immune-stimulator, and has anti-inflammatory and antiviral properties. *Typical dose:* 1/8 to 1 teaspoon of tincture, up to 3 times daily; or make a tea with 1 heaping teaspoon of chopped, dried licorice root steeped in 1 cup of water for 15 minutes, strain and drink up to 3 cups daily. Do not use longer than 6 weeks. Do not use if you have heart disease or high blood pressure, or if you are pregnant or taking drugs containing digitalis.

Mullein may help fight some of the viruses that a person with asthma may suffer from. Mullein is endorsed by the German Commission E for its expectorant, antispasmodic and anti-inflammatory properties. It is especially helpful if your cough is wet. It will also ease the pain of dry coughs. *Typical dose:* Make a tea with 2 teaspoons of dried flowers and 1 cup of hot water, steeped for 15 minutes and then strained. Take up to 6 cups per day.

Rosemary has been used as a traditional treatment for asthma. Its volatile oils may block the airway constriction that occurs in asthma and may accompany allergies. It is effective as an inhalant by adding 1/4 cup of the needles to 4 cups of hot water for 10 minutes and inhaling the steam. This concoction may also be used as a tea; drink up to 1 cup, 3 times daily. Do not ingest the volatile oil.

Turmeric's active ingredient, curcumin, has been shown to decrease the incidence of cell mutations in smokers. It is an anti-inflammatory herb that has several benefits for cardiovascular and overall health. *Typical dose:* 1 (450-mg) capsule, 3 times daily. Do not take if you are pregnant or lactating, or if you have gallbladder disease or gallstones.

Bronchitis

Bronchitis is an inflammation of the lining of the bronchial tubes (bronchi). These tubes connect the windpipe to the lungs. When the bronchi are inflamed and/or infected, it is more difficult for air to flow to and from the lungs, and a heavy mucus or phlegm is coughed up. Many people suffer a brief attack of acute bronchitis with cough and mucus production when they have severe colds. Sometimes, bronchitis is triggered by cigarette smoke or environmental pollutants.

Chronic bronchitis is defined by the presence of a mucus-producing cough most days of the month, 3 months out of the year, for 2 successive years without other underlying disease to explain the cough. The best treatment for chronic bronchitis is to quit smoking and avoid cigarette smoke and air pollution. As with asthma, some people with bronchitis may be sensitive to herbal preparations, so it is best to know if this is the case for you.

Helping Herbs

Eucalyptus oil from the leaves is an excellent expectorant and has benefits when applied externally or taken internally. Many commercial products are available for topical use that help loosen phlegm when the vapors are inhaled. There may be the possibility that a small amount taken internally may work because the volatile oil is excreted by the lungs. *Typical dose:* For commercially prepared products, read the label instructions; for a tea, steep 1 to 2 teaspoons of dried crushed leaves in 1 cup of boiling water for 10 minutes and drink 2 cups daily. Do not give the tea to children under age 2. Do not take the essential oil internally.

Echinacea is a natural when you think about diseases of the respiratory tract. It stimulates white blood cell activity, increases the body's own production of antiviral substances and enhances immunity. It may be effective against many of the viruses that cause bronchitis. *Typical dose:* Up to 9 (300- to 400-mg) capsules, taken in divided doses, daily. Echinacea is contraindicated in AIDS and other autoimmune diseases and in those allergic to members of the Asteraceae/ Compositae family, including marigolds and chrysanthemums.

Horehound has been used to relieve the symptoms of bronchitis and other respiratory infections for years. It is used in many cough and cold preparations. It can be effective as an expectorant and to soothe a sore throat. Try a prepared product if you are in a pinch, but make sure you read the label directions. *Typical dose:* Make a tea by steeping 2 teaspoons of dried leaves in 1 cup of hot water for 10 minutes. Strain. Take up to 3 cups daily.

Hyssop is a member of the mint family, so you might naturally think of it for relieving symptoms of bronchitis. It has several soothing ingredients and an expectorant. *Typical dose:* Steep 2 teaspoons of herb in 1 cup of boiling water for 10 minutes and strain. Drink up to 3 cups daily. Improve the flavor with a bit of honey.

Mullein is endorsed by the German Commission E for its expectorant properties. It is especially helpful if your cough is wet. *Typical dose:* Make a tea with 2 teaspoons of dried flowers to 1 cup of hot water, steeped for 15 minutes; strain. Take up to 6 cups per day; or try 25 to 40 drops of tincture every 3 hours.

Marsh mallow mucilage is the fiber that becomes gelatinous when soaked in water. It soothes the mucous membranes and protects them from bacteria and inflammation, and mildly stimulates the immune system while suppressing coughs. *Typical dose:* Take up to 6 (400- to 500-mg) capsules per day; or make a tea of 1 teaspoon dried root steeped in 1 cup of hot water for 10 minutes. Drink up to 3 cups per day.

Peppermint soothes coughs and sore throats. The menthol in peppermint is antibacterial and antiviral. It relaxes the airways, allowing for easier breathing. *Typical dose:* As a tea, made with 2 teaspoons of dried herb steeped in 1 cup hot, not boiling, water. Take as needed. Drink up to 3 cups per day.

Emphysema

When the elasticity of the fibers in the lungs that allow them to expand and contract is lost, a person develops emphysema. Emphysema comes on very gradually. Years of exposure to the irritation of cigarette smoke usually precede the development of emphysema. Some persons do develop emphysema from working in a lung-irritating environment, but 80 to 90 percent of the cases are related to smoking. Some persons may have had chronic bronchitis before developing emphysema.

Helping Herbs

Basil does contain expectorants that can be helpful in reducing phlegm production. It is also rich in antioxidants that are helpful for scavenging free radicals that may cause additional damage if left unchecked. For a hefty dose of basil, you might want to try pesto, which is also full of healthy olive oil (and calories). Persons with emphysema who are overweight may choose to limit pesto because of its high calorie value. Those persons who are underweight may benefit from the extra calories.

Eucalyptus oil from the leaves is an excellent expectorant and has benefits when applied externally or taken internally. Many commercial products are available for topical use that help loosen phlegm when the vapors are inhaled. There may be the possibility that a small amount taken internally may work because the volatile oil is being excreted by the lungs. *Typical dose:* For commercially prepared products, read the label instructions; for a tea, steep 1 to 2 teaspoons of dried crushed leaves in 1 cup of boiling water for 10 minutes and drink 2 cups daily. Do not give the tea to children under age 2. Do not take the essential oil internally.

Licorice is estimated to have nine compounds that act as an expectorant. These compounds may help relieve the excess secretions that are so common in the disease and help clear the airways. *Typical dose:* 1/8 to 1 teaspoon of tincture, up to 3 times daily; or make a tea with 1 heaping teaspoon of chopped, dried licorice root steeped in 1 cup of water for 15 minutes, strain and drink up to 3 cups daily. Do not use longer than 6 weeks. Do not use if you have heart disease or high blood pressure, or if you are pregnant or taking drugs containing digitalis.

Mullein is rich in mucilage, which has a soothing property that may be helpful in treating emphysema. *Typical dose:* Make a tea with 2 teaspoons of dried flowers in 1 cup of hot water, steeped for 15 minutes and then strained; take up to 6 cups per day.

Peppermint relaxes the airways, allowing for easier breathing. *Typical dose:* Make a tea with 2 teaspoons of dried herb steeped in 1 cup hot, but not boiling, water and take as needed, up to 3 cups per day.

Common Cold & Flu

Colds are minor infections of the nose and throat caused by several different viruses. Colds are highly contagious.

One to three days after a cold virus enters the body, symptoms begin, including:

- runny nose
- congestion
- sneezing
- weakened senses of taste and smell
- scratchy throat
- cough

Infants and young children are more likely than adults and teens to develop a fever. Smokers usually have more severe symptoms than nonsmokers.

The flu, on the other hand, is an infection of the respiratory system caused by the influenza virus. There are three types of influenza virus: A, B and C. Types A and B are the most severe. The viruses change constantly, and varying strains circulate around the world each year. It's impossible for the body's natural defenses to keep up with these changes. Type C causes either a very mild illness, or has no symptoms at all.

Flu symptoms are more severe than those of colds. They come on suddenly and include high fever, cough and body and muscle aches. Care must be taken with young children and the elderly to make sure that complications do not occur. Most people recover from the flu within 1 or 2 weeks, but others, especially those with other illnesses and the elderly, may feel weak long after most symptoms have gone away.
Herbal medications can minimize discomfort associated with flu symptoms.

Helping Herbs

Astragalus has long been known in Traditional Chinese Medicine for its immune-boosting and antiviral properties. Astragalus differs from echinacea in that it may be taken long term without depressing the immune system. It has long been used as a preventive for the common cold. It is helpful for building resistance to infection. *Typical dose:* up to 8 to 14 (400- to 500-mg) capsules of astragalus powder daily; or try 15 to 30 drops of a tincture daily.

Echinacea is effective for giving the immune system a boost. Use it for 2 weeks, then skip a week. Repeat the cycle using teas, tinctures or capsules. Avoid echinacea if you have an auto-immune disorder or are allergic to members of the Asteraceae/Compositae family, including daisies, marigolds and chrysanthemums.

Ephedra is effective for short-term treatment of diseases of the respiratory tract, including asthma, bronchitis and bronchospasms. However, doses for these ailments often exceed the safe limit. The active ingredient, ephedrine, helps relieve coughs, may control the reproduction of bacteria and is anti-inflammatory. *Typical dose:* 15 to 30 mg of the total alkaloids calculated as ephedrine. Maximum dose, according to some sources, is 300 mg per day. The general consensus at this writing is that the maximum safe dose is not more than 8 mg every 6 hours, not to exceed 24 mg daily. To ensure standard doses, a purchased product is recommended. Do not use if you have heart disease, an eating disorder, BPH (Benign Prostatic Hyperplasia), diabetes, thyroid conditions, high blood pressure, kidney stones or urinary retention, or if you are pregnant or lactating.

Ginger is well known for its ability to ease the discomfort of nausea that may accompany the flu. It has been used for thousands of years to relieve seasickness and morning sickness. It is an antispasmodic, meaning it is effective against spasms of the smooth muscle of the GI tract. It can be especially helpful for flu-like symptoms. Use whatever remedy sounds good. *Typical dose:* Up to 8 (500- to 600-mg) capsules daily. You may also choose to use raw or crystallized ginger or ginger ale that contains real ginger (not just the flavoring). A tea made with 1 to 2 teaspoons of fresh grated root, steeped in 1 cup of boiling water for 5 to 10 minutes, may be soothing and warming if you have the chills. Don't take ginger if you have gallbladder disease. If you are pregnant, contact your healthcare provider prior to taking ginger.

Goldenseal's active constituent berberine makes it an antiseptic and immune-stimulating herb. Although there is no reliable research that proves the effectiveness of goldenseal against the viruses that cause the common cold and flu, many people swear by it and take it the minute symptoms appear. *Typical dose:* Make a tea using ½ to 1 teaspoon of powdered root in 1 cup of boiling water; steep for 10 minutes and drink up to 2 cups daily. Commercial preparations are also available; follow label directions if you choose to use them.

Lemon balm acts as a digestive aid by relaxing the smooth muscle of the digestive tract. This can help relieve the nausea associated with the flu. *Typical dose:* Make a tea from 2 teaspoons of dried leaves in 1 cup of hot water; steep for 10 minutes. Take up to 4 times daily.

Licorice has been prescribed for hundreds of years for the relief of flu and flu-like symptoms. The herb acts as an expectorant, mucus inhibitor and immune stimulator, and has anti-inflammatory and antiviral properties. *Typical dose:* ⅛ to 1 teaspoon of tincture, up to 3 times daily; or make a tea with 1 heaping teaspoon of chopped, dried licorice root steeped in 1 cup of water for 15 minutes. Strain and drink up to 3 cups daily. Do not use longer than 6 weeks. Do not use if you have heart disease or high blood pressure, or if you are pregnant or taking drugs containing digitalis.

Marsh mallow mucilage is the fiber that becomes gelatinous when soaked in water, soothes the mucous membranes and protects them from bacteria and inflammation. It mildly stimulates the immune system while suppressing coughs in the flu. *Typical dose:* Up to 6 (400- to 500-mg) capsules per day; or make a tea of 1 teaspoon dried root steeped in 1 cup of hot water for 10 minutes.

Mullein appears to have expectorant, antispasmodic and anti-inflammatory properties that help relieve some of the coughing and excess mucus produced when you have the flu. Mullein is especially helpful if you have a wet cough, but it will ease the pain of a dry cough. *Typical dose:* Make a tea with 2 teaspoons of dried flowers in 1 cup of hot water steeped for 15 minutes. Strain and drink up to 6 cups per day.

Slippery elm, when taken as a tea or decoction, soothes the throat and digestive tract, relieving some annoying symptoms of the flu. *Typical dose:* Make a decoction blending 3 teaspoons of powdered herb in 1 cup of water; bring it to a boil and simmer for 15 minutes. Drink up to 3 cups per day.

Willow, with its active compound salicin, may be effective in relieving the aches, pains and fever of a cold or flu. *Typical dose:* Prepare a decoction with 1 teaspoon powdered bark soaked in 1 cup cold water for 8 hours, then strained. Drink up to 3 cups daily. Do not give to children under 16 with fevers related to colds, flu or the chicken pox. Do not take willow if you have GI upset including ulcers, nausea, vomiting or diarrhea. Do not take if you are pregnant or lactating. Use caution if you are taking other blood-thinning herbs or drugs.

Cough

A cough is your body's way of telling you that something is not quite right. A cold may be on the way, an allergen is in the air or it may be something more serious. Coughs are either non-productive (dry, hacking cough) or productive (mucus-producing). If herbal remedies don't take care of the symptoms, see your healthcare provider.

Helping Herbs

Hyssop is a member of the mint family, so you might naturally think of it for relieving a cough or cold. It has several soothing ingredients and an expectorant. *Typical dose:* Steep 2 teaspoons of herb in 1 cup of boiling water for 10 minutes and strain. Drink up to 3 cups daily. Improve the flavor with a bit of honey.

Mints act as a decongestant and are effective as a cough suppressant. The active ingredient, menthol, is popular in many commercially prepared cough drops. *Typical dose:* Steep 1 to 2 teaspoons of dried peppermint in 1 cup of boiling water for 10 minutes. Drink up to 3 cups per day.

Mullein's mucilage becomes a slippery gel when it absorbs water. This is what makes it soothing on the throat and the skin. *Typical dose:* Make a tea by steeping 1 to 2 teaspoons of dried flowers and leaves in 1 cup of boiling water for 10 minutes. Strain. Drink up to 3 cups daily.

Slippery elm is an ingredient in popular lozenges sold commercially for coughs and colds. Try it the next time you feel the tickle of a cough coming on. When taken as a tea or decoction, slippery elm soothes the throat and digestive tract. *Typical dose:* Make a decoction blending 3 teaspoons of powdered herb in 1 cup of water; bring it to a boil and then simmer for 15 minutes. Drink up to 3 cups per day. Commercial lozenges provide sustained release of mucilage to the throat and may be preferred to the powdered herb for coughs and sore throats.

Sore Throat

A sore throat is one of the first signs of a cold or the flu. Other environmental exposures, including chemical irritants, mouth-breathing while sleeping, shouting your favorite team on to victory or speaking to a large group without a microphone, can cause a sore throat. Before choosing an herbal remedy, evaluate a sore throat to determine if the origin is streptococcal bacteria or a virus. Untreated strep is the kind of bacteria that can cause heart damage.

Helping Herbs

Echinacea, with its immune-boosting properties, may kill some of the bacteria that cause upper respiratory tract infections. It may help numb an inflamed throat, but may also irritate it, depending on your symptoms. Take it as a tea so it can soothe the throat at the same time it is fighting off the bugs. Or, if you are looking for something a bit stronger, try the tincture. *Typical dose:* 50 to 60 drops of tincture every 2 hours during waking hours the first 2 days you are sick. Stop taking the tincture when your symptoms are gone. Use caution if you are allergic to members of the Asteraceae/Compositae family, including marigold, daisies and ragweed.

Eucalyptus is an ingredient found in many commercial mouthwashes that may be used as a gargle. You can make your own gargle by steeping 3 ounces dried, or 6 ounces fresh, eucalyptus in 2 cups of vodka. Steep for several weeks. Strain if desired. Use as you would any purchased mouthwash. You may combine several breath-freshening herbs in this concoction if you like. This keeps well when stored in a dark glass container so you can make it in the fall to have on hand the next time you get a cold.

Horehound is used in many cough and cold preparations. It can be effective as an expectorant and to soothe a sore throat. Try a prepared product if you are in a pinch, but make sure you read the label directions. *Typical dose:* Make a tea by steeping 2 teaspoons of dried leaves in 1 cup of hot water for 10 minutes. Strain. Take up to 3 cups daily.

Lemon balm has antiviral activity that treats a variety of viruses and bacteria, including streptococcus. *Typical dose*: As a tea, made from 2 teaspoons of dried leaves in 1 cup of hot water, steeped for 10 minutes and taken up to 4 times daily.

Marsh mallow is good for just about any respiratory condition. It mildly stimulates the immune system while suppressing coughs. *Typical dose:* Up to 6 (400- to 500-mg) capsules per day; or make a tea of 1 teaspoon dried root steeped in 1 cup of hot water for 10 minutes. Take up to 3 cups per day.

Mullein is endorsed by the German Commission E for its expectorant properties. It is especially helpful if your cough is wet or productive. It will also ease the pain of dry coughs. *Typical dose:* Make a tea with 2 teaspoons of dried flowers and 1 cup of hot water, steeped for 15 minutes and then strained; take up to 6 cups per day.

Slippery elm is an ingredient in popular lozenges sold commercially for coughs and colds. When taken as a tea or decoction, slippery elm soothes the throat and digestive tract. *Typical dose:* Make a decoction blending 3 teaspoons of powdered herb and 1 cup of water; bring to a boil, then simmer for 15 minutes. Drink up to 3 cups per day.

Tonsillitis

Tonsils, once thought a nuisance, are now considered important for fighting off infections. Inflammation of the tonsils, or tonsillitis, is most common in children under 9 years of age. Tonsillitis in adults is infrequent but does occur. Tonsillitis should be evaluated to determine if the origin is streptococcal bacteria or a virus. Untreated strep is the kind of bacteria that can cause heart damage.

Helping Herbs

Echinacea, with its immune-boosting properties, may help fight tonsillitis. It is best taken as a tea so it can soothe the throat at the same time it fights off the bugs. Do not use if you have an autoimmune disorder or are allergic to members of the Asteraceae/Compositae family.

Goldenseal may be useful in treating tonsillitis. The constituent berberine is thought to be responsible for its antiseptic and anti-inflammatory properties. *Typical dose:* Make a tea with ½ to 1 teaspoon of goldenseal root in 1 cup of boiling water and steep for 10 minutes. Because it is bitter, you may want to add a bit of honey. You might also try combining echinacea with goldenseal for more fighting power.

Gargling with **sage** is commonly prescribed for tonsillitis in Germany. The tannins in sage appear to have a soothing and astringent property. It also is antimicrobial. *Typical dose:* Add 2 teaspoons of dried sage to 1 cup of boiling water and steep 10 minutes. Use when barely warm as a gargle.

Laryngitis

When the mucous membranes lining the larynx become inflamed, the result is hoarseness or loss of voice, or laryngitis. Laryngitis may be caused by a cold, irritating fumes, talking more than usual, smoking or an allergic reaction. If your laryngitis is chronic, it may be a sign of a more serious disorder that requires medical attention.

Helping Herbs

Echinacea is useful for treating laryngitis. It may help numb an inflamed throat, but may also irritate it, depending on your symptoms. Take it as a tea so it can soothe the throat at the same time it fights off the bugs. Or, if you are looking for something a bit stronger, try the tincture. *Typical dose:* 50 to 60 drops of tincture every 2 hours during waking hours the first 2 days you are sick. Stop taking the tincture when your symptoms are gone. Use caution if you are allergic to members of the Asteraceae/Compositae family, such as daisies and marigolds.

Horehound is useful for treating laryngitis. Try a prepared product if you are in a pinch, but make sure you read the label directions. *Typical dose:* Make a tea by steeping 2 teaspoons of dried leaves in 1 cup of hot water for 10 minutes. Strain. Take up to 3 cups daily.

Marsh mallow mucilage, the fibers that becomes gelatinous when soaked in water, soothes the mucous membranes and protects them from bacteria and inflammation. *Typical dose:* Up to 6 (400- to 500-mg) capsules per day; or make a tea of 1 teaspoon dried root steeped in 1 cup of hot water for 10 minutes. Take up to 3 cups per day.

Mullein has constituents that can help relieve the symptoms of laryngitis. *Typical dose:* Steep 2 teaspoons of flowers in 1 cup of boiling water for 10 minutes. Drink 2 to 3 cups per day.

Earache

An earache may be a sign of an infection, which is most likely in children, of excess earwax, perforated eardrum or swollen lymph nodes in the neck because of a cold.

First relieve the pain of your earache, then determine the cause. This is important because some infections can cause dramatic reactions, severe dizziness, nausea, vomiting and vision problems. Herbal remedies may help treat the pain.

Helping Herbs

Astragalus can be taken long term for prevention of ear infections if you are susceptible to them. Children over age 2 may use astragalus safely, but you should check with your physician before your child takes it. *Typical dose:* 8 or 9 (400- to 500-mg) capsules daily for adults; 15 to 30 drops of tincture in a small amount of water daily for young children. Begin with the low dose for children and adjust as needed.

Echinacea is a natural immune-booster. It stimulates white blood cell activity, increases the body's own production of antiviral substances and enhances immunity. It may be effective against many of the viruses that cause bronchitis. *Typical dose:* Up to 9 (300- to 400-mg) capsules, taken in divided doses daily. Echinacea is contraindicated in AIDS and other autoimmune diseases. Persons with allergies to members of the Asteraceae/Compositae family, including daisies and marigolds, should not use echinacea.

Garlic has been used to treat earaches throughout history. Its antibacterial, antifungal and antiviral properties are believed to be the reason for its effectiveness for earaches and many conditions. Because raw garlic may leave you with strong breath and body odor, you may want to try a commercially prepared product. Long-term garlic use bestows the most health benefits. *Typical dose:* 600 to 900 mg of garlic powder, tablets or capsules daily; 4 mL of aged garlic extract; 10 mg of garlic oil "perles" daily; or 1 or more medium-size fresh cloves daily.

Native Americans have used **goldenseal** drops for several centuries to treat ear infections. Try a commercially prepared product and follow label directions if you would like to try this remedy.

Sinus Infections

A sinus infection, often referred to as sinusitis, is inflammation and infection of the air-filled bony cavities surrounding the passages to the nose. With swelling, the openings from the sinuses to the nose may be obstructed, resulting in an accumulation of secretions that cause pain, pressure, headache, local tenderness and fever. Sinusitis may be a complication of an upper respiratory tract infection, dental infection, allergy, change in atmospheric pressure or a defect in the nose itself.

Some people with chronic sinusitis can be debilitated for weeks or months at a time. The cure can often be worse than the disease if you are taking multiple courses of antibiotics that further depress the immune system.

Helping Herbs

Astragalus is an immune stimulant and may help keep the system at its fighting best. *Typical dose:* up to 8 to 14 (400- to 500-mg) capsules of dried powder daily.

Echinacea should come to mind when you think about sinusitis. It stimulates white blood cell activity, increases the body's own production of antiviral substances and enhances immunity. It may be effective against many of the viruses that cause sinusitis. Take it every 1 to 2 hours at the first sign of symptoms, because your immune system has already been confronted with a cold or allergy that caused it. *Typical dose:* Up to 9 (300- to 400-mg) capsules, taken in divided doses daily. Echinacea is contraindicated in AIDS and other autoimmune diseases. Persons with allergies to members of the Asteraceae/Compositae family, including daisies, chrysanthemums and marigolds, should not use echinacea.

Eucalyptus oil rubbed on the forehead and temples is a traditional treatment aromatherapists use for sinusitis. It is possible that a small amount taken internally may work by excreting the volatile oil from the lungs and by clearing the sinus and nasal cavity. *Typical dose:* Mix a drop or two of essential oil in 1 teaspoon olive oil before applying a few drops to your forehead and temples. For commercially prepared products, read the label instructions. For a tea, steep 1 to 2 teaspoons of dried crushed leaves in 1 cup of boiling water for 10 minutes; drink 2 cups daily. Do not give tea to children under age 2. Do not take the essential oil internally.

Feverfew may help ease the pain from headaches associated with sinus infections. *Typical dose:* Up to 3 (300- to 400-mg) capsules, daily, or 2 fresh leaves chewed, daily. If you are purchasing feverfew, look for whole leaf feverfew standardized to 0.6 to 0.7 percent parthenolind, feverfew's active compound. Caution: Fresh feverfew leaves may cause mouth ulcers in some persons. Do not use feverfew if you are allergic to members of the Asteraceae/ Compositae family.

Garlic has been used to treat respiratory problems throughout history. Its antibacterial, antifungal and antiviral properties are believed to be the reason for its effectiveness for many conditions. Long-term garlic use bestows the most health benefits. *Typical dose:* 600 to 900 mg of garlic tablets or capsules daily; 4 mL of aged garlic extract; 10 mg of garlic oil "perles" daily; or 1 or more medium-size fresh cloves daily.

Goldenseal's active constituent, berberine, makes it an antiseptic, antiviral, and immune-stimulating herb. Although there is no reliable research that proves the effectiveness of goldenseal against the viruses that cause the flu, many people swear by it and take it the minute symptoms appear. *Typical dose:* Make a tea using ½ to 1 teaspoon of powdered root in 1 cup of boiling water; steep for 10 minutes and drink up to 2 cups per day. Commercial preparations are also available; follow label directions.

Tinnitus

Tinnitis is a subjective noise sensation in the ear. It is often described as "ringing" and may be heard in one or both ears. Unless it is caused by trauma or disease, the cause of tinnitus is usually unknown.

Helping Herbs

Gingko is believed to be effective in some persons for the relief of tinnitis as one of the common symptoms of aging. *Typical dose:* 60 to 80 mg of a purchased extract standardized to 24 percent gingko flavone glycosides and 6 percent terpene lactones, 3 times daily.

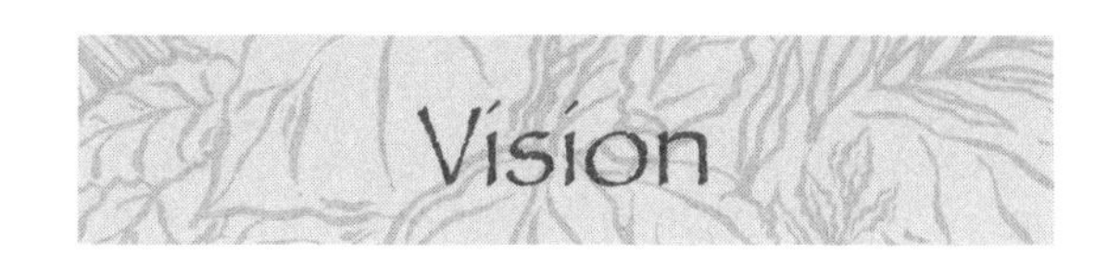

Vision is the capacity for sight. It brings the world closer by allowing us to see what is in our environment. Unfortunately, many people live with impaired vision. They either have difficulty seeing objects clearly or are unable to see at all.

Much of our ability to see is inherited. Whether and when we need glasses is often determined by our genes. Some eye diseases may also be hereditary. However, some diseases, such as macular degeneration and cataracts, may be prevented—or their symptoms lessened—by eating a diet rich in antioxidants. Herbs cannot cure vision problems once they have developed, but they may help reduce their severity and progression.

Age-Related Macular Degeneration

Age-related macular degeneration (AMD) is a degenerative disease that affects the macula, a small spot in the central area of the retina located at the back of the eye. The macula is responsible for sight in the center of the field of vision and is the most sensitive part of the retina.

As AMD progresses, symptoms will become more obvious. If you have AMD, you may notice that:

- straight lines in your field of vision, such as telephone poles or the sides of buildings, appear wavy.
- words in books, magazines and newspapers appear blurry.
- dark or empty spaces may block the center of your vision.

Age-related macular degeneration is the leading cause of visual impairment for persons age 75 and older. It is the most common cause of new cases of visual impairment among those over age 65.

AMD may be genetic or it may be associated with arteriosclerosis, eye trauma or other conditions that are not yet clearly understood. Recent speculation is that AMD may be preventable, or at least the symptoms lessened by a diet that is high in antioxidant vitamins and minerals.

Helping Herbs

Bilberry's antioxidant properties have a powerful effect on the health of the eyes. *Typical dose:* 3 (80- to 160-mg) extract capsules daily, in divided doses (total 240 to 480 mg).

Ginkgo contains antioxidants that may improve vision in some individuals with AMD. *Typical dose:* Take 3 (60-mg) capsules of extract, standardized to 24 percent gingko flavone glycosides and 6 percent ginkgolides, daily.

Cataracts

Cataracts were once thought of as an eye disease of old age. The lens becomes opaque and vision becomes impaired. If left untreated, a person will eventually go blind. Smokers face a greater risk of developing cataracts, as do those with diabetes, people who have been poisoned by heavy metals or those who have used steroids for a long time.

Cataracts happen because of oxidation within the cells of the eye. This results in the loss of transparency. It is believed that this process can be prevented with a diet rich in antioxidant fruits, vegetables and herbs.

Helping Herbs

Bilberry contains anthocyanosides that are believed to have a powerful effect on the eyes, possibly due to their capillary-strengthening properties. It has been used to stop the progression of early-stage cataracts when given in combination with vitamin E. Typical dose: 240 to 480 mg daily, divided into 2 or 3 doses of 80 to 160 mg capsules.

Rosemary is a multipurpose herb that is soothing but stimulating. Its powerful antioxidants may be helpful in reducing the risk of cataracts. *Typical dose:* As a tea, made by steeping 1 teaspoon of dried leaves in 1 cup of hot water for 15 minutes. Take up to 3 cups daily.

Turmeric's active ingredient, curcumin, is an antioxidant and anti-inflammatory herb that has several benefits for overall health. Turmeric may prevent the oxidative damage to the eye that occurs with cataracts. *Typical dose:* 1 (450-mg) capsule, 3 times daily; or make a tea with 1 teaspoon of turmeric powder in 1 cup of warm water and drink 3 times daily. Do not take if you are pregnant or lactating, or if you have gallbladder disease or gallstones.

Glaucoma

Glaucoma is a leading cause of blindness in the United States. Glaucoma is a group of diseases usually associated with increased pressure in the eye. This pressure causes damage to the cells that form the optic nerve, which is responsible for transmitting visual information from the eye to the brain. The damage is progressive with loss of peripheral vision first, followed by a decrease in central vision and, potentially, blindness. When diagnosed and treated, it can be easily controlled. It must be medically treated and controlled, but some herbs may help relieve some of the symptoms and possibly provide some treatment.

Helping Herbs

Bilberry contains anthocyanosides that are believed to have a powerful effect on the eyes, possibly because of its capillary-strengthening properties. Anthocyanosides prevent the breakdown of vitamin C, which is helpful for reducing pressure in the eye. *Typical dose:* 240 to 480 mg daily, divided into 2 or 3 doses of 80- to 160-mg capsules.

Ginkgo leaves may be beneficial for glaucoma because of their antioxidant and vasodilatory properties. *Typical dose:* 3 capsules daily, containing 60 mg of extract standardized to 24 percent flavone glycosides and 6 percent ginkgolides.

Sties (Sty)

Sties are a bacterial infection of the eyelash bed. Staphylococcal organisms often cause them. The typical treatment includes antibiotics and warm packs on the eyes. Herbal remedies focus on antibiotic herbs and ones that boost the immune system to prevent recurrence of the sty.

Helping Herbs

Echinacea's immune-enhancing capability stimulates white blood cell activity that helps battle the infection in sties. *Typical dose:* Up to 9 (300- to 400-mg) capsules, taken daily in divided doses. Echinacea is contraindicated in AIDS and other autoimmune diseases. Avoid echinacea if you are allergic to members of the Asteraceae/Compositae family, including chrysanthemums and daisies.

Musculoskeletal System

The musculoskeletal system is made up of the muscles and the skeleton.

Sore & Aching Muscles

Sore, aching muscles can be caused by many things. Often, it is just plain overdoing it, or doing more than your body is prepared to do. Herbs may help soothe aching muscles.

Helping Herbs

Ginger contains anti-inflammatory properties that may be beneficial for relieving muscle aches and pains. *Typical dose:* 2 cups of tea, made with 1 teaspoon of root or ½ teaspoon of dried root steeped in hot, not boiling, water for 10 minutes; or up to 8 (500-mg) capsules daily; or 10 to 20 drops of tincture daily; or for a topical application, mix 2 tablespoons of grated ginger with 3 tablespoons of olive oil or sesame oil and rub into affected area.

Horse chestnut helps relieve bruising, pain, swelling and inflammation. The tannins in horse chestnut are anti-inflammatory. Try a commercially prepared gel that contains horse chestnut for topical use. Follow label directions.

Peppermint contains compounds (menthols) that have been used for many years to treat muscle aches and pains, joint pain and backache. Menthols ease muscle tightness and may provide cooling relief to inflamed areas. These preparations may be purchased commercially. Use as directed.

Back Pain

Many of us suffer from back pain at one time or another. The root of the problem may be overuse; it may be chronic in people who are overweight or obese, or in those who have poor posture.

To solve the problem once and for all, it is necessary to find the cause. If it is excess weight, weight loss will help. Exercises to strengthen the back muscles work for many people because they help improve posture in addition to helping the muscles. While you are waiting for the positive results of weight loss and exercise, there are some herbal remedies that might help relieve your pain.

Helping Herbs

Capsicum (red pepper) may help relieve the pain of backache when applied topically. It is available commercially as creams called Capzasin-P and Zostrix. There may be some burning or skin irritation associated with their use. Make sure you wash your hands thoroughly after applying either and avoid touching your eyes as these products are made from hot peppers.

Peppermint contains compounds (menthols) that have been used for many years to treat muscle aches and pains, joint pain and backache. Menthols ease muscle tightness and may provide cooling relief to inflamed areas. These preparations may be purchased commercially. Use as directed.

Turmeric's active ingredient, curcumin, is an anti-inflammatory herb that may give relief to those suffering from backache. It is a natural COX-2 inhibitor. COX-2 inhibitors are a class of anti-inflammatory drugs that provide the same relief as NSAIDs, but with a potentially better safety profile. *Typical dose:* 1 (450-mg) capsule, 3 times daily. Do not take if you are pregnant or lactating, or if you have gallbladder disease or gallstones.

Willow has been found to be a safe and effective alternative treatment for lower back pain. The willow compound, salicin, is the precursor to aspirin, so it's no wonder that it is effective. *Typical dose:* Make a tea with 2 teaspoons bark in 1 cup of boiling water, steeped for 10 minutes; take up to 3 cups daily. Do not take willow if you have GI upset including ulcers, nausea, vomiting or diarrhea. Do not take if you are pregnant or lactating. Use caution if you are taking other blood-thinning herbs or drugs.

Sciatica

Sciatica is a painful inflammation of the sciatic nerve. Symptoms include pain and tenderness along the length of the nerve, which runs through the thigh and leg. In severe cases, the muscles of the legs may actually become wasted. Natural approaches, including mild exercise and visualization, along with herbal remedies, can help relieve the pain.

Helping Herbs

Dong quai is not only for female problems such as menstrual cramps, irregularity and symptoms of menopause. It may be effective as a mild sedative, pain reliever, anti-inflammatory and antispasmodic, and for the treatment of sciatica. Use dong quai cautiously as it may be carcinogenic/mutagenic. *Typical dose:* Up to 6 (500- to 600-mg) capsules daily (1 to 2 with meals); or 5 to 20 drops of a tincture, 3 times daily; or prepare dong quai as a tea, using 1 teaspoon of dried herb in ¾ cup of boiling water, steeped for 10 minutes. Drink 1¾ cups per day, a half-hour before each meal. Do not use if you are pregnant or lactating.

Ginger contains anti-inflammatory properties that may be beneficial for sciatica when taken internally or used externally. *Typical dose:* 2 cups of tea made with 1 teaspoon of root or ½ teaspoon of dried root, steeped in hot, not boiling, water for 10 minutes. Take up to 8 (500-mg) capsules daily; or 10 to 20 drops of tincture daily; or for a topical application, mix 2 tablespoons of grated ginger with 3 tablespoons of olive oil or sesame oil and rub into affected area.

White willow may be a safe and effective alternative treatment for sciatica. The willow compound, salicin, is the precursor to aspirin, so it's no wonder that it is effective. *Typical dose:* Make a tea with 2 teaspoons bark in 1 cup of boiling water, steep for 10 minutes and drink up to 3 cups daily, or try a commercially prepared supplement and use as directed. Do not take willow if you have GI upset including ulcers, nausea, vomiting or diarrhea. Do not take if you are pregnant or lactating. Use caution if you are taking other blood-thinning herbs or drugs.

Bursitis & Tendinitis

Bursitis and tendinitis can occur when you have placed unaccustomed demands on your body. Repetitive motions tend to inflame two joint structures, the tendons and the bursae.

Bursitis is an inflammation of the

bursae, the fluid-filled sacs that help lubricate the joints where muscles and tendons join. Tendinitis is an inflammation of the tendons, the tough fibrous but elastic tissues that connect the muscle to the bone.

Both bursitis and tendinitis respond to the same types of treatment, and are usually treated with rest and medications to relieve the pain and inflammation. This is where herbal remedies can provide an effective alternative to NSAIDs.

Helping Herbs

Echinacea is good for injured connective tissue. It helps reduce the pain and swelling of these conditions, often seen as tennis elbow, jogger's knee and swimmer's shoulder. *Typical dose:* Try a bit of tincture for fast relief: up to ½ ounce. Do not take for more than 2 weeks. The tincture may make your tongue tingly and numb, so you may want to opt for the tea. Echinacea is contraindicated in joint conditions related to autoimmune diseases and AIDS. Do not use if you are allergic to members of the Asteraceae/Compositae family, including marigolds and daisies.

Ginger has been used for pain and inflammation for centuries. Ginger tea may help with its anti-inflammatory powers. *Typical dose:* 2 cups of tea made with 1 teaspoon of root or ½ teaspoon of dried root steeped in hot, not boiling, water for 10 minutes. Or try a homemade massage oil using 2 tablespoons of grated fresh ginger in 3 tablespoons of olive oil or sesame oil; apply to affected area as needed.

Turmeric's active ingredient, curcumin, is an anti-inflammatory herb that may give relief to those suffering from bursitis and tendinitis. It is a natural COX-2 inhibitor. COX-2 inhibitors are a class of anti-inflammatory drugs that provide the same relief as NSAIDs, but with a potentially safer profile. *Typical dose:* 1 (450-mg) capsule, 3 times daily. Do not take if you are pregnant or lactating, or if you have gallbladder disease or gallstones.

White willow is worth trying for the pain of bursitis and tendinitis. It may be a safe and effective alternative to other pain relievers. The willow compound, salicin, is the precursor to aspirin, so it's no wonder that it might be effective. *Typical dose:* Make a tea with 2 teaspoons bark to 1 cup of boiling water; steep for 10 minutes and drink up to 3 cups daily, or try a commercially prepared supplement and use as directed. . Do not take willow if you have GI upset including ulcers, nausea, vomiting or diarrhea. Do not take if you are pregnant or lactating. Use caution if you are taking other blood-thinning herbs or drugs.

Multiple Sclerosis (MS)

Multiple sclerosis is a chronic, often disabling disease of the central nervous system. The protective myelin sheath around the major nerves breaks down, causing electrical malfunctions within the nerves. Most people with MS are diagnosed between the ages of 20 and 40, and a majority of those are women.

The symptoms of MS are highly variable, depending on where the central nervous system has been affected. Symptoms vary from one person to another and from day to day for any given individual. Symptoms include fatigue, tingling, numbness, painful sensations, blurred or double vision, muscle weakness, impaired balance, spasticity, tremor, changes in bladder, bowel and sexual function, cognitive changes such as forgetfulness or difficulty concentrating, speech and swallowing problems and mood swings. Symptoms may come and go, appear in any combination and be mild, moderate or severe.

Although the cause of MS is uncertain, several theories are being evaluated: Some think MS is caused by a virus, other researchers theorize that MS is an autoimmune disease and still others think MS might be linked to a high-fat diet.

Herbal remedies can't cure MS, but they may be able to provide some relief from the symptoms.

Helping Herbs

Evening primrose oil (EPO) contains omega-3 and omega-6 fatty acids that are beneficial for the myelin sheath surrounding the spinal cord. Long-term use of the oil may help control symptoms and extend remission. *Typical dose:* 3 to 4 grams daily taken in capsule form.

Ginkgo contains ginkgolides. They are powerful antioxidants that may reduce flare-ups of MS. *Typical dose:* 60 to 80 mg 3 times daily of a product standardized to 24 percent flavone glycosides and 6 percent terpene lactones. Do not take with anticoagulant/antiplatelet herbs or drugs.

Osteoporosis

Osteoporosis is a disease in which bones become fragile and more likely to break. If not prevented or if left untreated, osteoporosis can progress painlessly until a bone breaks. These broken bones typically occur in the hip, spine and wrist.

Women are more than four times more likely to get osteoporosis than men. Usually thought of as a disease of older women, osteoporosis can strike at any age. A woman's risk of hip fracture is equal to her combined risk of breast, uterine and ovarian cancer.

Helping Herbs

Alfalfa has been used more for livestock than for humans. We may have overlooked an important source of many essential nutrients. It is rich in minerals that help to maintain bones—calcium, magnesium and selenium. Use alfalfa cautiously if you are taking blood-thinning drugs or herbs. *Typical dose:* Up to 9 (400- to 500-mg) capsules daily; or make a tea by steeping 2 teaspoons of dried leaves in 1 cup of boiling water for 10 to 20 minutes; strain and drink up to 3 cups daily.

Red clover is an herb with weak estrogenic properties. The isoflavones in red clover are similar to those in other plants, including soybeans. Foods that are rich in isoflavones are being studied for their ability to reduce the risk of osteoporosis. A commercially available supplement, Promensil, is available in supermarkets and pharmacies. *Typical dose:* Make a tea by steeping 1 to 3 teaspoons of dried flowers in 1 cup of boiling water for 10 to 15 minutes; strain and drink up to 3 cups daily. For commercially available supplements, follow instructions on label. Do not use supplemental red clover if you have estrogen-sensitive cancers or are at risk of blood clots and/or inflammation of blood vessels.

Soy has become popular for the treatment of menopause and its related side effects. It is effective because of its weak estrogenic properties that limit the uptake of estrogen produced by the body. Soy's isoflavones are thought to contribute to its effectiveness in treating and preventing high cholesterol and possibly osteoporosis. *Typical dose:* 25 to 50 grams of soy protein, obtained from food, daily.

Risk Factors for Osteoporosis

Certain people are more likely to develop osteoporosis than others. The following risk factors increase the likelihood of developing osteoporosis:

- Being female
- Thin and/or small frame
- Advanced age
- A family history of osteoporosis
- Postmenopausal, including early or surgically induced menopause
- Abnormal absence of menstrual periods (amenorrhea)
- Anorexia nervosa
- A diet low in calcium
- Use of certain medications, such as corticosteroids and anticonvulsants
- Low testosterone levels in men
- An inactive lifestyle
- Cigarette smoking
- Excessive use of alcohol
- Being Caucasian or Asian (although African Americans and Hispanic Americans are also at significant risk)

Women can lose up to 20 percent of their bone mass in the 5 to 7 years following menopause, making them more susceptible to osteoporosis.

Arthritis

Arthritis is any inflammatory condition of the joints characterized by pain, swelling, heat, redness and inability to move easily or without discomfort. There are more than 100 different types of arthritis, and the cause of most types is unknown. Investigations are currently underway on the roles three major factors play in certain types of arthritis. These include the genetic factors, what happens to you during your life and your lifestyle.

Since many of the same herbal remedies are used in the various arthritic conditions, they will be discussed at the end of the descriptions of each. If a particular remedy is better for one condition than another, it will be pointed out.

Osteoarthritis (OA), or degenerative joint disease, is one of the most common types of arthritis. It is characterized by the breakdown of the joint's cartilage. Cartilage is the part of the joint that cushions the ends of bones. When cartilage breaks down, bones rub against each other, causing pain and loss of movement.

OA is most common in middle-aged and older people, and can range from very mild to very severe. It affects hands and weight-bearing joints such as knees, hips, feet and the back.

Rheumatoid arthritis (RA) is an inflammation in the lining of the joints and/or other internal organs. RA typically affects many different joints. It can be chronic, meaning it lasts a long time, or it can flare up, then go into remission.

RA is a systemic disease, meaning that it affects the entire body. It is one of the most common forms of arthritis, characterized by the inflammation of the membrane lining the joint, which causes pain, stiffness, warmth, redness and swelling. The inflamed cells of the joint lining, the synovium, release enzymes that may digest bone and cartilage. The involved joint can lose its shape and alignment, resulting in pain, disfigurement and loss of movement.

Although the cause is not known, it is known that RA is an autoimmune disease. The body's natural immune system does not operate as it should, and produces antibodies against its own body's cells. These antibodies attack healthy joint tissue, causing inflammation and subsequent joint damage.

Systemic Lupus Erythematosus (lupus) is a chronic rheumatic disease affecting joints, muscles and other parts of the body. Systemic lupus erythematosus involves chronic inflammation that can affect many parts of the body, including heart, lungs, skin, joints, spleen, kidneys and nervous system. The cause is unknown, although it is thought that it may be inherited. Lupus affects 8 to 10 times more women than men and can occur at any age. African Americans appear to get lupus more often than Caucasians.

Gout (sometimes referred to as gouty arthritis) causes sudden, severe attacks of pain and tenderness, redness, warmth and swelling in usually one joint at a time. Often, the big toe is the first place it is noticed.

Gout happens when too much uric acid builds up in the body and forms crystals that deposit in joints and cause inflammation. Uric acid is a substance that normally forms when the body breaks down waste products called purines. Gout can be inherited or be a complication of another condition. It is more common in men over the age of 40, but can happen to anyone.

Helping Herbs

Bosweilla is a resin that has been shown to relieve arthritis in laboratory animals. These studies look promising for bosweilla's effectiveness in treating arthritic conditions in humans. It also inhibits inflammation and improves circulation to joints. *Typical dose:* 300 to 400 mg daily of an extract containing 65 percent bosweillic acid.

Capsicum (red pepper) may relieve the pain of gout when applied topically. It is available commercially as creams called Capzasin-P and Zostrix. There may be some burning associated with their use. Make sure to wash your hands thoroughly after applying either and avoid touching your eyes, because these products are made from hot peppers.

Devil's claw may lower blood uric acid, which is responsible for gout. It has been used over time as an anti-inflammatory agent and pain reliever. Its digestive stimulant properties may interfere with the production of uric acid crystals that build up in the joints. *Typical dose:* 600 to 800 mg daily of a product standardized to 1.5 percent harpagoside. Do not use if you have ulcers or if you are pregnant or nursing. If you have heart disease, talk with your physician before taking devil's claw.

Ginger has been used for the pain and inflammation of arthritis for centuries. Ginger tea may help with its anti-inflammatory powers. *Typical dose:* 2 cups of tea made with 2 teaspoons of gingerroot (or

1 teaspoon of dried root) steeped in 1 cup hot (not boiling) water for 10 minutes.

Turmeric's active ingredient, curcumin, is an anti-inflammatory herb that may give relief to those suffering from arthritis. It is a natural COX-2 inhibitor. COX-2 inhibitors are a class of anti-inflammatory drugs that provide the same relief as NSAIDs but with a potentially safer profile. *Typical dose:* 1 (450-mg) capsule, 3 times daily. Do not take if you are pregnant or lactating, or if you have gallbladder disease or gallstones.

Fibromyalgia

Fibromyalgia is a common form of generalized muscular pain and fatigue. Fibromyalgia was once considered a catchall term for a disease with vague non-specific complaints that were thought to originate in the head. We now know different as more and more individuals, usually women, are diagnosed with it. The name "fibromyalgia" means pain in the muscles and fibrous connective tissues (ligaments and tendons). This condition is considered a "syndrome" because it's a set of signs and symptoms that occur together: pain, fatigue, change in mood, depression, anxiety and difficulty concentrating. It also involves feelings of numbness and tingling in the hands, arms, feet and face. Additionally, migraine headaches, abdominal pain, bloating or alternating constipation and diarrhea are common.

Fibromyalgia is especially confusing and often misunderstood because symptoms are common in other conditions. It is a form of soft-tissue or muscular rheumatism rather than arthritis of a joint.

Helping Herbs

Capsicum (red pepper) may relieve the pain of sore muscles and boost circulation when applied topically. It is available commercially as creams called Capzasin-P and Zostrix. There may be some burning associated with their use, so begin with a small amount of medium-to-low strength cream and add more cream or a higher strength cream as tolerated and as needed. Make sure to wash your hands thoroughly after applying either and avoid touching your eyes, because these products are made from hot peppers.

Devil's claw has been used over time as an anti-inflammatory agent and pain reliever. Its digestive stimulant properties boost digestion, increase nutrient absorption and improve overall health. *Typical dose:* 600 to 800 mg daily of a product standardized to 1.5 percent harpagoside. Do not use if you have ulcers or if you are pregnant or nursing. If you have heart disease, consult your physician before taking devil's claw.

Ginkgo is a vasodilator that helps improve peripheral circulation and oxygenation of body tissue. It also has anti-inflammatory properties that help ease the pain of the disease. *Typical dose:* 60 to 80 mg 3 times daily of a product standardized to 24 percent flavone glycosides and 6 percent terpene lactones.

Grapeseed extract contains powerful antioxidants that are anti-inflammatory and may be beneficial for persons with fibromyalgia. *Typical dose:* 75 to 300 mg daily for 3 weeks followed by a maintenance dose of 40 to 80 mg daily.

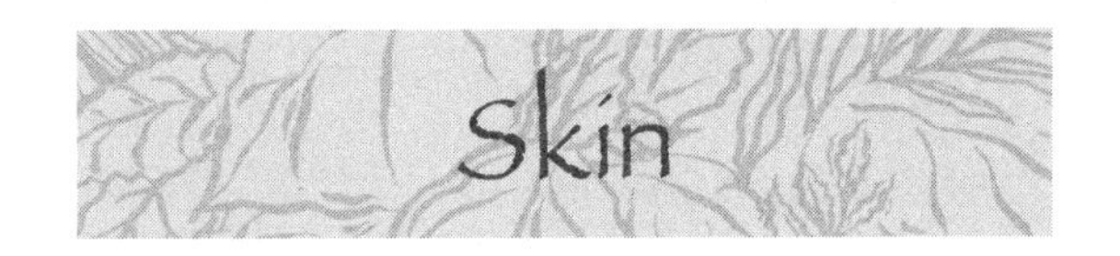

The skin is the covering of our body that protects our muscles, bones and internal organs from the environment. It is actually fairly tough and is composed of numerous layers of connective tissue. Because it is susceptible to the many organisms that might assault it, there are numerous problems that can occur. Let's look at some of these and what herbal remedies might provide relief.

Acne

Acne doesn't plague just teenagers; it can affect adults as well. Acne is a skin disease that affects areas where oil-producing glands are found—face, chest and back. The glands become plugged with excess dead skin cells, creating the telltale bumps known as pimples. Sometimes, the bacteria that reside in the hair follicles around the glands contribute to the infection.

Adult acne is seen in women more than men and is often linked to hormonal changes. Despite what your mother—or even your doctor—told you, milk and chocolate do not cause pimples.

Helping Herbs

Calendula, with its antibacterial and anti-inflammatory properties, is used to treat many skin conditions. *Typical dose:* Make a tea wash by steeping 1 teaspoon dried flowers in 1 cup boiling water for 10 minutes; cool in the refrigerator. Apply the tea to a clean face with a cotton ball.

Chamomile is a popular treatment for skin problems. You can purchase it commercially or make a skin wash using 1 tablespoon of dried flowers in 1 cup of hot water. Steep for 10 minutes, strain, cool and apply to a clean face with a cotton ball. Do not use chamomile if you are allergic to members of the Asteraceae/Compositae family (daisies, marigolds).

Dandelion root helps rid the body of toxins and impurities. The leaves contain numerous vitamins and minerals, which help maintain healthy skin. *Typical dose:* 3 to 4 cups of root tea daily; or 2 (400- to 500-mg) capsules, 3 times daily. Enjoy the leaves in salads.

Lavender oil is antibacterial and may be applied in a small amount to the affected area using a cotton swab.

Chaste tree, or vitex, is helpful if your pimples are hormonal or menstrual period–related. *Typical dose:* 40 drops of liquid extract or 1 capsule of dried extract daily. Do not use during pregnancy or if nursing. Chasteberry's effects are not immediate—it may take up to 7 months to see any obvious effects.

Eczema

Eczema is a superficial skin condition of unknown origins. It does seem to occur along with other allergic conditions like asthma and hay fever. In the early stages, it is a weepy patch of skin that later becomes crusted, scaly and sometimes infected.

Helping Herbs

Evening primrose oil is approved in Great Britain for eczema. Its oil is rich in gamma-linolenic acid (GLA), which is known to help numerous skin and other conditions by reducing inflammation and itching. *Typical dose:* The easiest way to take it is in 8 to 12 commercially prepared capsules of 500 mg daily; follow label directions.

Licorice has anti-inflammatory properties that seem to relieve eczema when applied topically. *Typical dose:* Make a tea wash using 2 tablespoons of ground root in 2 cups of water; simmer for 15 minutes. Apply cooled wash with a clean cloth to the affected areas. Licorice may be taken internally, but not in amounts greater than 1 teaspoon powdered root as a tea in 1 cup water 3 times daily or for more than 6 weeks. Do not use internally if you are pregnant, have high blood pressure, heart or liver disease, diabetes or severe kidney disease.

Psoriasis

Psoriasis is a skin disorder characterized by red, scaly patches of varying sizes, usually on the scalp, lower back, elbows, knees and knuckles. It often first appears in teenagers or young adults and continues throughout life. The cause is unknown; it is not hereditary or caused by an allergic reaction. Stress and trauma to the skin may make it worse.

Helping Herbs

Capsicum (red pepper) may help psoriasis when applied topically. It is available commercially as creams called Capzasin-P and Zostrix. They relieve pain and the red scaly skin of psoriasis. There may be some burning associated with their use. Make sure you wash your hands thoroughly after applying either; avoid touching your eyes, because these products are made from hot peppers.

Flaxseed may benefit persons with psoriasis by supplying some essential omega-3 fatty acids. *Typical dose:* 2 tablespoons of seeds, which can be ground and added to cereals, salads and other foods. Because flaxseed also acts as a bulk-forming laxative, it is important that you drink plenty of water to aid in its elimination. Take 1 hour before or after taking medication or eating in order to prevent interference with the absorption of drugs or nutrients.

Lavender is praised for its ability to treat numerous skin conditions. Apply a drop of it to the affected area, followed by almond oil cream. Do not take lavender oil internally.

Licorice has anti-inflammatory properties that may relieve psoriasis when applied topically. Purchase licorice extract and apply it directly to the affected area with a cotton ball or clean cloth. Do not take licorice oil internally.

Dry Skin

Dry skin is often seen in the winter when the furnace is turned on and the humidity drops. People living in dry climates can experience it year-round.

Helping Herbs

Aloe is a time-tested remedy for dry skin and for cuts and burns as well. Because of the amount required to cover your body, rather than deplete your home-grown supply, you may want to try one of the many commercial preparations made especially for dry skin.

Evening primrose oil (EPO) may also be helpful for dry skin conditions, both internally or topically. *Typical internal dose:* up to 12 (500 mg) capsules of EPO daily.

Oily Skin

Oily skin is a result of overactive oil glands in the face and upper body. There is nothing like a shiny nose to give away an oily complexion.

Helping Herbs

Witch hazel has potent astringents, in the form of tannins, that are helpful in closing pores and toning the skin. Apply a commercially prepared solution, as directed, to a clean face with a cotton ball.

Dandruff

No one seems to know what causes that telltale white stuff that falls on our collars. Dandruff is an excessive amount of flaking skin that usually comes from the scalp. Dandruff can be found on the face, back, stomach and folds of the body and is usually confused with psoriasis.

Helping Herbs

Evening primrose oil may be used internally for dandruff, or may be rubbed into the scalp. *Typical dose:* up to 12 (500 mg) capsules daily. May be taken in split doses of 2 (500 mg) capsules 4 to 6 times daily.

Flaxseed oil is high in anti-inflammatory omega-3 fatty acids. *Typical dose:* 1 teaspoon oil or 1 to 2 tablespoons ground seed daily. The seeds are tough to digest, so it is best to grind them as you use them to make their beneficial oils more available. The oil may also be rubbed into the scalp. Store oil and any ground seeds in the refrigerator or freezer; the oil is not stable and breaks down if stored improperly.

Tea tree oil is a potent antifungal but is also very drying. If you want to try it, start with a few drops in either flaxseed oil or primrose oil, rubbed into the scalp at bedtime and washed out in the morning.

Dry Scalp

Dry scalp is much like dry skin except it's on the top of your head. It differs from dandruff in that it is related more to the environment than an inflammation of the skin. Dry scalp is treated the same as dry skin, and some of the remedies for dandruff may work as well.

Sunburn

Who has not experienced the pain of sunburn at least once in their life? Most people have, regardless of their skin color. Sunburn is a skin injury characterized by redness, tenderness and sometimes blistering as a result of the skin being exposed to ultraviolet (UV) rays. Excessive sun exposure puts us at risk for more than just wrinkles: risk of skin cancer rises exponentially with excessive exposure to the sun.

Helping Herbs

Aloe gel, from the inner leaf of the plant, has been shown to be effective in the healing of burns of all types. Aloe sunburn relief products can usually be found next to the sunscreen in stores. Aloe is anti-inflammatory, antibacterial and antifungal. It may be applied directly from the plant as needed (up to several times daily), or purchased commercially.

Calendula is astringent, antibacterial, anti-inflammatory and cooling to many types of burns. *Typical dose:* Make a tea wash with 1 teaspoon dried flowers in 1 cup boiling water. Steep for 10 minutes, then cool in the refrigerator. Apply cooled wash to a clean face with a cotton ball.

Tea has been known for centuries for its cooling properties. Either black or green teas may be used. The simplest way to apply it is to wet a tea bag with cool water and apply it to a small area. For larger areas, steep the tea bag for 5 to 10 minutes, remove it and cool the tea in the refrigerator. Apply with a cotton ball or a clean cloth several times daily.

Witch hazel is effective as an astringent, tightening swollen tissues and reducing inflammation. Apply a commercially purchased witch hazel with a cotton ball or clean cloth as often as needed.

Insect Bites & Stings

Insects are an inevitable part of our environment ... or are we an essential part of their environment? We all have to live together and must risk the occasional bite or sting. Mosquitoes, chiggers, lice, bedbugs, fleas and flies all bite, while fire ants, bees, hornets and wasps sting. Stings, and some bites, can cause allergic reactions that require immediate attention. When either happens, the result is an inflammatory response by our body that results in swelling, redness, sometimes warmth and itching. There are numerous herbal remedies that can help relieve the pain and itching. There are also preparations that may help repel those pesky little critters as well.

Helping Herbs

Aloe accelerates healing. Apply the gel from the plant directly to the bite or sting.

Calendula works for insect bites. Use the same recipe for bites as used for sunburn. If you are growing it in your garden, you may apply fresh flowers directly to the bite or sting.

Comfrey is an antiseptic and hastens wound-healing. Fresh or dried leaves or root can be mixed with a small amount of water and applied as a poultice to a bite or sting. An effective tea can also be made using 1 heaping teaspoon of the dried plant in 1 cup of boiling water. Steep for 10 minutes, strain, cool and apply to insect bites with a clean cloth. Some commercially prepared herbal salves contain comfrey. Do not take comfrey internally.

Lavender oil, an anti-inflammatory, may be applied directly (undiluted) to the affected area with a cotton swab. Do not take lavender oil internally.

Tea, either black or green, helps shrink swollen tissues. Dampen a tea bag with cool water and apply directly to the bite or sting.

Witch hazel is soothing to bites and stings. A commercial concentrate may be applied directly, following label directions.

Repellant Herbs

Basil might work in a pinch if you're in the garden and being chased by insects. Break off a few of the leaves and rub it on your skin.

Pennyroyal is considered a powerful insect repellent. It was first documented as a flea repellant in the first century C.E. Pick the leaves and rub a small amount on your skin. Do not use if you are pregnant or lactating.

Tea tree oil can be applied directly to the skin as an insect repellant.

Hives

Hives are an allergic reaction. They are itchy, red, raised patches of skin with whitish centers. Hives are a result of histamine, a substance that is released by special cells called mast cells. The histamine makes the surrounding cells leak, resulting in localized swelling and itching. Many things can cause hives, including medications, food and insect bites.

Helping Herbs

Aloe, once again, comes to the rescue. Use a purchased gel or apply aloe directly from the plant as needed.

Chamomile acts as an anti-inflammatory when applied topically or enjoyed as a relaxing tea. *Typical dose:* 3 to 4 cups of tea daily, made with 1 teaspoon of dried flowers in 1 cup of hot water, steeped for 10 minutes and strained. For a bath, brew a gallon of tea and pour it into a lukewarm, not hot, bath. (Hot baths will only aggravate the itching.) Do not use if you are allergic to other members of the Asteraceae/Compositae family, including daisies, marigolds and echinacea.

Ginger tea may help with its anti-inflammatory powers. *Typical dose:* 2 cups of tea made with 1 teaspoon of fresh gingerroot (or ½ teaspoon of dried root) steeped in hot, not boiling, water for 10 minutes.

Nettle tea, taken internally, appears to have an anti-allergy property. *Typical dose:* 1 to 2 cups of tea daily, made with 1 teaspoon of dried leaves in 1 cup of boiling water. Or, carefully pick fresh nettles, using heavy gloves, and steam the leaves, eating them as a vegetable.

Cuts & Abrasions

Cuts and scrapes don't need a description; we all experience these minor wounds on a regular basis. These are skin abrasions that do not require medical attention.

Helping Herbs

Aloe to the rescue once more. It reduces inflammation, soothes minor cuts and protects from infection with its antibacterial properties. Apply gel directly from the plant, or use a commercial preparation as needed.

Calendula encourages new skin growth and has antiseptic and anti-inflammatory properties. It is endorsed by the German Commission E for reducing inflammation and promoting wound-healing. You can purchase commercial creams or make a simple wash using 1 teaspoon dried herb in 1 cup boiling water. Soak for 10 minutes; cool and apply with a clean cloth.

Comfrey contains a substance called allantoin, which speeds healing, and tannins that act as an astringent. To apply comfrey externally as a poultice, wrap fresh leaves in a clean, wet cloth. Commercial preparations may also be purchased and used according to directions. Do not take comfrey internally.

Garlic can be applied directly to a boil or abscess. Cut a clove in half, apply it and leave it for about 2 hours. The antibiotic properties of garlic are also found in its relatives, onions and chives. Garlic can irritate the skin when applied directly. If this happens, discontinue use immediately.

Echinacea is a fine immune stimulant, but it is also an antiseptic that improves wound-healing, decreases inflammation and has a numbing effect. Applying it directly may sting a bit, so add it to glycerin to reduce the sting. Take echinacea internally as a complement to its external use. *Typical dose:* Apply tincture directly to the affected area up to 3 times daily. Persons with autoimmune diseases or with allergies to other members of the Asteraceae/Compositae family should not use echinacea internally. Members of the family include daisies, chrysanthemums and chamomile.

Plantain can be applied "out in the field" if necessary. It contains antibiotic and anti-inflammatory substances as well as allantoin, which speeds wound-healing. Mash a leaf or two to release its gooey healing substances and apply directly to the wound.

Tea tree oil is another excellent antiseptic that can be applied directly by diluting 5 or so drops in 2 tablespoons of vegetable oil. If this preparation is irritating, dilute it more. Discontinue if irritation persists. Do not take tea tree oil or any other essential oils internally.

Burns

Burns can, and do, happen to everyone at some time or another. Burns are measured by degree—first, second and third, depending on the severity. First-degree burns happen on the surface of the skin and result in mild redness and pain. Second-degree burns extend to the deeper skin layers, producing blisters, dark redness, swelling and pain. Third-degree burns destroy the layers of skin that are affected, resulting in pain surrounding the burn, but not within the burn itself.

Third-degree burns, and second-degree burns over an area larger than the palm of your hand, require immediate medical attention. Only small first-degree burns may benefit from the herbs discussed here. If you have severe blistering of the skin, seek immediate medical attention.

Helping Herbs

Aloe has long been known as a treatment for burns. The gel from the split leaves has been shown to be helpful in common kitchen burns as well as burns received during radiation therapy for cancer. Just cut open a leaf and apply the gel directly, several times a day.

Calendula, once again, is a treatment of choice, this time for burns. Buy an over-the-counter product or make a tea wash with 1 teaspoon dried herb in 1 cup boiling water, soaked for 10 minutes. Apply cooled wash with a clean cloth to the affected area.

Comfrey leaves and root contain the healing substance allantoin. Look for commercial products or make a poultice or tea from fresh leaves. For a tea, use 1 teaspoon of dried herb in 1 cup of hot water. Steep for 10 minutes, strain and cool. For a poultice, mash fresh leaves, or soak 1 cup of dried leaves in enough water to cover. Place the poultice in a clean cloth and apply to the burn as needed. Do not take comfrey internally.

Lavender oil may be applied directly to the affected area. It has been shown to relieve pain and enhance healing. If you find the scent unpleasant or think the essential oil may irritate your skin, mix it with a tablespoon of olive oil. Do not take lavender oil internally.

Plantain, with its allantoin and other healing properties, works well for burns when the juice of the leaves is applied directly.

St. John's wort is often forgotten for its topical healing properties. Commercially prepared salves appear to speed healing and reduce scarring, but they may not be widely available in the United States. You can make your own using a few drops of tincture, or steeping 2 teaspoons of dried herb in 1 or 2 tablespoons of olive oil. Do not use this oil if you plan to be out in the sun.

Warts

Warts are unsightly and embarrassing growths that are caused by a virus from a family called papillomavirus. Warts commonly occur on the hands and feet. People with suppressed immune systems appear to be more susceptible to warts. It may take several weeks to completely remove a wart, regardless of whether you use a traditional preparation or an herbal treatment.

Helping Herbs

Bloodroot contains substances that irritate the skin and enzymes that help dissolve the proteins of the wart-infected tissue. Commercially prepared bloodroot preparations, rather than homemade concoctions, may be the most effective for wart removal.

Dandelion latex is the white milky substance produced from the stem when the dandelion is picked. Dab a bit of the white stuff on the wart several times a day until it disappears.

Willow is found in many over-the-counter preparations for removing warts. Purchase one of the prepared removers, or make your own by taping a piece of moistened inner bark to the affected area. Change every 5 to 7 days until the wart disappears.

Athlete's Foot

Athlete's foot is a fungus that can infect not just the feet, but other parts of the body as well, in the form of ringworm or jock itch. The fungus requires moisture and darkness, just the right combination for any of these areas. It's important to keep the area(s) dry.

Helping Herbs

Garlic is an excellent antifungal and antiseptic for athlete's foot and other fungal infections. Tape a cut clove to the infected area, making sure it does not irritate the surrounding skin. This is probably not the best choice if you are planning a big night out, but it's probably safe for watching Sunday afternoon football. Or try a footbath made with 5 or more crushed garlic cloves, enough warm water to submerge your foot or feet and 2 to 4 tablespoons of rubbing alcohol. Or try the Chinese method of crushing 3 cloves of garlic in olive oil to cover (about 1 tablespoon) for 3 days. Strain the oil and apply it with a cotton ball to the affected area.

Goldenseal contains berberine, a very powerful antifungal and antibacterial compound. Make a strong decoction with 5 to 7 teaspoons of herb to 1 cup of water; simmer for 20 minutes, then strain, cool and apply it using a clean cloth or cotton ball.

Licorice may complement the garlic footbath, not just by masking some of the odor, but also by contributing antifungal properties to the mixture. This same solution could be used to treat any one of the athlete's foot–type fungi and applied with a clean cloth. Licorice as a strong decoction—5 to 7 teaspoons of dried herbs boiled in 1 cup of water for 20 minutes—can be applied directly to the affected area once it has cooled.

Tea tree oil, with its antiseptic properties, works very well for athlete's foot. Dilute the tea tree oil with an equal amount of olive oil and apply directly to the affected area, 3 times daily. Do not take tea tree oil internally.

Scabies

Scabies are microscopic mites that burrow into the surface of the skin and lay their eggs. The result is small, itchy bumps, sometimes all over the body, but more often between the fingers, on the wrists, at the waist and in the groin area. Infected clothing and bedding transmit scabies from person to person. It is imperative that all clothing and bedding is cleaned thoroughly during treatment to prevent reinfection. Herbs have been used for centuries to treat scabies, but their effectiveness has not been measured. They are worth a try.

Helping Herbs

Aloe applied directly to the scabies rash can help relieve the itch.

Clove oil has traditionally been used for scabies. The essential oil has an analgesic and anti-inflammatory effect, which helps to reduce the constant itching of the lesions and prevent bacterial infections. Clove oil can be irritating, so it should be tested on a small patch of skin first. Combine 10 drops of the essential oil with 1 cup of olive oil and apply it to the rash at bedtime. Do not use clove oil during pregnancy, while nursing or on open or broken skin.

Tea tree's essential oil fights not only insects, but also parasites like the mite that causes scabies. Combine 1 teaspoon of tea tree oil with 5 teaspoons of vegetable oil and apply liberally to the skin before bedtime. Do not use tea tree oil internally and discontinue use if irritation develops.

Body Odor

Body odor is a result of several factors. Perspiration produced from the eccrine and apocrine glands are two major contributing factors. When we are under environmental or psychological stress, these glands produce sweat. Sweat is a perfect breeding ground for bacteria that contribute to the odor, especially if we do not bathe regularly. Health conditions such as skin infections, diabetes, liver disease and zinc deficiency can contribute to body odor.

Helping Herbs

Fennel has been used since early times as a treatment for body odor. Fennel seeds, when chewed, can help treat bad breath and body odor that comes from the intestines. *Typical dose:* Take whole seeds after each meal as desired, or make a tea using 2 to 3 teaspoons crushed fennel seeds simmered for 10 minutes in 1 cup of water. Take 1 cup of tea daily.

Rosemary is a wonderful culinary herb with antiseptic and antibiotic properties. Rosemary tea, made with 1 teaspoon of dried leaves steeped in 1 cup of hot water for 15 minutes, may be used as a body wash. The herb may also be used as a body powder to treat skin odor caused by bacteria or fungus on the skin. Combine 1 tablespoon ground, dried rosemary with 1 tablespoon ground, dried sage, ½ cup baking soda and ½ cup cornstarch; store in an airtight container. Use on the body and underarms. Do not continue using if irritation occurs.

Sage can dry perspiration and sage oils act as an antiseptic and antibiotic. A tea made from sage, using 2 teaspoons dried herb steeped for 5 to 10 minutes in 1 cup of hot water may be used as a body wash to help reduce excessive sweating. Dried sage may be used as a body powder. Combine 1 tablespoon ground, dried sage with 1 tablespoon ground, dried rosemary, ½ cup baking soda and ½ cup cornstarch; store in an airtight container. Use on the body and underarms.

Bruises

Bruises result from damage to the soft tissue of the skin and muscles. The result can be a rainbow of colors from blue and black to red and yellow. Bruises can originate from very noticeable trauma or from a mild, barely noticeable bump, especially in older people. If you bruise often and without obvious injury, there may be an underlying disorder that needs to be medically evaluated.

Helping Herbs

Sometimes excessive use of anticoagulant/antiplatelet herbs may contribute to bruising. If you are taking several of these, discontinue or decrease amounts and see if they disappear.

Calendula is good not only for other skin problems, but for bruises as well. Make a compress by steeping 2 teaspoons of calendula flowers in 1 cup of hot water for 10 minutes, strain and cool. Wet a clean cloth with the solution and apply to the bruise.

Comfrey contains a substance called allantoin that helps knit body cells back together and has anti-inflammatory properties. Look for commercial products or make a poultice or tea from fresh leaves. *Typical dose:* Make a tea with 1 teaspoon of dried herb in 1 cup of hot water. Steep for 10 minutes, strain and cool. For a poultice, mash fresh leaves, or soak 1 cup of dried leaves in enough water to cover. Place the poultice in a clean cloth and apply to the bruise as needed. Do not take comfrey internally.

St. John's wort flowers are anti-inflammatory and are effective when applied topically to bruises. You can make your own oil for topical application by using 5 to 10 drops of tincture in 1 tablespoon oil, or steeping 2 teaspoons of dried herb in 1 or 2 tablespoons of olive oil. Apply the oil as needed. Do not use this oil if you plan to be out in the sun.

Tea, once again, has been found to act as a remedy for a skin problem. Both green and black tea work equally well as an anti-inflammatory agent. Moisten a tea bag and apply it directly to the bruised area as needed.

Wrinkles

Wrinkles appear when skin begins to lose its elasticity. With continued exposure to sun, cigarette smoke, air pollution and normal aging comes oxidative damage to the skin. When this happens, skin can no longer absorb moisture. The result is wrinkles. Many creams on the market—some expensive ones, too—profess to be able to return skin to its youthful appearance. Herbal products can probably do just as well, for less.

Helping Herbs

Aloe is an ingredient in many skin-care products. No one knows for sure if it works, but it can't hurt to try. It has been reported that Cleopatra used aloe for her skin every day.

Horse chestnut and **witch hazel**, combined as an astringent salve, appear to have some promise. The witch hazel is astringent, toning the skin. Both contain powerful antioxidants. Look for salves with these herbs, combined with rosemary and sage in natural foods stores. Use as directed.

Rosemary tea, made with 1 teaspoon of dried herb in 1 cup of hot water, can provide a soothing antioxidant tea that may provide beneficial antioxidants that protect the skin.

Infections

An infection is a pathogenic organism (virus or bacteria) that invades your body. Sounds serious, huh? Well, it may be. That is why you should seek a medical diagnosis before you begin treatment with an herbal remedy, just to make sure you know what you are dealing with.

Viral Infections

Viral infections have no cure. Antibiotics are useless against them. There are just a few prescription medicines that are effective against viruses, and those are for herpes and AIDS. This is where herbal remedies come in handy. There are several that have been used effectively for centuries and are worth a try.

Helping Herbs

Astragalus is an immune-boosting stimulant used in Traditional Chinese Medicine for centuries. It is believed to protect the body by keeping the system at its fighting best. *Typical dose:* up to 8 (400- to 500-mg) capsules of dried powder daily.

Echinacea is one of the most popular antiviral herbal therapies. It contains three compounds with specific antiviral properties. Roots are believed to act like the body's own antiviral compound, interferon. No matter what is responsible for its beneficial action, it is worth a try if you have a viral infection. *Typical dose:* Up to 9 (300- to 400-mg) capsules daily. Take for 2 weeks, stop for 1 week, then resume. Repeat this cycle as needed. Do not take if you are allergic to members of the Asteraceae/Compositae family including daisies and marigolds. It is contraindicated in AIDS/HIV.

Garlic has been used to treat viruses throughout history and is safe for most persons when taken as directed. Its antibacterial, antifungal and antiviral properties are believed to be the reason for its effectiveness against viruses. Because garlic may leave you with strong breath and body odor, you may want to try a commercially prepared product. Long-term garlic use bestows the most health benefits. *Typical dose:* 600 to 900 mg of garlic powder, tablets or capsules daily; 4 mL of aged garlic extract daily; 10 mg of garlic oil "perles" daily; or 1 or more medium-size fresh cloves daily.

Goldenseal may be effective in a number of infections, including viral and fungal. The active constituent, berberine, has been used to treat yeast, fungal and viral infections. It can be used externally as a decoction and internally to complement its external use. *Typical dose:* Make a decoction by simmering 5 to 7 teaspoons of dried goldenseal to 1 cup of water for 20 minutes; cool and apply to the affected area. Take up to 6 (500- to 600-mg) capsules daily. Do not use internally if you are pregnant or lactating.

Juniper contains a potent antiviral called deoxypodophyllotoxin, which may be effective in inhibiting several viruses. *Typical dose:* Try some juniper tea the next time you feel under the weather; add 1 teaspoon of crushed berries to 1 cup of boiling water. Steep for 10 to 20 minutes, then strain; drink up to 2 cups daily.

Lemon balm has antiviral activity that may be beneficial in all types of viruses, including herpes virus sores. *Typical dose:* Make a tea with 2 teaspoons of dried leaves in 1 cup of hot water. Steep for 10 minutes and drink up to 4 times daily.

Urinary & Bladder Infections

Many adults know the feeling: the urge to urinate, but the inability to expel more than a few painful dribbles. Bladder or urinary tract infections (UTIs) can develop in men or women, but are more common in women. The main culprit for women is usually an *Escherichia coli* bacterium that invades from the anal area. Men get UTIs as well, often because of an enlarged prostate gland.

UTIs can possibly be prevented and treated effectively using herbal remedies. However, if you think you have a UTI and it is accompanied by back pain and/or blood in your urine, take the shortest route to your physician. These more serious symptoms, if left untreated, can result in kidney damage or worse.

Helping Herbs

Cranberry is one of the most widely respected and used remedies for preventing recurring UTIs and helping to reduce the odor of urine, particularly in long-term care residents. Cranberry juice is the most common prescription, but may not be the best treatment because of the sugar and calories you get with the recommended dose. Cranberry juice extract capsules will suffice and save you upwards of 100 calories a day. *Typical dose:* 1 (300- to 400-mg) capsule, 2 to 3 times daily. If you choose to use cranberry juice, 3 ounces of cranberry juice cocktail daily may help prevent infections; 12 to 32 ounces may help treat infections. If you have diabetes, opt for capsules instead of cranberry juice cocktail, which may have too much sugar in therapeutic amounts.

Echinacea's immune-enhancing properties can help people with recurrent bladder infections. *Typical dose:* Up to 9 (300- to 400-mg) capsules daily. Do not take if you are allergic to members of the Asteraceae/Compositae family, including daisies and chrysanthemums.

Dandelion doesn't cure a UTI, but it can help flush out urine and, along with it, bacteria. *Typical dose:* 1 cup of tea, made with 1 to 2 teaspoons dried root in 1 cup of hot water, steeped for 15 minutes. Take 2 times daily.

Marsh mallow plant roots, with their mucilage properties, can coat the urinary tract and prevent additional inflammation, thus easing pain. *Typical dose:* As a tea, made with 2 teaspoons of dried root in 1 cup of hot water, steeped for 10 to 15 minutes. Take 1 cup 3 times daily.

Fungal Infections

Individual fungal infections were discussed earlier, but this is a more generic approach to treating those organisms that like dark, moist places. If you are not sure you have a fungal infection, call your physician or healthcare provider to make sure you know what you are treating. If home remedies don't work after 2 to 4 weeks, you may need medical treatment.

Helping Herbs

Chamomile, besides being an anti-inflammatory and antibacterial herb, is a fungicide that is very effective against fungal infections like candida. It can be taken internally or used externally. *Typical dose:* 3 to 4 cups of tea, daily, made with 1 teaspoon of dried flowers in 1 cup of hot water, steeped for 10 minutes and strained. For a bath, brew a gallon of tea and pour it into a lukewarm bath (hot baths will only aggravate the itching). For a compress, apply damp tea bags. Do not use internally if you are allergic to other members of the Asteraceae/Compositae family, including marigolds, echinacea or chrysanthemums.

Garlic has antifungal properties that make it effective for treating fungal infections. Because garlic may leave you with strong breath and body odor, you may want to try a commercially prepared product. Long-term garlic use bestows the most health benefits. *Typical dose:* 600 to 900 mg of garlic powder, tablets or capsules daily; 4 mL of aged garlic extract daily; 10 mg of garlic oil "perles" daily; or 1 or more medium-size fresh cloves daily. A fresh cut garlic clove may be applied directly for up to 1 week. If your skin becomes irritated, discontinue use. If the infection does not go away in 7 to 10 days, seek medical attention.

Tea tree oil is a powerful antiseptic that has many uses and is a good topical remedy for fungal skin infections. Candida albicans is easily destroyed by tea tree oil. There are commercially prepared products available for treating vaginitis caused by yeast. *Typical dose:* For skin infections, mix equal amounts of tea tree oil and olive oil and apply it directly to the affected area 3 times a day. It may be especially effective for thrush in skin folds and in the groin area. Do not use the oil or oil preparation directly on the vaginal area, as it may be irritating. Tea tree oil taken internally may aggravate skin rashes.

Human Immunodeficiency Virus

Human Immunodeficiency Virus (HIV) is a devastating virus that causes acquired immunodeficiency syndrome (AIDS). HIV infects beneficial cells of the immune system and causes infection with a long incubation period, averaging 10 years. With the immune system destroyed, opportunistic infections are more likely. Anyone with HIV or AIDS should be under medical care. Use of herbs in either condition remains controversial, especially the use of immune-boosting herbs, as they may cause a flare-up of the condition. There are some herbs, however, that can provide relief for some symptoms and may be worth considering. If you are interested in using herbal therapies, discuss your options with your healthcare provider before using them.

Helping Herbs

Evening primrose oil (EPO) may provide some essential components that increase the quality and possibly the quantity of life in patients with HIV. EPO contains gamma-linolenic acid and provides beneficial omega-3 and omega-6 fatty acids thought to contribute to improved quality and possible increased length of life. *Typical dose:* 8 to 12 commercially prepared capsules of 500 mg daily, or per label directions.

Garlic has antiviral properties that boost the immune system and are believed to be the reason for its potential use in HIV. *Typical dose:* 600 to 900 mg of garlic powder, tablets or capsules daily; 4 mL of aged garlic extract daily; 10 mg of garlic oil "perles" daily; or 1 or more moderate-size fresh cloves daily.

Hyssop is a member of the mint family that has antiviral properties. The antiviral compound has been found in laboratory tests to inhibit the replication of the HIV virus with no toxicity to healthy cells. Effectiveness in humans is uncertain at this time. *Typical dose:* Make a tea with 2 teaspoons of herb in 1 cup of boiling water; steep for 10 minutes; strain. Drink up to 3 cups daily. Improve the flavor with a bit of honey.

Appendix A

HERBAL FIRST AID KIT

When we have minor bumps, bruises or sprains, we are more likely to head for the medicine chest rather than the emergency room. Most of us have an assortment of pain relievers and antiseptics that we apply to wounds that do not need medical attention. Herbs can offer effective alternatives to OTC preparations. Make sure, however, that you know what you are using and its safety for your particular use.

Also remember that herbs are natural products and many of them will not have the shelf life that OTC preparations have. If you decide to make your own, make sure the batches are small enough that they can be used within a few months. Some of these are also suggestions that can be taken to the field with you: If you have a minor scrape, there may be something in the wild that can be safely picked and used. Many of these are available commercially and a list of these is provided here as well.

Homemade Remedies

Many of the following are ingredients commonly found in the kitchen. It's a good idea to get to know them for their culinary as well as their medicinal uses. For additional herbs that you might use in your home or in the field, refer to Chapter 3.

Aloe is useful for minor burns, scrapes or sunburn. To use, just break off a leaf from the aloe vera plant, split it open and apply the gel to the cleaned, affected area immediately.

Chamomile tea soothes the nerves but may also be beneficial for canker sores, indigestion and insomnia. When applied externally, it is an anti-inflammatory and antiseptic for wounds and hemorrhoids.

Cloves are helpful for motion sickness and bad breath. Brew a tea using 1 or 2 teaspoons of clove or make a homemade mouthwash with its powerful aromatic oil and alcohol. To make mouthwash, mix 1 cup of vodka and 1 tablespoon of clove oil (or to taste) in a glass container. Use 1 tablespoon of the mixture in about 1/4 cup of water as a mouthwash. Do not take the oil internally without diluting it properly.

Dill seeds are helpful for gas and to freshen breath. Try a teaspoon if you are in need of a remedy for either of these.

Fennel is effective in treating motion sickness, indigestion and gas. Try chewing 20 seeds or make a tea and drink 1 cup per day. To make tea, steep 1 to 2 tablespoons of fennel in 1/2 cup (150 mL) of water for 10 minutes; strain.

Feverfew can help relieve a headache or migraine, or other minor aches and pains. Try chewing 1 to 4 fresh leaves or take up to 3 (300- to 400-mg) capsules daily. Fresh feverfew may cause mouth sores when chewed, so you may opt for the commercially prepared capsules. If you are allergic to members of the Asteraceae/Compositae family, feverfew is probably not for you.

Ginger is helpful for nausea and for minor aches and pains. Chew a bit of crystallized ginger to ease nausea or motion sickness. Small amounts in foods or beverages may safely be used for morning sickness as well. Use the ginger topically as described on page 281 for minor muscle strains and sprains.

Lemon balm can be soothing from the inside out. Lemon balm is calming to frayed nerves and may be helpful in relieving symptoms of nausea associated with the flu. It also offers some anti-inflammatory benefits. Tea bags, either homemade or purchased, may be used as instant compresses for muscle spasms.

Peppermint, both fresh and dried, is helpful for indigestion. If you have GERD or other diagnosed stomach disorders, check with your physician before taking peppermint or any of its family members.

St. John's wort–infused oil is useful when used externally for treating first-degree burns, varicose veins and cuts, and to speed the healing of bruises. If your wounds do not heal quickly, seek medical attention. This remedy is not for serious wounds.

Tea tree oil is an anti-inflammatory, antiseptic oil that is indispensable for treating fungus and wounds. Blend equal amounts of the essential oil with olive oil and apply. It may be effective as an insect repellant and can be applied topically to warts and herpes blisters. Do not take this oil internally.

Remedies to Use in the Field

A few bruised **basil** leaves can be applied as an instant remedy for a bump or scrape.

Lemon balm, if you are lucky enough to find some, or if you have some in your garden, can be applied for insect bites.

Plantain can be applied directly to burns, insect bites, stings, poison ivy and sunburn. Make sure you know how to identify plantain before using it. Bruise a few leaves and apply directly to the area.

Remedies to Buy

Bach Rescue Remedy is a popular mixture that advocates say will treat a full range of illnesses by stabilizing emotions, promoting a general sense of well-being, and stimulating and speeding healing. It is touted for its ability to reduce stress, induce sleep, calm fears and ease muscle and arthritic pains. There are no scientific studies to support the claims, but the remedy of aromatherapy from the flower essences may be helpful in itself.

Capsicum creams and ointments are beneficial for sore muscles and arthritic pain. Follow label directions for use.

Chamomile creams and ointments can provide natural relief similar to that afforded by hydrocortisone creams, to help fade age or sun spots, and for soothing minor scrapes and bumps. Use as directed on the label.

Either fresh or frozen **cranberries**, or cranberry juice, can be used when you feel the onset of minor urinary tract irritations or infections. Be sure you know that what you are treating is not a serious infection. If you have diabetes, do not use the sugar-sweetened juice. Cranberry capsules may also be purchased. Drink 12-32 ounces of cranberry juice daily or take 1 (300- to 400-mg) capsule in the morning and evening.

Evening primrose oil capsules have been touted to help relieve a hangover if taken in 2- to 3-gram doses, possibly because of its known use for headaches and pain. It also may be used on a regular basis to help relieve menstrual cramps, PMS and to keep your skin healthy and glowing.

Lavender oil is used at the first signs of a tension headache. It is the only oil that may be applied safely without being diluted. It may also relieve minor burns, scalds, insomnia and psoriasis.

Witch hazel is a common treatment for minor burns, sunburn, minor cuts, insect bites, bruises and sprains.

Approximate Metric Equivalents

Metrics are rounded to the nearest decimal point in most cases.

Liquid Measurements

Volume (mL= milliliter)

U.S.	Metric
1/4 teaspoon	1 mL
1/2 teaspoon	2.5 mL
3/4 teaspoon	4 mL
1 teaspoon	5 mL
1 1/4 teaspoons	6 mL
1 1/2 teaspoons	7.5 mL
3/4 teaspoons	8.5 mL
2 teaspoons	10 mL
1 tablespoon	15 mL
2 tablespoons	30 mL
1/4 cup	59 mL
1/3 cup	79 mL
1/2 cup	118 mL
2/3 cup	158 mL
3/4 cup	78 mL
1 cup	237 mL
1 1/2 cup	355 mL
2 cups (1 pint)	473 mL
3 cups	710 mL
4 cups (1 quart)	.95 liter
1.06 quarts	1 liter
4 quarts (1 gallon)	3.8 liters

Solid Measurements

U.S.	Metric
.035 ounce	1 gram
1/4 ounce	7 grams
1/2 ounce	14 grams
3/4 ounce	21 grams
1 ounce	28 grams
1 1/2 ounces	42.5 grams
2 ounces	57 grams
3 ounces	85 grams
4 ounces	113 grams
5 ounces	142 grams
6 ounces	170 grams
7 ounces	198 grams
8 ounces	227 grams
16 ounces (1 lb.)	454 grams
2.2 lb.	1 kilogram

GLOSSARY

Acquired Immunodeficiency Syndrome (AIDS): an HIV-infected person receives a diagnosis of AIDS after developing one of the CDC-defined AIDS indicator illnesses. A positive HIV test result does not mean that a person has AIDS. A physician using certain clinical criteria (e.g., AIDS indicator illnesses) makes a diagnosis of AIDS. Infection with HIV can weaken the immune system to the point that it has difficulty fighting off certain infections. These types of infections are known as "opportunistic" infections because they take the opportunity a weakened immune system gives to cause illness.

Adaptogens: substances that help the body return to a normal state while increasing resistance to viruses, exercise and environmental and psychological stress.

Age-related macular degeneration (AMD): a degenerative disease that affects the macula, a small spot in the central area of the retina located at the back of the eye.

Allantoin: used for wound healing, skin regeneration and skin softening.

Alopecia areata: an autoimmune skin disease that results in the loss of hair from the head and elsewhere on the body. Visit www.alopeciaareata.com for more information.

Anti-inflammatories: used to calm inflamed tissues and swelling.

Antioxidants: components of plants, including herbs, which prevent or delay the oxidation process in cells that results in damaging free radicals.

Antispasmodics: help relieve spasms and are often used for respiratory and intestinal problems.

Aromatherapy: the use of therapeutic oils distilled from plants and used externally for treating headaches, anxiety and tension.

Arrhythmia: irregular beating of the heart.

ASA: acetylsalicylic acid; aspirin

Ayurveda: believed to be the oldest healing science, originating in India more than 5,000 years ago, with written information dating back to about 2500 B.C.E. Ayurveda is a Sanskrit word that means the "Knowledge of Life."

Benign: not cancerous; does not invade nearby tissue or spread to other parts of the body.

Benign prostatic hypertrophy (BPH): a non-cancerous condition in which an overgrowth of prostate tissue pushes against the urethra and the bladder, blocking the flow of urine. Also called hyperplasia.

Bitters: used as a "tonic" after a meal to help improve digestion and absorption of food.

Body mass index (BMI): a measure that takes into account one's weight in relation to height and gauges body fatness. Being overweight (a body mass index of 25 to 29.9) or obese (a body mass index over 30) is linked to increased incidence of diabetes, heart disease and some types of cancer. Visit www.nhlbisupport.com/bmi for more information.

Botanicals: the Food and Drug Administration prefers this term for herbs. It allows for the broader definition consisting of plant-based products including trees, shrubs and herbs.

Capsaicin: may provide temporary pain relief for arthritis and some neuralgias. It is also considered a digestive stimulant and may inhibit production of cancer-causing substances. Capsaicin is a purified compound from red peppers.

Carcinogenic: a substance that has the ability to cause cancer.

Carminatives: relieve cramping and bloating caused by gas that builds up in the intestine.

Central Nervous System (CNS): includes the brain and the spinal cord; processes sensory information, integrating it with past experiences to produce appropriate responses to external stimuli.

Chronic Fatigue Syndrome (CFS): a debilitating syndrome characterized by profound fatigue that is not improved by bed rest and that may be worsened by physical or mental activity. The cause or causes behind CFS have not been determined and no specific diagnostic tests are available. It may include numerous symptoms including insomnia, general weakness, impaired memory and ability to concentrate and inability to recover from physical exertion within 24 hours. Visit www.chronicfatigue.about.com for more information.

CNS Depression: a condition in which the reactions that are normal to the CNS are depressed. Messages from the brain to the extremities may take longer than normal; reaction time to stimuli may be decreased.

Complementary and Alternative Medicine (CAM): treatment modalities used in addition to (complementary) or instead of (alternative) standard treatments. These practices are not considered standard medical approaches. CAM includes dietary supplements, megadose vitamins, herbal preparations, special teas, massage therapy, magnet therapy, spiritual healing and meditation.

Congestive heart failure (CHF): a condition in which the heart can't pump enough blood to the body's other organs; heart failure.

COX-2 inhibitor: can block pain and inflammation by blocking the activity of the COX-2 enzyme, which is present in each cell in the body and is responsible for pain and inflammation.

Daily Values (DV): a dietary reference value on food labels used to help consumers use this information to plan a healthy overall diet. DVs serve as a basis for declaring on the label the percent of the Daily Value for each nutrient that a serving of the food provides.

Deglycyrrhizinated (DGL): licorice with the natural compound, glycyrrhizin, removed. Glycyrrhizin is believed to be related to fluid retention and possibly high blood pressure.

Demulcents: believed to soothe the mucous membranes and digestive system by coating the tissues and protecting them from further irritation.

Diastolic pressure: the pressure between heartbeats (the pressure when the last sound is heard).

Dietary Supplement Health and Education Act (DSHEA): defines dietary supplements and forbids FDA from treating them as chemicals or drugs; allows and defines health claims for supplements. DSHEA's goal is to ensure the safety of supplements and the accuracy of health claims and labeling. Passed in 1994.

Dihydrotestosterone (DHT): synthesized primarily by the liver from free testosterone. Levels of DHT, not free testosterone, are proportionally correlated to sex drive and erectile potential. DHT has been associated with both benign prostate hypertrophy and prostate cancer.

Edema: swelling of tissues and accumulation of fluid in the body.

Expectorants: reduce the viscosity of secretions from or decrease the persistence with which mucus adheres to the respiratory system, allowing them to be expelled more easily.

Extract: sometimes called tinctures and are most commonly made by steeping a quantity of herb in alcohol. The alcohol will extract the water and oil-soluble compounds from the herb.

Federal Trade Commission (FTC): regulates the advertising of dietary supplements.

Fibromyalgia: a chronic syndrome characterized by widespread musculoskeletal pain, fatigue, and multiple tender points. Persons with fibromyalgia may also experience sleep disturbances, morning stiffness, irritable bowel syndrome, anxiety, and other symptoms.

Flavonoids: have antioxidant properties. They are members of the phenolic family thought to protect tissue from free-radical damage that can lead to heart disease and some types of cancers. Many people became familiar with flavonoids (but did not know that's what they were) when resveratrol, found in wine and grape juice, was touted for a healthy heart.

Food and Drug Administration (FDA): does not require proof from clinical trials regarding the safety and effectiveness of herbal products before they are put on the market. The FDA does limit, however, the claims that can be made regarding the use and efficacy of supplements. They also require that health problems associated with herbal products be reported, but this happens all too infrequently.

Free radicals: molecules produced by cellular oxidation that can interact with the DNA in cells and may factor into the development of heart disease, cancer and diseases related to diabetes.

Gamma-linolenic acid (GLA): a constituent of a few plants (Evening Primrose, Borage and Black Currant oils) that is a building block for anti-inflammatory substances within the body.

Gastrointestinal (GI): pertains to the gastrointestinal tract as defined below.

Gastrointestinal (GI) Tract: includes all organs that are involved in the ingestion and digestion of food, the esophagus, stomach, duodenum, small and large intestine, liver, and pancreas.

Generally Recognized as Safe (GRAS): food additives that have been submitted to the US Food and Drug Administration (FDA) and have been determined to be "generally recognized as safe" for human consumption. Many additives are on the list due to their long history of use as culinary herbs and spices.

GERD: gastric esophageal reflux disease. It is the flow of the stomach's contents back up into the esophagus.

German Commission E: an expert panel of European healthcare professionals and researchers who examined existing research evidence and used their expertise to develop the German Commission E Monographs (see below). The committee evaluates the safety and efficacy of herbs and herb combinations sold in Germany.

German Commission E Monographs: provides information on more than 300 herbs that are, with "reasonable certainty," safe and effective. Thought to be the most authoritative information sources available worldwide on herbs, their uses, doses, safety, side effects and interactions.

Giardia: *Giardia lamblia* (intestinalis) is a single-celled animal that is the most frequent cause of non-bacterial diarrhea in North America.

Good Manufacturing Practices (GMPs): GMPs are regulations that describe the methods, equipment, facilities and controls required for producing botanical, pharmaceutical, food and medical device products that are intended for human use. GMP guidance suggests ways in which manufacturers, packagers, labelers, importers and distributors of these products can meet the GMP requirements.

GRAS: a designation (Generally Recognized As Safe) given to substances that are considered safe for human consumption and can be added to foods by manufacturers without establishing their safety through rigorous studies and research.

Healthcare provider: a licensed provider, trained in the area of expertise they are practicing in. Licensing or registration varies from state to state, but generally helps to assure that the person is qualified to treat you. Persons with licensing usually must meet certain educational and experiential requirements before becoming licensed or registered. Among practitioners that are licensed: chiropractors, doctors of osteopathy (D.O.), naturopaths (in some states), physicians (M.D.), physician assistants (P.A.), registered dietitians (R.D.), registered nurses (R.N.), certified clinical nutritionists (C.C.N.), certified nutritionists (C.N.), Licensed Acupuncturists and specialists in Traditional Chinese Medicine.

Herbal Medicinals: products that are derived from plant parts and have a pharmacologic effect (sometimes used interchangeably with phytopharmaceuticals).

HDL cholesterol: the blood fat that picks up cholesterol in the bloodstream and returns it to the liver to be recycled. HDL is considered the "good" cholesterol because of its protective effects against heart disease.

High Blood Pressure (HBP): HBP is defined in an adult as a systolic pressure of 140 mm Hg or higher and/or a diastolic pressure of 90 mm Hg or higher. Blood pressure is measured in millimeters of mercury (mm Hg). High blood pressure directly increases the risk of heart disease and stroke, especially along with other risk factors. High blood pressure can occur in children or adults. High blood pressure usually has no symptoms. It's truly a "silent killer."

HIV: human immunodeficiency virus; the virus that causes AIDS. This virus is passed from one person to another through blood-to-blood and sexual contact. In addition, infected pregnant women can pass HIV to their baby during pregnancy or delivery, as well as through breast-feeding. People with HIV have what is called HIV infection. Most of these people will develop AIDS as a result of their HIV infection.

HMO: Health Maintenance Organizations.

Hypothyroidism: a low thyroid function that may cause symptoms that include lethargy, depression and weight gain.

***In vitro*:** biological testing and reactions within the test tube.

***In vivo*:** occurring in a living organism, not necessarily human.

Infusions: similar to teas and can be made with water or oil. This method is used mostly for the flowers and leafy parts of herbs and should be made fresh each time you want to use it.

Inflammatory bowel disease (IBD): an incurable chronic disease of the intestinal tract. It includes Crohn's disease and ulcerative colitis, which have similar symptoms. The most common symptoms of IBD include abdominal pain, weight loss, fever, rectal bleeding, skin and eye irritations and diarrhea.

Irritable bowel syndrome (IBS): a disorder that does not show evidence of disease when tested diagnostically; there are no inflammation or ulcers present. It is believed that in a person with IBS, the muscles of the gastrointestinal tract (predominantly the intestines) are exceptionally sensitive to stimuli, or triggers. While the stimuli would not normally affect those without IBS, triggers such as food or stress can provoke a strong response in a person with IBS.

Lignans: fibers that are believed to give flax its cholesterol-reducing properties. Lignans found in flaxseed may also act as a bulk-forming laxative.

LDL cholesterol: the "bad" cholesterol that gets incorporated into the plaque that forms deposits on artery walls, causing hardening of the arteries.

Monoamine Oxidase Inhibitors (MAOI): a class of antidepressant medications.

Mucilage: a substance that is soothing on the mucous membranes.

Mutagenic: any chemical or physical environmental agent that has the ability to induce a genetic mutation (an unusual change in genetic material) that results in changes in future generations and possibly in the individuals themselves.

National Sanitation Foundation (NSF): NSF International, The Public Health and Safety Company™, is a not-for-profit, nongovernmental organization that focuses on standards development, product certification, education, and risk-management for public health and safety. NSF provides for third party assessment of food, water, environment, air and dietary supplements.

NSAIDs (non-steroidal anti-inflammatory drugs): possess anti-inflammatory actions as well as other properties. These drugs inhibit the synthesis and actions of certain substances that are widely distributed in body tissues and are integral to the inflammatory process, blood clotting and many more metabolic pathways.

Nutrition Labeling and Education Act of 1990 (NLEA): requires that there be pre-market approval of all health claims by the FDA. Claims fall under two categories: structure/function claims and disease claims. The final rule enacting labeling standards for dietary supplements was published in 2000.

OCD: oral contraceptive drug.

Office of Dietary Supplements (ODS): responsible for coordinating funding for scientific studies on the relationship between dietary supplements and disease prevention.

Organosulfurs: are responsible for the onion or allium cepa family's distinctive taste and odor. They have been found to boost the immune system, reduce cholesterol production in the liver and assist the liver in neutralizing carcinogens.

Osteoarthritis (OA): degenerative joint disease; one of the most common types of arthritis.

OTC: over-the-counter.

PC-SPES: contains eight Chinese herbs including saw palmetto, licorice, reishi mushroom, skullcap and ginseng. Due to processing irregularities, PC-SPES is currently not available.

Phytoestrogens: may reduce the risk of hormone-sensitive cancers, such as breast and prostate, by substituting weak plant estrogens for human estrogen. They may help reduce cholesterol levels, prevent bone loss after menopause and suppress the spread of existing cancer cells. They are most commonly referred to as isoflavones and are found in largest amounts in soy products and flaxseed.

Phytopharmaceuticals: plant-based medicines that have been standardized for key compounds, or active constituents, and adjusted to ensure that the levels of these compounds are consistent.

Phytosterols: inhibit intestinal absorption of cholesterol by about 50 percent. Some phytosterols are also thought to enhance immunity, reduce inflammation and may reduce the risk of cancer. Phytosterols are compounds found naturally in a wide variety of plants including nuts, seeds, fruits and vegetables.

PID: pelvic inflammatory disease.

Polyphenols and phenols: part of the largest category of phytochemicals—phenolics—and among the most widely distributed in the plant kingdom. They may protect the body from some diseases by blocking the formation of nitrosamines that are believed to cause some types of cancers. Tea, coffee, cranberries, turmeric, mustard, curry and parsley all contain beneficial phenolic compounds.

Prostate Specific Antigen (PSA): a substance produced by prostate cells, which increases if prostate cancer is present. PSA is a screening tool for the potential for prostate cancer or its spread, not a diagnosis. For diagnosis, consult your primary care provider.

Prothrombin Time/Internationalize Normalized Ration (PT/INR): the protime (or prothrombin time) is a method of measuring how well the blood clots. INR is a ratio that helps physicians monitor patients taking anticoagulant medications. It is applied to the results of a protime blood test in order to adjust for the different conditions in labs performing the test. INR/PT measures the time it takes for a person's blood to clot. Patients taking medications that inhibit the formation of blood clots (anticoagulants) often have these tests done routinely.

Qigong: exercises known in a system of Chinese healthcare that also includes acupuncture, massage, meditation, concentration, cupping and moxibustion.

Recommended Daily Intake (RDI): The value established by the Food and Drug Administration (FDA) for use in nutrition labeling. It was based initially on the highest 1968 Recommended Dietary Allowance (RDA) for each nutrient, to ensure that nutritional needs were met for all age groups.

Rheumatoid arthritis (RA): an inflammation in the lining of the joints and/or other internal organs.

Rhizomes: root-like underground stems that produce roots below ground and send up shoots.

Saponins: a type of carbohydrate, found in ginseng and soy, that neutralizes enzymes believed to cause cancer in the intestine. Wound-healing and immune-boosting properties may also be credited to saponins.

Specifics: are for a particular condition and should be taken only for a short time, just as a prescription medicine might be used.

SSRIs: selective serotonin reuptake inhibitors are antidepressant drugs.

Standardized extracts: processed to ensure that they contain minimum levels of one or more of the active ingredients.

Systemic Lupus Erythematosis: a chronic rheumatic disease affecting joints, muscles and other parts of the body.

Systolic pressure: the pressure of the blood flow when the heart beats (the pressure when the first sound is heard).

Teas: (also referred to as tisanes) are infusions made from herbs. All of the usable portion of the plant may be used for teas, but generally they are made with leaves, flowers and sometimes fruit. They are a weaker solution and are usually steeped for 5 minutes.

Tinctures: similar to fluid extracts and decoctions. Use an alcohol–water mix (generally one part herb to four parts solution) and steep for at least 12 hours.

Tonics: are for general health enhancement and are taken for longer periods of time, sometimes with a break.

Traditional Chinese Medicine (TCM): for prevention and treatment of "disharmony" or imbalances in the body—disease concepts that are foreign to Western healthcare. The basic idea is that energy flows through the body along pathways called meridians, or *qi*. In TCM, disease is recognized as an imbalance in qi and therapies are focused on balancing the qi. To balance the person, practitioners use the principles of the five elements and yin-yang as described below. TCM has been used for more than 3,000 years.

United States Pharmacopoeia (USP): the United States Pharmacopoeia (USP) and the National Formulary (NF) are the official compendia of the United States for drugs, excipients (non-drug ingredients), dietary supplements and other therapeutic products.

Urinary tract infections (UTIs): an infection of any part of the urinary tract, which is the path that urine takes to exit the body.

Vasodilator: any agent that causes blood vessels to dilate. It is usually a drug including botanical, but dilation may also happen because of nervous stimulation.

Vinegars: a delicious but limited alternative to alcohol-based tinctures. Most suited for salads and cooking, herbal vinegars can be made using the same ratios as for tinctures by simply steeping the herbs in vinegar instead of alcohol.

Wildcrafting: harvesting plants from the wild rather than cultivating them.

World Health Organization (WHO): the United Nations' special agency for health. Its goal is the attainment of the highest possible level of health for all people worldwide. WHO published Guidelines for the Assessment of Herbal Medicines in 1991. These guidelines were developed to help regulatory agencies evaluate the quality, safety and effectiveness of herbal medicines, and have expanded to include information about commonly used medicinal plants in China, the South Pacific, Korea and Viet Nam. A collection of 28 monographs covering the quality control and traditional and clinical uses of selected widely used medicinal plants was published in 1999.

Selected References

Chapter 1

Berman BM, Singh BB, Hartnoll SM, Singh BK, Reilly D: Primary care physicians and complementary-alternative medicine: training, attitudes, and practice patterns. *J Am Board Fam Pract.*1998;11:272-281.

Considering Complementary and Alternative Therapies? http://nccam.nih.gov/fcp/faq/considercam.html

Gallo M, Sarkar M, Au W, Pietrzak K, Comas B, Smith M, Jaeger TV, Einarson A, Koren G: Pregnancy outcome following gestational exposure to echinacea. *Arch Intern Med* 2000;160:3141-3.

A Healthcare Professional's Guide to Evaluating Dietary Supplements. Chicago: American Dietetic Association, American Pharmaceutical Association; 2000.

Herbs to Avoid During Pregnancy http://www.healthy.net/asp/templates/article.asp?pageType=article&Id=1586#rice

Hutchens Alma R. *A Handbook Of Native American Herbs.* Boston: Shambhala Publications Inc; 1992.

Integrative Medicine. Wisconsin Medical Journal. 100;7: 2001.

http://www.mdheal.com/

Morton, Mary & Michael: *Five Steps to Selecting the Best Alternative Medicine: A Guide to Complementary & Integrative Health Care.* Quality Paperback excerpted at: http://www.healthy.net/

http://nccam.nih.gov/health/whatiscam/#6

Ody Penelope. *The Complete Medicinal Herbal.* New York: Dorling Kindersley Limited; 1993.

www.plantsavers.org

Quillin, Patrick & Noreen: *Beating Cancer with Nutrition.* Nutrition Times Press. Tulsa, OK; 2001.

www.supplementquality.com/testing/USP_revsup_0203.html

Workman Jennifer. *Stop Your Cravings.* New York: The Free Press; 2002.

Chapter 2

Blumenthal Mark, Goldberg Alicia, Brinckmann Josef. *Herbal Medicine Expanded Commission E Monographs.* Newton, MA: Integrative Medicine; 2000.

Brown Deni. *The Herb Society Of America—New Encyclopedia of Herbs & Their Uses.* New York: Dorling Kindersley Limited; 2001.

Castleman Michael. *The New Healing Herbs.* Emmaus, PA: Rodale Press; 2001.

Constantine George H. *Tyler's Tips: The Shopper's Guide for Herbal Remedies.* Binghamton, NY: The Haworth Herbal Press; 2000.

Dewey Laurel. *Plant Power—The Humorous Herbalist's Guide to Finding, Growing, Gathering & Using 30 Great Medicinal Herbs.* East Canaan, CT: ATN/Safe Goods; 1999.

Jellin Jeff M, Editor. *Natural Medicines Comprehensive Database,* 3rd edition. Stockton, CA: Therapeutic Research Facility; 2000.

Kavasch Barrie E, Baar Karen. *American Indian Healing Arts—Herbs, Rituals, and Remedies For Every Season Of Life.* New York: Bantam Trade Paperback; 1999.

McCaleb Robert S, Leigh Evelyn, Morien Krista. *The Encyclopedia of Popular Herbs.* Roseville, CA: Prima Health; 2000.

Miller, Lucinda G, Murray Wallace J. Herbal *Medicinals: A Clinician's Guide.* New York: Pharmaceutical Products Press; 1998.

Moore Michael. *Medicinal Plants Of the Desert And Canyon West.* Santa Fe: Museum of New Mexico Press; 1989.

Moore Michael. *Medicinal Plants Of The Mountain West.* Santa Fe: Museum of New Mexico Press; 1979.

Ody Penelope. *The Complete Medicinal Herbal.* New York: Dorling Kindersley Limited; 1993.

Rotblatt Michael, Ziment Irwin. *Evidence-Based Herbal Medicine.* Philadelphia: Hanley & Belfus; 2002.

Chapter 3

Blumenthal, Goldberg, Brinckmann. *Herbal Medicine Expanded Commission E Monographs.* Newton, MA: Integrative Medicine; 2000.

Castleman Michael. *The New Healing Herbs.* Emmaus, PA: Rodale Press; 2001.

Constantine George H. *Tyler's Tips: The Shopper's Guide for Herbal Remedies.* Binghamton, NY: The Haworth Herbal Press; 2000.

Jellin Jeff M, Editor. *Natural Medicines Comprehensive Database*, 3rd edition. Stockton, CA: Therapeutic Research Facility; 2000.

McCaleb Robert S, Leigh Evelyn, Morien Krista. *The Encyclopedia of Popular Herbs.* Roseville, CA: Prima Health; 2000.

Rotblatt Michael, Ziment Irwin. *Evidence-Based Herbal Medicine.* Philadelphia: Hanley & Belfus; 2002.

Chapter 4

American Lung Association http://www.lungusa.org/

Arthritis Foundation http://www.arthritis.org/

Castleman Michael. *The New Healing Herbs.* Emmaus, PA: Rodale Press; 2001.

Constantine George H. *Tyler's Tips: The Shopper's Guide for Herbal Remedies.* Binghamton, NY: The Haworth Herbal Press; 2000.

Duke James A. *The Green Pharmacy.* Emmaus, PA: Rodale Press; 1997.

A Healthcare Professional's Guide to Evaluating Dietary Supplements. Chicago: American Dietetic Association, American Pharmaceutical Association; 2000.

McCaleb Robert S, Leigh Evelyn, Morien Krista. *The Encyclopedia of Popular Herbs.* Roseville, CA: Prima Health; 2000.

National Cancer Institute http://www.nci.nih.gov/

National Heart Lung and Blood Institute http://www.nhlbi.nih.gov/

National Institute of Diabetes and Digestive and Kidney Disorders http://ndep.nih.gov/

National Multiple Sclerosis Society http://www.nmss.org/

National Osteoporosis Foundation http://www.nof.org/

National Parkinson Foundation http://www.parkinson.org/

Prevent Blindness America http://www.preventblindness.org/

White Linda B, Foster Steven. *The Herbal Drugstore.* Emmaus, PA: Rodale Press; 2000.

Web Resources

American Herbal Pharmacopoeia and Therapeutic Compendium 2002 http://www.herbal-ahp.org/

ConsumerLab.com http://www.consumerlab.com/

Dietary Supplement Information Bureau http://www.supplementinfo.org/

Herb Research Foundation http://www.herbs.org/

Longwood Herbal Taskforce http://www.mcp.edu/herbal/

National Center for Complementary and Alternative Medicine http://nccam.nih.gov/

NSF International http://www.nsf.org/

The United States Pharmacopeial Convention http://www.usp.org/

World Health Organization http://www.who.int/

F

G

H

I

J

K

L

M

N

O

P

R

S